Springer Japan KK

H. Asakura, Y. Aoyagi,
S. Nakazawa (Eds.)

Trends in Gastroenterology and Hepatology

Millennium 2000

With 90 Figures, Including 5 in Color

Springer

Hitoshi Asakura, M.D.
Professor
Third Department of Medicine
Niigata University School of Medicine
1-757 Asahimachi-dori
Niigata 951-8122, Japan

Yutaka Aoyagi, M.D.
Associate Professor
Third Department of Medicine
Niigata University School of Medicine
1-757 Asahimachi-dori
Niigata 951-8122, Japan

Saburo Nakazawa, M.D.
Consulting Director, Yamashita Hospital
1-3-5 Naka-machi, Ichinomiya
Aichi 491-8531, Japan

Library of Congress Cataloging-in-Publication Data

Trends in gastroenterology and hepatology : millennium 2000 / H. Asakura, Y. Aoyagi, S. Nakazawa, eds.
p. ; cm.
Includes bibliographical references and index.
ISBN 978-4-431-67993-6 ISBN 978-4-431-67895-3 (eBook)
DOI 10.1007/978-4-431-67895-3

1. Digestive organs—Diseases—Congresses. I. Asakura, Hitoshi. II. Aoyagi, Y. (Yutaka), 1948- III. Nakazawa, Saburo. IV. Nihon Shokakibyo Gakkai. Sokai (86th : 2000 : Niigata-shi, Japan)
[DNLM: 1. Digestive System Diseases—Congresses. WI 140 T794 2001]
RC799 .T74 2001
616.3′3—dc21

2001020615

Printed on acid-free paper

SPIN: 10784698

Preface

It is our great pleasure and honor to present the proceedings of the 86th annual congress of the Japanese Society of Gastroenterology. This book contains distinguished papers presented at the congress, which took place in April 2000 in Niigata City. The congress included the presentation of some 1064 papers, with 9 symposiums, 9 panel discussions, and 10 workshops on the basic and clinical aspects of recent advances in gastroenterology, hepatology, and biliary and pancreatic diseases in Japan. This book includes selected papers from 2 symposiums, 3 panel discussions, and 5 workshops in the fields of basic and clinical research of digestive diseases.

In the history of the science of digestive diseases in Japan, from 1945 to 1960, new clinical findings in pathological, radiographic, and biochemical studies were the main topics of presentations at the Japanese Congress of Gastroenterology. From 1960 to 1985, with the discovery of the hepatitis B virus and development of endoscopic procedures, the congresses covered hepatological findings regarding hepatitis B, relating chronic hepatitis, cirrhosis, and hepatocellular carcinoma. Concepts of early gastric and colonic cancers were also reported. From 1985 to the present, molecular, cellular, and immunological studies using polymerase chain reaction (PCR), gene analysis, and other new techniques were the subjects of the main presentations, especially for hepatitis C virus-related liver diseases, *Helicobacter pylori*-related diseases, and inflammatory bowel diseases. Recent advances in the fields of helical CT, MRI, angiography, and echography, and their capacity for three-dimensional graphic demonstration in biliary and pancreatic diseases, have contributed to the further development of the congress.

This proceedings includes Professor D. Podolsky's special lecture on gastroenterology in the new millennium, and two additional special lectures, one of which is by Professor S. Nakazawa on life style-related diseases. Also included are excellent papers on apoptosis in digestive organs, NO, transcription factors in digestive organs, antigen-presenting cells, the pathophysiology of inflammatory bowel disease, NSAID-induced gastric lesions, microcirculation in digestive diseases, hepatic regeneration, and hepatic fibrosis.

We hope that this book will contribute to 21st-century research in digestive diseases in commemoration of Millennium 2000.

Hitoshi Asakura, M.D.
Yutaka Aoyagi, M.D.
Saburo Nakazawa, M.D.

Contents

Contents

Part 5 Is Nitric Oxide Friend or Foe?

Part 6 Transcription Factors in Digestive Organs

Part 7 The Role of Antigen-Presenting Cells in Pathophysiology

Part 8 The Pathophysiology of Inflammatory Bowel Disease

Part 9 NSAID-Induced Gastric Lesions

Part 10 Prevention of Disease by Modulation of Microcirculation

Part 12 Hepatic Fibrosis Research and Its Application to Therapy

Contributors

Part 1
Gastroenterology and the New Millennium

Reflecting Forward: Gastroenterology in the New Millennium

Daniel K. Podolsky*

As Nobel Prize-winning physicist Niels Bohr first said, "Prediction is difficult, especially when it concerns the future." Anticipating where trends in clinical gastroenterology and research may lead in the new millennium is therefore fraught with danger. However, it is at least apparent that a number of forces will result in a very different field of gastroenterology.

Predicting the future is best begun with an appreciation of the remarkable advances that have been accomplished in the first hundred years since gastroenterology emerged as a distinct field. During the early years, attention focused on a better understanding of the structure and function of the major organs of the gastrointestinal tract and related accessory glands including the liver and pancreas. Progress was based on the sciences of anatomy, pathology, histology, and physiology. Additional progress was made through identification of the infectious agents responsible for many of the major disorders that affect the gastrointestinal tract, including the viral agents that cause hepatitis and many of the bacterial and nonbacterial agents that cause diarrhea—still among the most prevalent of all gastrointestinal (GI) disorders. More recently, approaches to the management of peptic ulcer disease have been transformed by our recognition of the central role that *Helicobacter pylori* plays in this highly prevalent disorder. Progress in genetics has begun to provide even more fundamental understanding of the basis of GI disease. The genes responsible for many disorders have now been identified. These are well illustrated by the several genes that confer risk for the polyposis syndromes (e.g., *APC*), the gene for hemochromatosis (*HFE*), and the gene responsible for cystic fibrosis (*CFTR*), admittedly a more systemic disorder but one that nonetheless affects the GI tract.

In addition to this impressive set of accomplishments, a number of ancillary developments that define the practice of modern gastroenterology have had an equally important impact. The successive development of rigid, then fiberoptic, and now digital endoscopy has been instrumental in making more precise diagnoses and the

Gastrointestinal Unit GRJ719, Massachusetts General Hospital and Harvard Medical School Center for the Study of Inflammatory Bowel Disease, 32 Fruit Street, Boston, MA 02114-2696, USA
* e-mail: podolsky.daniel@mgh.harvard.edu

development of more specific therapeutic strategies possible. Advances in endoscopy have been complemented by those of other imaging modalities, which are essential for the daily practice of gastroenterology and contribute to more precise diagnosis and treatment. They include conventional forms of radiology, computed tomography (CT) scanning, and more recently magnetic resonance imaging (MRI) and related techniques.

Today, a hundred years after the emergence of gastroenterology, effective therapeutics are now available for many disorders. Many of these agents are truly impressive in their effectiveness, perhaps no better exemplified by the proton pump inhibitors, antibiotics for the treatment of specific infections, a variety of antiinflammatory drugs, and vaccines that have changed the landscape for the future because of their ability to prevent disease.

Notwithstanding these many developments, considerable challenges remain to meet the needs of patients. Although the basic structures and functions of the GI tract have been characterized, understanding has still not been reduced to its most fundamental level (i.e., the nature of the genes responsible for GI tract function). Understanding of the fundamental basis of function can make possible an understanding of the basic etiology of disease and dysfunction for the many disorders that remain enigmas. Although much better understanding of the causation of peptic ulcer disease has been achieved, the causation of inflammatory bowel disease remains uncertain. Similarly, there is no definitive understanding of the causes of the most common forms of GI malignancy, which now dominate—and will continue to dominate—the clinical arena of gastroenterology.

Given that understanding of disease mechanism or even normal function is not yet at its most fundamental level, it is perhaps not surprising that definitive therapies for most of the disorders that comprise the object of the practice of gastroenterology are lacking. Indeed, even if definitive therapies that could reliably treat the full range of GI diseases were available, it would still have achieved only half the goal of medicine: It is of paramount importance to develop the means to prevent disease rather than treat its aftermath.

Large unmet needs persist, prompting the question: What are the future possibilities of meeting these needs? Before attempting to answer that question, it is useful to outline the issues that will shape the specific way in which those questions are addressed. First, it is important to recognize that the landscape of clinical problems the gastroenterologist encounters has changed over the years and likely will continue to change. So that prediction making about the future of gastroenterology should begin with consideration of the nature of the major clinical problems that will confront the practitioner in the year 2050, compared to present-day gastroenterology. A number of factors are causing significant changes in the variety of diseases with which the gastroenterologist contends. While as the past 30 to 40 years have been dominated by the important, ongoing problems related to viral hepatitis, in the distant future that may no longer be the case because of the eventual impact of widespread vaccination leading to decreases in the frequency of hepatitis B, and hopefully hepatitis A, in conjunction with better hygiene and overall socioeconomic development. Thus chronic hepatitis and its consequent cirrhosis and hepatocellular carcinoma which—certainly in Japan and in many parts of the world—are common today, may become much less common. In addition to the import of specific developments such as vaccines, there are the more general effects of what hopefully will be improving socioeconomic conditions throughout most of the world. The impact of the latter cannot be exaggerated because many GI conditions have a basis of risk related to socioeconomic conditions: the quality of the water supply and the quality of the food supply. In developed countries, improving sanitation has certainly already had an impact on the frequency of hepatitis A. It is reasonable to expect that the same will be true for *H. pylori*-related disease. Remarkable changes in the frequency of a hugely prevalent disorder can be anticipated.

Unfortunately, decreases in disorders that are generally associated with low socioeconomic development, will likely be offset by increases in the problems associated with development. Inflammatory bowel disease—which is increasing in Japan as well as in North America and Europe—and most importantly colon cancer offer just two examples of problems that loom larger in the future. In addition, medical interventions will cause changes in the spectrum of disease. This is illustrated by the many reports that demonstrate an increased frequency of symptomatic gastroesophageal reflux disease (GERD) following eradication of *H. pylori* as a result of the unmasking effect of the beneficial effect of acid suppression by *H. pylori*. Finally, demographic trends will have a significant impact on the prevalence of GI disorders. The population, in association with improving socioeconomic conditions, is aging. As a consequence, the problems associated with aging will be more common for the gastroenterologist. Comparative profiles of the relative frequency of disorders that fell within the domain of gastroenterology between 1950 and 1999 illustrate the dynamic nature of this clinical landscape. The projected evolution in these trends will result in a different clinical field by 2030. Proportionally, colon cancer and GERD will dominate the clinical specter in developed countries, compared to a different picture of a mere 50 years ago.

Thus the clinical landscape of gastroenterology will be different. How then, will the practice of gastroenterology change? It is likely that four forces will determine the further evolution of the field: (1) the impact of the full elucidation of the human genome; (2) the ability ultimately to cross the immune identity barrier without toxic drugs; (3) the development of increasingly more sophisticated engineering tools that allow new approaches to bioengineering and microdevices; and (4) the development of the capacity for high through-put screening, which will allow more powerful approaches to drug development. Although it is likely that none of these four forces would have been considered as defining the future as recently as 5 years ago, it is likely that they will indeed determine the practice of gastroenterology in this new millennium sooner than expected.

Human Genome

Complete determination of the human genome will have an almost immediate impact, most obviously through identification of disease-associated genes. It is reasonable to assume that identification of the genes associated with diseases will enable better understanding of the mechanisms for disorders that have remained a puzzle, such as inflammatory bowel disease. In addition, gene identification will almost immediately allow subclassification of patients on the basis of genetic profiles. Most important, full delineation of the genetic basis of disease will result in a profound change for medicine generally. Definition of the association between specific genes and later disease development will permit diagnosis before individuals are actually patients—a presymptomatic diagnosis. In the future the time spent treating disease may be equally balanced by the time treating people before they have disease, resulting in a fundamentally different type of medicine.

The challenges for gastroenterology after benefiting from this genomic revolution are considerable because most GI disorders do have some genetic component. However, most are not simple monogenic disorders like hemochromatosis. Rather, most of the common problems of gastroenterology result from the interactions of the products of many genes. The future ability to realize the promise of the identification of disease genes also depends on a more sophisticated understanding of the mechanisms through which multiple genes interact to cause one disease in a given individual. Identification of disease genes should allow better appreciation of the common elements in disease, as exemplified by the *CFTR* gene. As noted above, mutations in this gene are responsible for cystic fibrosis. Although the classical manifestations of cystic fibrosis are well known, since identification of *CFTR* it has become clear that mutations in the same gene may be associated with disorders quite distinct from classical cystic fibrosis. Perhaps as many as 20% of individuals with idiopathic chronic pancreatitis have mutations of the *CFTR* gene without other signs of cystic fibrosis. It is possible that a background mutation may contribute to the development of chronic pancreatitis in some individuals who consume large amounts of alcohol, reflecting the determining interaction between an environmental agent and an underlying genetic susceptibility. Indeed, many other disorders we never suspected clinically may also be associated with this gene now that we can study its mutations in different patient groups.

What can be expected in the reasonable near future from knowing the various components of the human genome? Within the next few years it may be possible to identify the genes associated with inflammatory bowel disease, celiac disease, and GI cancer and therefore understand who is at risk before they develop the disease. One can guess that this predisposition is, in fact, more broadly important than their role in these purely genetic disorders. For example, there is reasonable evidence to support the supposition that the nature of the outcome from hepatitis C virus infection in a given individual will be determined by the nature of the underlining genetically determined host characteristics. It is already apparent that the response to a drug and the risk of a toxic reaction to the drug in most instances are determined by specific genetic loci, including those responsible for drug metabolism. Within the near future, genetic tests may be available to assess risk of toxicity and likelihood of drug response prior to administration of the agent. In general terms, this is illustrated by testing for thiopurine methyltransferase (TPMT) prior to using 6-mercaptopurine.

What are the implications of this determining factor of the genomic revolution? As noted, physicians will be in a position to diagnose illness (actually, the risk of illness) before they have disease. It also means that gastroenterologists will need additional skills and different approaches or perspectives than have been necessary in the past. In particular, greater sophistication will be needed to counsel patients about genetic risk, an issue fraught with many potential ethical implications. In addition, if the diseases we treat have some genetic basis, and we identify genes that confer the likelihood of developing that disease in an index patient, there are also broader implications for involving the entire family in understanding what those genes mean to them. Hence the nature of what it means to be a gastroenterologist may go beyond what it means to take care of the single patient to now include the entire family.

Crossing the Immune Barrier

A second force determining the future of gastroenterology is the eventual ability to circumvent the immune barrier, which has constrained the treatment of many disorders and the entire area of transplantation. With a full understanding of the complexity of the immune system, it is reasonable to expect that highly targeted immunosuppression will become possible, allowing such currently radical notions as xenotransplantation to become a reality. As a result, the future will offer the possibility of treating end-stage GI disease, which is, at best, imperfect for our patients with end-stage liver disease, pancreatic disease, or even intestinal disease.

Crossing the immune barrier is part of a broader set of possibilities, as the molecular and cellular basis of GI tract function and disease are finally understood. There is already evidence of innovative approaches that will deal with end-stage disease by variations on the theme of transplantation and without the use of whole-organ transplantation as we currently think about it. For example, efforts are under way to fabricate organs through the combined use of specific cell populations and artificial matrices. Furthermore, organs that can be fabricated can also be engineered to have specific functional capabilities (e.g., to express a protein that would be therapeutically important in a given patient so they no longer have to take a drug on an intermittent basis in the usual way it is administered to a patient). A whole host of exciting possibilities will emerge once the immune barrier, which prevents easy transplantation across individuals and across species, has been breached. In addition to overall xenotransplantation, the possibilities include the development of cloned organs and extracorporeal, liver-assist devices, which are truly practical. Which will turn out to be the most powerful approach(es) remains to be seen, but broadly they will offer the opportunity to treat patients with end-stage diseases that are currently managed with palliative and empiric measures at best.

Microengineering

The third factor that will transform our future is microengineering. This should be viewed in the context of the present applications of endoscopy, which currently dominates the field. If the development of endoscopy continues on its current, natural path, what can be expected? Eventually, the technological development of endoscopes will allow, in a convenient way, comprehensive endoscopic inspection of the entire luminal GI tract, which is a reasonably close possibility now. In addition, endoscopy will be coupled to some of the other specific capabilities already mentioned for even more precise diagnosis, either in vivo through special spectroscopic and other means of metabolic scanning or through more sophisticated analysis of mucosal and organ biopsies obtained through the endoscope. It is also reasonable to assume that the therapeutic uses of endoscopy itself will continue to expand. Although there are already an impressive variety of interventions in use (e.g., management of hepatobiliary disease), it is reasonable to assume that these scopes will permit therapies, such as chemopharmaceuticals, to be directed more precisely or to deliver constructs of genes to transfect specific areas of the GI tract.

There is certainly room for further sophistication in endoscopy; and with the innovation and creativity being displayed currently by members of our field their development is inevitable. However, it is still reasonable to ask: Is there no other transforming event that could, in fact, change the landscape for endoscopy in a more fundamental way? The question is important for a number of reasons: first, because it is always a mistake not to appreciate the possibility of whole new technologies. Also, in some practical terms, it is difficult not to wonder about limits to existing trends of expanding endoscopy.

The latter point is illustrated by considering the trends in the number of endoscopy procedures done at one hospital (Massachusetts General Hospital) during the last 8–9 years. The shape of the curve is quite telling and is typical, I believe, of most hospitals in the United States and in many other countries as well. In 1989 only 2500 procedures were performed, but the curve percentage is almost hyperbolic, increasing at 30% per year, so that last year we performed about 15,000; indeed, this year we are on a pace to do about 20,000 procedures in our endoscopy suite. Can that continue? If you project these same trends for just a few more years, you arrive at seemingly astronomical numbers of procedures. Indeed, if everything continued without change, it would suggest that by the year 2004 we would do 70,000 procedures, which is practically inconceivable. The question posed is whether other factors will change the shape of this curve, will at least tend to stabilize it because many of the patients currently undergoing endoscopy will be treated in other ways. What might be an intervening force?

The third defining factor that will transform GI is the incredible vigor of new, sophisticated microengineering that is being applied at major institutions to problems of biology. In general terms, these innovations will result in remote-serving diagnostics, remote disease monitoring, and regulation of drug administration. Real prototypes already exist for each of these areas now, so in the next several years it is reasonable to expect the availability of microdiagnostics: small capsules that can traverse the GI tract and transmit physiologic data (pressures, sampling of luminal contents) to a remote receiver (outside the body). The process of microminiaturization of cameras has already allowed internal visualization from a capsule after it has been swallowed. As the engineering challenges are resolved and these techniques become widely available, it could have a transforming effect on the need to perform endoscopy, at least as conventionally defined. This will also be coupled with the enablement of continuous monitoring of disease and drug levels by subcutaneous, small sensors that can transmit the data about the current drug level (e.g., the level of insulin and blood glucose in the diabetic) to a remote station, while the patient is going about his or her daily activities. Prototypes already exist. Taken one step further, it should be possible to transmit instructions back to a subcutaneous drug delivery depot vehicle to release more or less insulin; or instructions could be given in a patient with GI dysmotility that more or less of a drug is to be released to regulate motility on a real-time basis while the patient is going about his or her daily activities.

Although these modalities may seem like science fiction, each exists at least in experimental form. The future offers the potential for convergence of engineering with medicine, specifically gastroenterology. Telemetry and the ability to measure motility on an ongoing basis may finally provide insight into the alterations present in patients with irritable bowel syndrome. The ability to measure portal pressure would provide a means for precisely treating the patient with advanced liver disease to control portal hypertension in a more effective way than is presently possible. In the short term, engineering should facilitate more precise use of endoscopy as increasingly better scopes are made. The same kind of microcapsulization that can make telemetry possible will also allow in vivo "metabolic biopsy" (e.g., current status of hepatic or mucosal oxygenation to assess potential ischemia).

Developments of this sort will make gastroenterology a very different field than is seen today. With implantable delivery modules, telemetry monitoring, and continual feedback, disease treatment will not be intermittent, with adjustments occurring only when the patient comes to an appointment at the clinic, but on an ongoing basis. These possibilities prompt the question: Is it possible that 20 years from now endoscopy will be something we read about in a historical textbook? Although that is unlikely because of the overall power of the technique, it is likely that the curve of increasing usage may not continue in the same exponential fashion because newer technologies will supersede many of the current uses of endoscopy.

High Through-Put Screening

Finally, though perhaps not as obvious, the fourth transforming factor that will determine the future of gastroenterology is the ability (already available) to carry out through-put screening. Pharmaceutical companies now can evaluate many tens of thousands of compounds for their ability to interact with a receptor in a matter of a few days. This capability suggests that as soon as all human genes have been identified, it will be possible to apply this incredible power to develop or identify agents that might be useful for treating disease rather than the slow trial and error method that was possible when only one drug candidate could be tested at a time. As much as this may be looked at as a simple, technical footnote to drug development, this capability should accelerate development of the medications that will be available to provide to patients. Thus, the process of drug development itself will be a major determining factor in the future of gastroenterology. The ability to do high through-put screening will enable the development of new categories of therapeutics that are now only beginning to emerge, such as bioactive proteins and biologicals. A number of these agents are already entering treatment for GI disorders (e.g., interleukins for the treatment of inflammatory bowel disease). Indeed, although gene therapy holds great promise, high through-put screenings by their sheer scale to evaluate many compounds to find the best small molecule with the desired therapeutic effect without the unintended pharmacological effects that might cause adverse reactions will leapfrog over the development of gene therapy. As a result, better treatments should be available for many of the disorders treated essentially empirically today. Treatment is largely empiric because presently the causes of disease are mostly unknown and because current drug development, which has depended on evaluation of one compound at a time is remarkably tedious. The convergence of molecular biology, identification of target genes, and the ability to develop new drugs is already leading to new effective therapies that are specific for a given type of receptor (e.g., irritable bowel syndrome). Potent ways to develop better chemotherapeutic agents for GI cancers and specific agents to treat some of the more important aspects of liver disease for which currently there is no effective treatment (e.g., fibrosis in the patient with chronic hepatitis) will become therapeutically accessible.

Miscellaneous Changes

Having summarized four areas that may result in a very different type of gastroenterology, it is worth noting some more general ways in which the experiences of the future will differ. Not only will there be change in clinical care, but there will also be important changes in GI research and training. Research is likely to evolve through a number of phases. The first, as already described, will be the definition of the genetic basis of each of the major GI disorders. After that, the challenge will be to understand how the products of those genes interact with environmental factors to cause the disease. For example, although it is clear there are predisposing genes in inflammatory bowel disease, this disorder does not develop consistently even in identical twins, indicating that environmental factors must determine which susceptible individual develops the disease.

Furthermore, the rapid evolution of technology and the magnitude of the problems are changing the way research is performed. For the most part, research in the past has been accomplished by relatively small groups of individuals: a senior scientist or physician scientist working with a group of students and fellows. Increasingly, the tools described briefly above require an intensive use of resources and large amounts of money, equipment, and space. As a result, small research group efforts will be, in part, overtaken by larger research consortiums, which can bring together all these resources. Investigators working in groups of three, five, or ten, or even twenty, may soon be superseded by much larger collaborative interrelated groups. Many will involve further collaborations between academic and commercial interests with academic investigators partnering with industry scientists. Thus, in the future, scientific investigations will be done on a bigger scale.

Interesting and paradoxical new challenges will also emerge in the clinical investigation arena. The aggregate effect of powerful high through-put screening, the identification of genes related to most of the GI diseases, and a better understanding of the mechanisms of diseases will present a challenge for clinical investigators: to select those agents that deserve a priority for clinical trials. It is easy to list several dozen potential targets for pharmacologic intervention in inflammatory bowel diseases, and even today it is possible that for each one of those targets there may be ten drugs that could be used to obtain a pharmacological effect. However, it would be impractical to launch 500 clinical trials in IBD patients simultaneously. Therefore selection of the best drug candidates to commit to treating patients will be a central challenge for GI clinical research. One factor that will offset this challenge is the ability to pursue clinical investigation in a more efficient way because surrogate markers based on gene responses permit rapid assessment of the effect of a compound in the patient rather than necessarily requiring prolonged treatment to determine the overall clinical benefit. If it is clear that blocking a disease-causing gene will eventually cause a clinical benefit, it should be possible to determine quickly if a candidate therapeutic agent is useful. Nonetheless, these challenges will conspire to promote movement to larger networks of collaboration, particularly international collaboration for drug development in a way that has only begun during the last 10 years.

Finally, all these changes will have a major impact on the training of gastroenterologists. If we will be seeing a different spectrum of patients, and if we are to have different sets of tools, we must learn different skills than are needed for medicine today. First, there will be a larger foundation of science to understand to be an effective clinician. There will, at least in the short term, be a broader spectrum of endoscopic skills that will require expertise if physicians are to offer their patients everything possible in modern gastroenterology. Finally, because gastroenterology will expand into new territory in terms of some of the effects of the genomic revolution and the other factors discussed above, trainees will need to gain experience in areas that have not traditionally been a part of GI training, including skills to interpret genetic tests and provide genetic counseling.

Consideration of the future of any field would be incomplete without mentioning the role of the rapid escalation in communication made possible by the Internet. The latter is already having an impact in several ways. Certainly, as a result of the Internet, there is now virtually global access to physicians. Although computer access is still scarce in some parts of the world, with its rapid dissemination many physicians are already being contacted for advice by a patient in a remote country. An international marketplace of access to care is becoming a reality. As a consequence, physicians may be forced to adapt to realities that will redefine the very essence of medicine: from direct patient–physician interaction to decision-making at a distance. Another way in which the Internet is already having an impact is through the immediacy by which new advances become disseminated to patients and the general lay public. Many physicians find themselves being confronted with a rash of e-mails from patients about the latest *New England Journal of Medicine* report (perhaps before the physician has received the journal), wanting to know, "Does this apply to my disease?" Hence physicians will be running faster to obtain the same information as our patients, certainly a turnaround in the historical doctor–patient relationship.

Some of these changes will come with new challenges of a different sort as well: Ethical issues must be met in a thoughtful way. The impact of a genetic diagnosis is profound. If we can make a genetic diagnosis (or have the ability to make it) while a child is still developing, particularly if definitive treatment is not yet available for that disorder (e.g., polyposis), the possibility of genetic discrimination is especially worrisome.

Once you can identify someone who is at risk of a disease, will she or he be given equal opportunity for jobs? These advances will also challenge the notion of the essence of the very uniqueness of human life. With this resource-intensive development of medicine, the ethics of access to care will be increasingly at the forefront of society's dilemmas. The treatment of end-stage disease becomes more and more sophisticated at the very time society is confronting the difficult problem of determining when intervention is no longer appropriate in an aging population.

All of these considerations highlight a certain irony. If you accept even part of the described vision for future gastroenterology, it is reasonable to expect "smarter," or at least more precise, diagnosis and knowledge of the causes GI disorders and more sophisticated equipment for diagnosis and treatment. As more and more sophisticated telemetry and other tools are available that permit almost automatic management by computers, what is the role for the gastroenterologist? The paradox is that the true value of the physician will increasingly return to the historical value of the physician: the ability to care for patients, to advise them as someone interested in their humanity and their well-being, not simply in the management of a specific problem. The role of the physician historically was as much counselor as healer in the broad sense.

With all of these changes, it is interesting to speculate on the nature of the visit to the gastroenterologist of the future in contrast to the present reality. In the future, a patient may arrive, and instead of a blood test for a blood count, their full genotype will be assessed. Instead of sending patients to the endoscopy suite when they have complained of abdominal pain, the gastroenterologist will give the patient a small capsule to swallow that will automatically transmit the pattern of motility to a machine, which will analyze the data to provide a (suggested) diagnosis, and with it a recommendation for a specific receptor antagonist, which has been proven to treat that particular disorder of motility. The drug will be monitored, not necessarily by having the patient come in to see the gastroenterologist every 6 months, but by implanting a subcutaneous sensor unit that detects the drug and may also deliver it by communicating with a computer in the physician's office or somewhere else in the health care system.

The gastroenterologist will be at the center of that interaction by virtue of his or her ability to provide something irreplaceable: The physician can talk to patients and ask them how they are feeling. With ultimate progress in diagnostic technology and self-correcting automated therapy, the primary value of the gastroenterologist will be the intangible value of the physician as humanist caring for the patient—the same as that at the threshold of modern scientific medicine. Although any one of these predictions or assumptions may prove mistaken, one thing is clear: Gastroenterology will not be the same 20 or 40 years from now. As a pundit once said, "The future is not what it once was." Indeed, it will be quite different.

Part 2
Ulcerative Colitis Pathophysiology and Therapy

Pathophysiology of and New Treatment for Ulcerative Colitis

Hitoshi Asakura*

Summary. Ulcerative colitis (UC) is a chronic inflammatory disease affecting the mucosa of the colon and rectum. The inflammation seen with UC is an acute-on-chronic type with marked infiltration of lymphocytes, plasma cells, neutrophils, and macrophages induced by interleukin-8 (IL-8) and other cytokines. There was a significant correlation between IL-8 and myeloperoxidase levels in the colonic mucosa of UC tissue. Activated platelets were involved in increased production of reactive oxygen metabolites released from neutrophils, soluble phospholipase II, and platelet microparticles. Cytokine balance, which consists of proinflammatory and immunosuppressive cytokines, is important for provoking the mucosal inflammation. In UC, production of proinflammatory cytokines such as IL-1β, IL-6, IL-8, and tumor necrosis fector-α in the colonic mucosa was more increased than that of immunosuppressive cytokines such as IL-10, transforming growth factor-β, and interleukin-1 receptor antagonist. The number of $CD45RO^{+}CD4^{+}$ and $CD45RO^{+}CD8^{+}$ T cells expressing Fas ligands in UC mucosa was significantly increased compared to that in the controls. We succeeded in establishing an experimental ulcerative colitis model in mice (MAIDS colitis). A double color-staining immunofluorescence study showed that Mac-1 cells were positive for interferon-γ (IFNγ) or IL-10 (or both), and CD4 T cells were positive for IL-10. The susceptible genes for inflammatory bowel disease are being assessed. The carriage ratio of allele K in codon 469 of ICAM-1 and allele A6 of MICA was higher in UC than the controls. There are three kinds of leukocytapheresis for treatment of UC: the leukocyte removal filter method, centrifugal leukocyte apheresis, and granulocyte apheresis (G-column). These treatments were effective for 60%–70% of patients with steroid-resistant and steroid-dependent UC.

Key words. Ulcerative colitis, HLA, Cytokine, Treatment, Susceptibility gene

Ulcerative colitis (UC) is a chronic disease of unknown etiology that affects the mucosa of the colon and rectum. The disease is thought to begin usually in the rectum

---

Third Department of Internal Medicine, Niigata University School of Medicine, 1-757 Asahi-machi-dori, Niigata 951-8122, Japan
* e-mail: asakura@med.niigata-u.ac.jp

and then extend to involve parts of the remaining colon. The histopathological features of UC are characterized by two major features. One is diffuse inflammation with mucosal infiltration of lymphocytes, plasma cells, histiocytes, neutrophils, and eosinophils; and the other is architectural distortion of the colonic crypts with frequent depletion of goblet cells. Clinical patterns are classified by the extent of the diseased portion of the large intestine, disease severity, and disease course. When 234 patients with UC we treated were grouped by clinical patterns, the disease extent was as follows: entire colitis 52.1%, left-sided colitis 29.1%, proctitis 15.8%, and segmental colitis 3.0%. The disease severity was as follows: mild type 31.6%, moderate type 46.1%, severe type 21.8%, and fulminant type 0.4%. The disease course was as follows: intermittent type 63.7%, continuous type 18.8%, acute fulminant type 6.0%, and only one attack type 11.5%. Most of the UC we encountered had a chronic and intermittent course.

Acute-on-Chronic Inflammation

Studies of Neutrophils, Free Radicals, and Interleukin-8

During the active stage of UC, marked infiltration of neutrophils near and invading the epithelial line forms crypt abscesses and infiltration of neutrophils in the colonic mucosa affected by chronic inflammation in UC. This may indicate acute-on-chronic inflammation resembling the features of chronic active gastritis induced by *Helicobacter pylori*. To clarify these histopathological findings, we measured myeloperoxidase levels, which are indicative of infiltrating neutrophils, free radical expression and interleukin-8 (IL-8) with the capacity to infiltrate neutrophils into the inflamed mucosa and release reactive oxygen metabolites. IL-8 and myeloperoxidase levels measured by enzyme-linked immunosorbent assay (ELISA) and electroimmunoassay (EIA), respectively, in 24-hour organ cultures of the biopsy specimens from active UC were significantly higher than those from inactive UC tissue and controls [1]. Reactive oxygen metabolites from biopsy specimens in active UC measured by luminol-dependent chemiluminescence were also markedly increased when compared with those of inactive UC tissue and controls. Interestingly, IL-8 levels were closely correlated to luminol-dependent chemiluminescence and myeloperoxidase levels. These findings suggest that IL-8 plays an important role in the acute-on-chronic inflammation of UC. The expression and localization of IL-8 mRNA were examined in the colonic mucosa of patients with UC using an in situ hybridization technique [2]. IL-8 mRNA expression was clearly augmented in most active UC mucosa; and the cell count positive for IL-8 mRNA per unit area was markedly increased in moderate and severe UC compared with that in mild UC and controls (Fig. 1). The epithelial cells of the colonic mucosa obtained from patients with active UC revealed expression of IL-8 mRNA. The colonic epithelial cells are thought to have antenna against the antigens in the intestinal cavity.

Role of Activated Platelets in Colonic Inflammation

Production of reactive oxygen metabolites was markedly increased in the peripheral blood and colonic mucosa of patients with active UC. Most of these metabolites were released from granulocytes. We found that activated platelets were involved in the pro-

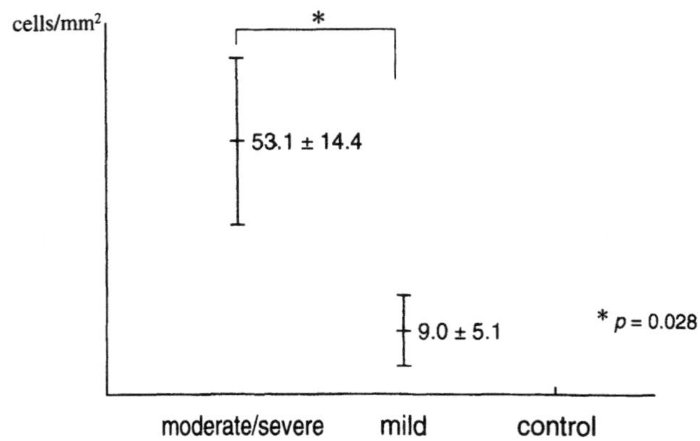

FIG. 1. Population of interleukin-8 (IL-8) mRNA-positive cells in colonic mucosa of ulcerative colitis (UC)

duction of reactive oxygen metabolites from granulocytes in the inflammation of UC. As activated platelets express P-selectin, they were assessed by flow cytometry using fluorescein thiocyanate (FITC)-labeled anti-P-selectin antibody. The population of P-selectin-positive activated platelets was markedly increased in the peripheral blood of patients with UC compared with that of controls [3]. When polymorphonuclear neutrophils (PMNs) obtained from healthy controls were incubated with platelets obtained from patients with UC or normal controls, stimulated by phorbol 12-myristate 13-acetate (PMA), and measured by luminol-enhanced chemiluminescence, production of reactive oxygen metabolites by the PMNs was markedly enhanced in UC compared with that of controls. These reactions between activated platelets and PMNs occurred via P-selectin. The activated platelets also released more microparticles in UC than in healthy controls.

Soluble phospholipase II is an enzyme with the capacity to convert phospholipid to arachidonic acid, resulting in the production of leukotrienes and prostaglandins, which are involved in inflammation. The soluble phospholipase II levels were increased in the peripheral blood of patients with UC compared with those of controls and were closely correlated with the total amount of intestinal inflammation (assessed by histological activity of the biopsy specimens obtained from each segment of the large intestine during colonoscopy). Interestingly, the total amount of histological activity was closely correlated with the number of platelets in peripheral blood (Fig. 2). Soluble phospholipase II is released from platelets, colonic epithelial cells, and others. The above-mentioned findings may support the idea that reactive oxygen metabolites produced by the combined reactions of PMNs and activated platelets play an important role in the acute-on-chronic inflammation of UC.

Cytokine Balance

Proinflammatory cytokines such as IL-1, IL-6, IL-8, IL-12, IL-18, tumor necrosis factor-α (TNFα), and interferon-γ (IFNγ) may accelerate inflammatory reactions in the colonic mucosa. On the other hand, cytokines such as IL-10, transforming growth

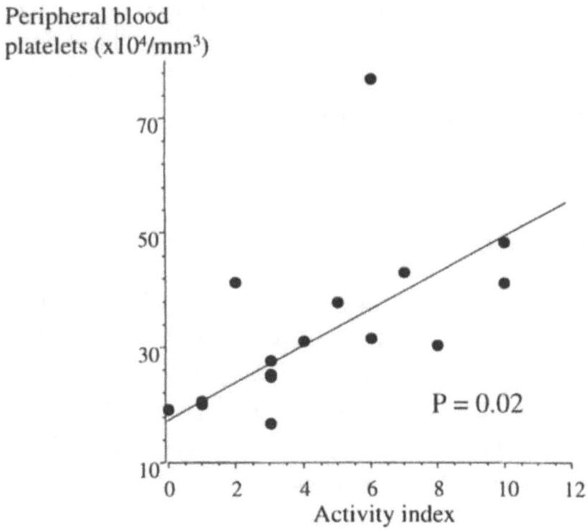

FIG. 2. Correlation between peripheral blood platelet counts and the activity index of colonic mucosa in UC. The activity index was determined as follows: active = 1, inactive = 0. The total of each histological score from 10 segments of colon was regarded as disease activity

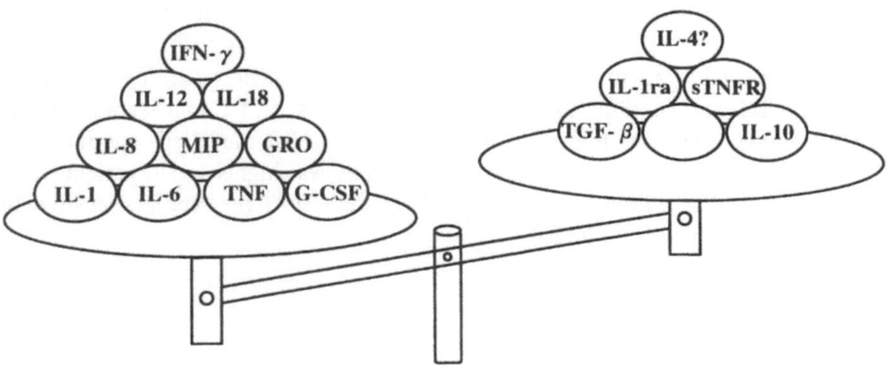

FIG. 3. Cytokine balance in the inflammation of UC. Balance beam declines to the proinflammatory cytokines. *IFN-γ*, interferon-γ; *IL*, interleukin; *MIP*, macrophage inflammatory protein; *TNF*, tumor necrosis factor; *G-CSF*, granulocyte colony-stimulating factor; *STNFR*, soluble TNF receptor; *TGF-β*, transforming growth factor-β; *GRO*, growth related oncogene; *IL-1ra*, interleukin-1 receptor antagonist

factor-β (TGFβ), IL-1 receptor antagonist (IL-1ra), sometimes IL-4, and high doses of soluble TNFα receptor (sTNFR) may suppress the inflammatory response. Therefore, cytokine balance is important to understand in terms of the inflammatory processes in UC (Fig. 3) [4].

Levels of proinflammatory cytokines such as IL-1, IL-6, IL-8, and TNFα in the active colonic mucosa of patients with UC were markedly increased compared with those of inactive UC tissue and healthy controls. However, production of such cytokines as IL-10, IL-1ra, sTNFR, and TGFβ to suppress the inflammatory reactions did not increase in the active stage of UC but increased at the resolving stage compared to levels during the remission stage of UC and of controls [5]. Enhanced expression of IL-1, IL-6, IL-8, and TNFα mRNA, but not IL-10 mRNA, of mononuclear cells obtained from the colonic mucosa [assessed by reverse transcriptase-polymerase chain reaction (RT-PCR) using appropriate primers] was found in the active stage of UC [6]. These findings may support the idea that cytokine balance between proinflammatory cytokines and cytokines to suppress inflammation inclines to induce the mucosal inflammation of UC.

Role of Lymphocytes and Macrophages

Numerous lymphocytes infiltrated the colonic mucosa of UC. $CD4^+$ T cells more than $CD8^+$ T cells infiltrated the active mucosa [7]. $CD4^+$ T cells had a median 23.5% HLA-DR expression, indicating activation of CD4 T cells. The Fas/Fas ligand (FasL) system is a mechanism responsible for activation-induced cell death (AICD), which maintains homeostasis of the mucosal immune system. Fas/FasL expression on activated colonic T cells of UC patients was assessed to clarify the role of activated colonic T cells in the long-standing inflammation of UC.

Fas, FasL, and CD45RO expression on peripheral blood and colonic T lymphocytes of patients with UC were assayed by flow cytometry using each antibody. Most colonic T cells expressed both CD45RO and Fas antigen, a situation different from that in peripheral blood [8,9]. The number of $CD45RO^+CD8^+$ and Fas^+CD8^+T cells was significantly lower in patients with UC than in the controls. However, the number of $CD45RO^+CD4^+$ and $CD45RO^+CD8^+$T cells expressing FasL in UC mucosa was significantly higher than in the controls. In addition, Fas-mediated apoptosis of $CD45RO^+CD8^+$ T cells, but not $CD45RO^+CD4^+$ T cells, was higher in UC patients than in the controls. These findings suggest that $CD45RO^+CD4^+$T cells are less sensitive to apoptotic signals mediated by Fas.

Experimental Colitis

Many kinds of experimental colitis are available for studying the immunological states of colitis (e.g., IL-2-deficient mice, IL-10-deficient mice, TGFβ1-deficient mice, SCID mice transferred with $CD45RB^{high}$ T cells, and so on) (Fig. 4). The LP-BM5 murine leukemia virus (MuLV) is a retrovirus known to induce profound immunodeficiency with splenomegaly and generalized lymphoadenopathy in B6 mice, resulting in an acquired immunodeficiency syndrome (AIDS)-like syndrome (MAIDS). Sjögren's syndrome-like exocrinopathy occurred in these mice; and nude mice that underwent adoptive transfer of spleen cells from these mice developed ulcerative colitis-like colitis (MAIDS colitis) and Sjögren-like exocrinopathy [10] (Fig. 5). There were numerous $CD4^+$ T cells and Mac-1^+ cells in the colonic mucosa of these MAIDS colitis mice. However, few Mac-1^+ cells infiltrated the salivary glands. The MAIDS colitis had enhanced expression of IFNγ and IL-10 mRNA assessed by RT-PCR. A double color-staining immunofluorescence study using several antibodies (e.g., CD4, CD8, Mac-1, IFNγ, IL-10) showed that Mac-1^+ cells were positive for IFNγ, IL-10, or both; and that most $CD4^+$ T cells were positive for IL-10, although the population of IFNγ-positive $CD4^+$ T cells was low [11]. These results suggest that Mac-1^+ macrophages producing IFNγ and IL-10 might play a crucial role in the pathogenesis of MAIDS colitis in combination with $CD4^+$ T cells.

1. Chemical model
   - (1) Acetic acid
   - (2) Ethanol
   - (3) Sulfated polysaccharides
     - ① Carrageenan
     - ② Dextran sulfate sodium (DSS)
2. Immunological model
   - (1) T cell model
     - ①2,4-dinitro-chlorobenzene (DNCB)
     - ②Trinitrobenzene sulfonic acid (TNBS)
   - (2) Cell transfer model
     - ①$CD4^{+}CD45RB^{high}T \rightarrow$SCID mice
     - ②MAIDS colitis
3. Genetic engineering model
   - (1) Transgenic animal model
     - ① HLA-B27 transgenic rat
     - ② IL-7 transgenic mice
     - ③ Bone marrow reconstituted tg ε 26 mice
   - (2) Gene targeting animal model
     - ① IL-2-deficient mice
     - ② IL-10-deficient mice
     - ③ T cell-receptor mutant mice
     - ④ TGF-β 1-deficient mice
     - ⑤ Gαi2-deficient mice

FIG. 4. Experimental colitis model

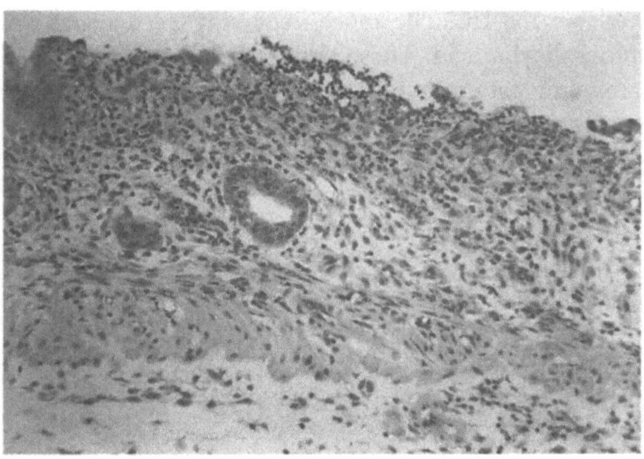

FIG. 5. Histopathological findings of chronic nonspecific colitis in our model. H & E

Gene Polymorphism and Disease Susceptibility

An increased frequency of inflammatory bowel disease (IBD) in families may implicate genetic factors in the etiology of these diseases. The susceptible genes for IBD are being assessed using twins suffering from IBD. Genetic analysis of IBD in a large European cohort showed linkage to chromosomes 12 and 16 [12]. We analyzed single nucleotide polymorphism (SNP) on IL-1α and IL-1β, and intercellular adhesion molecule-1 (ICAM-1). The carriage ratio of allele K in codon 469 of the ICAM-1 gene was significantly higher in patients with UC and Crohn's disease than in the controls.

The association of HLA with UC was studied merely as a genetic marker in the early stage of the HLA study. An increased incidence of HLA-B35 in UC was shown in a Jewish population. However, in Japanese patients with UC, the increased incidence of HLA-B52 and DR2(DRB1* 1502) and conservation of B52 and DR2 haplotype were reported by us [13,14]. There is a class III antigen in HLA between a class I antigen (HLA-A, B, and C) and class II antigen (DR, DP, and DQ). The MICA [major histocompatibility complex class I (MHC-I) chain-related gene A] is the nearest neighbor of the HLA-B locus. The MICA gene has the α1, α2, and α3 extracellular domains and a transmembrane region, which has a triplet repeat microsatellite polymorphism of $(GCT/AGC)_n$. This consists of four, five, six, and nine repetitions of GCT (alanine) or five repetitions of GCT with one additional nucleotide insertion (GGCT). These alleles are designated A4, A5, A6, A9, and A5.1 alleles, respectively. MICA and MICB were recognized by intestinal epithelial T cells expressing γδ T cell receptors. The MICA gene is strongly expressed on the gastrointestinal epithelial cells. Analysis of microsatellite polymorphism in the transmembrane region of the MICA gene in Japanese UC revealed a high frequency of MICA allele A6 when compared with the controls. Interestingly, the patients with UC who had homozygous allele A6 had an early onset of UC (second to third decade of life); those having no allele A6 had a late onset of UC (fourth to fifth decade) [15].

New Treatment

Many treatments are now available for UC. The most frequently used drugs are salazosulfapyridine and 5-aminosalicylic acid. These drugs are effective for mild and moderate UC, but there are many patients with UC who are steroid-resistant or steroid-dependent. Immunosuppressive drugs such as 6-mercaptopurine, azathio-

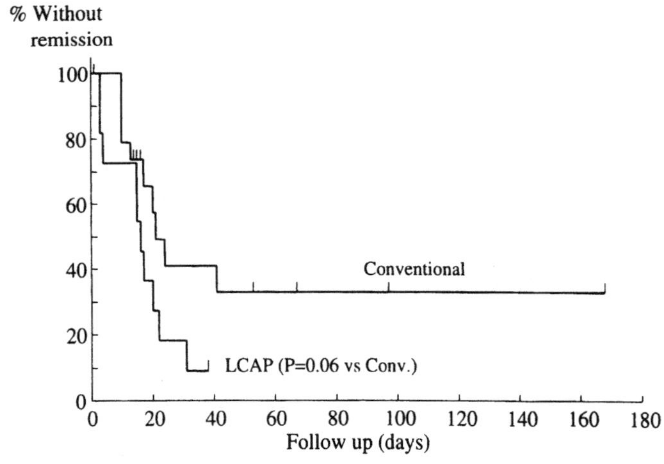

FIG. 6. Remission rates of UC in steroid-resistant patients undergoing leukocytapheresis and patients receiving only conventional treatment with prednisolone and salazosulfapyridine. *LCAP*, leukocytapheresis; *Conv.*, conventional

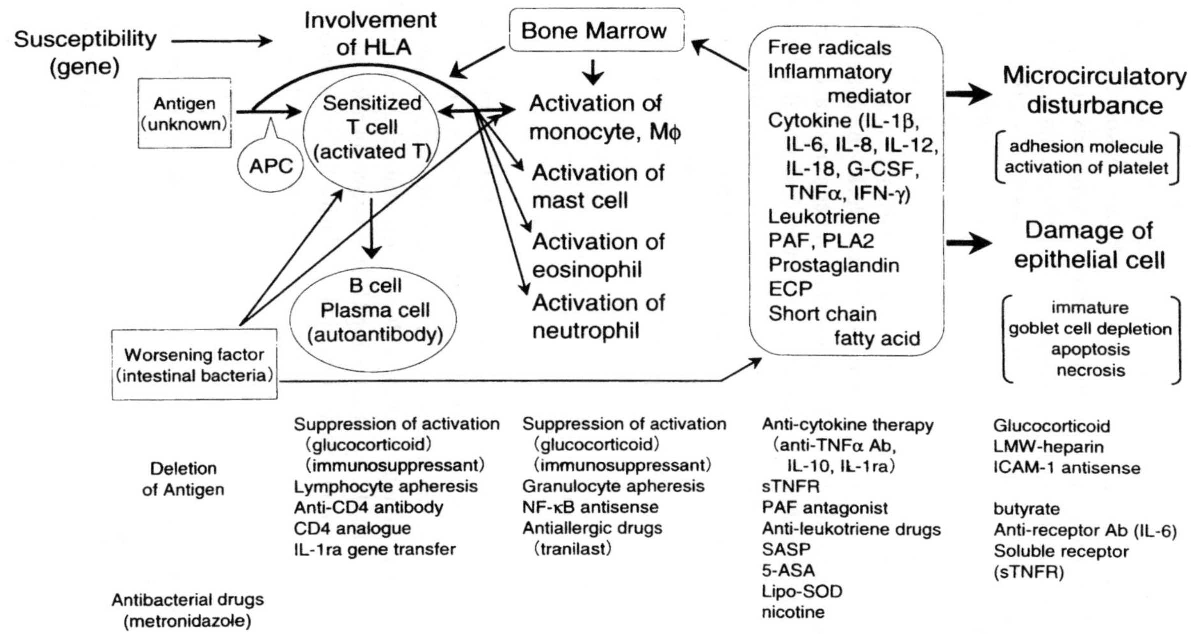

Fig. 7. Schema of the pathophysiology of UC and treatments corresponding to each of its immunological states. *APC*, antigen-presenting cells; *Mø*, macrophages; *PAF*, platelet-activating factor; *ECP*, eosinophilic cationic protein; *SASP*, salazosulfapyridine; *5-ASA*, 5-aminosalicylic acid; *Lipo-SOD*, superoxide dismutase; *LMW*, low molecular weight; *ICAM-1*, intercellular adhesion molecule-1, *Ab*, antibody

prine, cyclosporine, and methotrexate are available for steroid-dependent or steroid-resistant UC. Recently, three white blood cell apheresis methods have become available for treatment of UC and Crohn's disease in Japan: leukocytapheresis with leukocyte removal filter (LCAP), centrifugal leukocyte apheresis, and granulocyte apheresis (G-column, Adacolumn). We performed these three treatments for steroid-dependent or steroid-resistant patients with UC once a week. More than 90% of the patients receiving the treatment with leukocyte apheresis by LCAP and centrifugal leukocyte apheresis achieved clinical remisson within 4 weeks after starting leukocyte apheresis (Fig. 6). Some of the patients in whom remission had been induced had exacerbations when they were treated with apheresis only once a month. Therefore, we treated them again with leukocyte apheresis once a week. The patients in whom remission was not induced with these treatments had undergone total colectomy with a W-type ileal pouch procedure. One female patient who had a total colectomy with W-type of ileal pouch procedure developed severe pouchitis and ileitis a few years after the operation that did not respond to metronidazole. It was reported that pouchitis developed in patients with UC but not in those with familial adenomatous polyposis. Patients who undergo the pouch procedure should be carefully followed.

Conclusions

Ulcerative colitis is an intractable, nonspecific inflammatory disease of the colon and rectum with acute-on-chronic inflammation. The pathophysiology of UC, including the immunological state, is summarized in Fig. 7. Many treatments that respond to each step of the pathophysiological states of UC are now available. However, because we have no way to eliminate the agent inducing UC, the above-mentioned treatments are only symptomatic. Further study is needed to clarify the immunological and pathophysiological states of UC for the development of new treatments.

References

1. Anezaki K, Asakura H, Honma T, et al (1998) Correlation between interleukin-8, and myeloperoxidase or luminol-dependent chemiluminescence in inflamed mucosa of ulcerative colitis. Intern Med 37:253–258
2. Arai F, Takahashi T, Furukawa K, et al (1998) Mucosal expression of interleukin-6 and interleukin-8 messenger RNA in ulcerative colitis and in Crohn's disease. Dig Dis Sci 43:2071–2079
3. Suzuki K, Sugimura K, Hasegawa K, et al (in press) Activated platelets in ulcerative colitis enhance the production of reactive oxygen metabolites by polymorphonuclear cells. Scand J Gastroenterol
4. Asakura H (1999) Proinfammatory cytokines in IBD. J Gastroenterol 34:149–151
5. Ishizuka K, Sugimura K, Honma T, et al (2001) Influence of interleukin-10 on the interleukin-1 receptor antagonist (IL-1ra)/interleukin-1β (IL-1β) ratio in the colonic mucosa of ulcerative colitis. Digestion 63(suppl 1):22–27
6. Funakoshi K, Sugimura K, Anezaki K, et al (1998) Spectrum of cytokine gene expression in intestinal mucosal lesions of Crohn's disease and ulcerative colitis. Digestion 59:73–78
7. Sasakawa T, Takizawa H, Bannai H, et al (1995) Activated $CD4^+$ and $CD8^+$ cells in the colonic mucosa of ulcerative colitis patients: their relationship to HLA-DR antigen

expression on the colonic epithelium and serum soluble CD25 levels. Digestion 56:516–522

8. Asakura H, Suzuki A, Ohtsuka K, et al (1999) Gut-associated lymphoid tissues in ulcerative colitis. J Parent Enter Nutr 23:S25–28
9. Suzuki A, Sugimura K, Ohtsuka K, et al (2000) Fas/Fas ligand expression and characteristics of primed CD45RO^{+} T cells in the inflamed mucosa of ulcerative colitis. Scand J Gastroenterol 35:1278–1283
10. Suzuki K, Narita T, Tui R, et al (1997) Induction of intestinal lesions in nu/nu mice induced by transfer of lymphocytes from syngeneic mice infected with murine retrovirus. Gut 41:221–228
11. Suriki H, Suzuki K, Baba Y, et al (2000) Analysis of cytokine production in the colon of nude mice with experimental colitis induced by adoptive transfer of immunocompetent cells from mice infected with a murine retrovirus. Clin Immunol 97:33–42
12. Curran ME, Lau KF, Hampe J, et al (1999) Genetic analysis of inflammatory bowel diseases in a large European cohort supports linkage to chromosomes 12 and 16. Gastroenterology 115:1066–1071
13. Asakura H, Tsuchiya M, Aiso S, et al (1982) Association of the human leukocyte DR2 antigen with Japanese ulcerative colitis. Gastroenterologty 82:413–418
14. Asakura H, Sugimura K (1995) HLA, antineutrophil cytoplasmic autoantibody, and heterogeneity in ulcerative colitis. Gastroenterology 108:597–599
15. Sugimura K, Ota M, Matsuzawa J, et al (2001) A close relationship of triplet repeat polymorphism in MHC class I chain-related gene A (MICA) to the disease susceptibility and behavior in ulcerative colitis. Tissue Antigens 57:9–14

Part 3
Life Style-Related Diseases and Gastroenterology

New Target of Gastroenterology: Overcoming Life Style-Related Diseases

Saburo Nakazawa*

The world population is now over six billion. In addition, we are in the middle of an unprecedent aging society, and medical practice is starting to focus on age-related diseases. The pathogenesis, early diagnosis, research, and development of treatments and prophylaxis are highlighted as an issue not only in the medical field but also in society. The target has shifted from secondary prevention via early diagnosis and early treatment to primary prevention before symptoms and signs are apparent.

Looking as far back in medical history as the era of Galileo Galilei (1564–1643), René Descartes (1596–1650), and Sir Isaac Newton (1642–1727), the basics of modern Western medicine were established during the nineteenth century by pursuing specific pathogeneses, with the medical targets infectious diseases or acute diseases. By the second half of the twentieth century most of these diseases were under control.

Discovery of the double helical structure of DNA by James Watson and Francis Crick in 1953 was followed by drastic advances in molecular biology and genetics, and these technologies have been applied clinically. Research studying the masses and medicine based on statistical analysis are no longer suitable. Detailed genetic analysis of individuals, or "tailor made" technology, draws our attention.

On the other hand, though the genes determine the personal primary condition and have only indirect effects on acquired life style, it is difficult to determine the physiological activity and function based on one's personal life style by looking at genes. Hereafter, we can consider disease as an issue of personal misadaptation to the environment. It is the chronic disease or life style-related disease we should study.

Disease never derives from a single pathogenic cause. (1) Genetic factors interact with the nervous system, immune system, and endocrine system. (2) Genetic factors, pathogens that invade the human body directly, and social, economic, and mental factors interact. The consequence is disease. Life style-related diseases may be caused by misadaptation to the drastic changes of environmental factors though changes at the genetic level that take thousands or tens of thousands of years to develop. The

---

President of the Japanese Society of Gastroenterology
Department of Internal Medicine, Second Teaching Hospital, Fujita Health University School of Medicine, 3-6-10 Otobashi, Nakagawa-ku, Nagoya 454-8509, Japan
* e-mail: nakazawas@muh.biglobe.ne.jp

negative aspects of various industries have continued since the industrial revolution including industrial wastes and public nuisances. Obesity due to excessive food intake is followed by diseases that include atherosclerosis, diabetes mellitus (DM), ischemic heart disease, cerebrovascular disease, and cancer.

Human genetic factors no longer control the changes. According to Yoshinori Hiroi, the focus is now "genes and culture." Human genes have not changed since the Cro-Magnon era. However, the culture humans have established affects our food life and has forced us to spend huge amounts of money to improve the environment and medical caw in Japan. The rapid increase in the aged population falls also into the category of "genes and culture."

Looking at the changes in mortality in Japan, cerebrovascular disease took the place of tuberculosis as the most common cause of death in 1951. In 1958 cerebrovascular disease, cancer, and heart disease were in a higher rank. Now cancer, heart disease, and cerebrovascular disease are responsible for 60% of deaths. In parallel with these changes, the number of outclinic patients increased, reaching 7.49 million with hypertension, 2.18 million with diabetes mellitus (DM), 2.04 million with heart disease, 1.73 million with cerebrovascular disease, and 1.36 million with cancer.

Genetic factors, external environmental factor, and life style are major causes of the diseases or determinant factors of prognosis. Typical factors in the life style and their related diseases are as follows.

1. Smoking—lung cancer or pulmonary emphysema
2. Excessive fat intake—colon cancer
3. Excess sodium intake—apoplexy
4. Obesity—diabetes mellitus (DM)
5. Alcohol excess—liver cirrhosis

We could, then, prevent life style-related disease or its progression by changing our life style. The present situation with major life style-related diseases and their pathogenic mechanisms are as follows.

Diabetes Mellitus

Most DM in Japan is non-insulin-dependent diabetes mellitus (NIDDM). DM is the ninth most common cause of death in Japan. In 1997 the people whose hemoglobin A1c level was over 5.6% numbered 13.7 million. About 26.9%–29% of the total population have obesity of more than 20% over standard body weight. The DM patients numbered 6.9 million and people in a pre-DM condition numbered 6.8 million. About 3000–4000 people became blind annually.

Hypertension

The number of patients with hypertension is rapidly increasing in those over 40 years of age. The associated mortality rate was 11.9/100 000 population) in 1950 and 17.7/100 000 in 1970. It decreased to 5.4/100 000 in 1998.

Atherosclerosis

Atherosclerosis derives from an abnormality in lipid metabolism. It is the most important cause of life style-related disease.

Hyperlipidemia

According to the guidelines of the Japanese Society for Atherosclerosis, hyperlipidemia is defined as total cholesterol >220 mg/dl, low density lipoprotein (LDL) cholesterol >140 mg/ml, and triglycerides >150 mg/dl. M.G. Marmot and colleagues compared the prevalence of cardiovascular disease in 11 900 Japanese individuals (age 45–69 years) who lived in Japan, Hawaii, and California. The prevalence of definite coronary heart disease was 5.3/1000 population in Japan, 5.2/1000 in Hawaii, and 10.8/1000 in California. These numbers correlated positively with the serum cholesterol level.

Apoplexy

Apoplexy is the third most common cause of death. The number of patients increased from 1 144 000 in 1987 to 1 729 000 in 1996.

Obesity

According to the census of national nutrition in 1998 (published in 2000), one in four males (13 millions) and one in five females (10 millions) are obese (defined as weight of more than 25% of standard body weight). A follow-up of the Framingham study after 26 years by Helen B. Hubert and colleagues showed that obesity is an independent risk factor for cardiovascular disease, even in the absence of other risk factors, including age, serum cholesterol, systolic blood pressure, and smoking.

Tadasu Tsujii investigated the causes and complications of fatty liver in 209 patients in 1996. He reported that excessive nutrition, DM, and excessive drinking are common causes of fatty liver; and hypertension, gout (hyperuricacidemia), angina pectoris, and gallbladder stones are common complications. There are two types of fatty liver, one of which tends to be accompanied by complications indicating that fatty liver should not be neglected. Fat cells store energy and secrete various substances including leptin, tumor necrosis factor-α (TNFα), PAI-1, angiotensinogen, lipoprotein lipase, cholesterol ester carrier protein, and adipsin (complement factor D). Leptin is a protein coded by the *ob* gene; it binds receptors in the ventromedial hypothalamus and inhibits appetite. It also increases the metabolic rate and controls body weight. Abnormalities in leptin or its receptor (in target organs or cells?) result in obesity. TNFα decreases the action of insulin by inhibiting insulin receptor kinase, or it induces insulin resistance by inhibiting the production of glucose carrier.

Ischemic Heart Disease

After World War II an increase of atherosclerotic disease was predicted in the United States, and the Framingham study was undertaken in 1948. The Framingham study revealed the positive correlation of the serum cholesterol level with coronary heart disease and showed that a high serum cholesterol level (>220 mg/ml) increased mortality due to coronary heart disease. In 1975 the Ni-HO-San study reported that the general population has high serum cholesterol levels because of high fat intake in Western countries and so has a high mortality rate due to coronary heart disease. In Japan 2 039 000 people have coronary heart disease. The mortality rate due to coronary heart disease in Japan was 57.5/100 000 in 1935 and has increased year by year. It was to up 106.2/100 000 in 1980 and had almost doubled in 1998 (i.e., 114.3/100 000).

Cancer

The prevalence of cancer increases with aging. Aging is an inevitable phenomenon as an effect of natural selection. Cancer cells are those that escape from the natural selection process. Thus, aging and cancer are closely related.

The oncogene was discovered during the early twentieth century. In 1910 Rous found that an RNA virus infection in chickens causes sarcoma, and he designated this gene *src*. Later study demonstrated that normal cells have cellular oncogenes, called proto-oncogenes. When a proto-oncogene is mutated by a carcinogen (e.g., radiation, aging) it causes cancer.

Free radicals, O_2^- (superoxide anion), and oxidative stress (such as that caused by a peroxidated lipid) cause DNA fragmentation, chromosome abnormalities, and mutation, resulting in cancer. For example, hepatitis B (HBV) and C (HCV) viruses and alcohol induce chronic hepatitis and adenoma. Inactivation of the *p53* and *Rb* genes or deletion of the 16q chromosome results in liver cancer. In the colon, inactivation of the *APC* gene or the *ras* gene is related to adenoma, and inactivation of the *p53* gene is related to cancer. Inactivation of the *DCC* gene and deletion of 13q/14q are also related to carcinogenesis.

Among the more than 100 000 human genes, several hundred cancer-related genes are expected. As described above, genetic abnormalities cause cancer, and each cancer has a different combination of genetic abnormalities. Genetic abnormalities are affected by foods, smoking, excess drinking, O_2^-, and free radicals, to many of which we are exposed during daily life. Hence cancer is a life style-related disease.

Oxidative stress is related to various pathogeneses. Oxidation-facilitating agents that induce oxidative stress are as follows.

1. Intrinsic factors: oxygen produced by leukocyte and macrophage: oxygen produced by enzyme reaction
2. Extrinsic factors: food/nutrition; tobacco/alcohol; radiation; drugs/hormones; carcinogens; inflammation.

The *duration* of oxidative stress is more closely related to abnormalities in the human body than is the *degree* of oxidative stress.

In conjunction with cancer and oxidative stress such as O_2^-, the Notional Cancer Institute reported a correlation of 50% with foods in 1975. In 1981 Richard Doll reported that carcinogenic factors are food/nutrition (35%), tobacco (30%), alcohol (3%), radiation and sunlight (3%), food additives (1%), medicines (1%), and others. He emphasized the importance of foods. The incidence of gastric cancer and liver cancer was decreased among immigrants from Japan to the United States. In contrast, the incidence of colon cancer, prostate cancer, and breast cancer was increased. It is not fully understood what substances in foods are related to cancer production. Nitroso compounds, decreased diet fiber, shortage of vitamin A, overnutrition, and obesity may be related to cancer. In addition, peroxidated lipid radicals derived from the peroxide reaction induce DNA damage, resulting in cancer. The amount of peroxidated lipid radicals in daily foods is more than 1000 times that of carcinogens in foods. Such large oxidative stress affects carcinogenesis.

Oral lipid intake in Japan was increased from 24.7 g/day in 1960 to 58.4 g/day in 1992. Along with this rapid increase, which has more than doubled during the past 30 years, breast cancer, colon cancer, and prostate cancer increased in Western society. Thus, it is interesting to elucidate the relation between genetic factors and environmental factors (i.e., nature and nurture).

Cancer is a phenomenon of aging. Genomic abnormalities are closely related to aging. The aged population has many more mutations in the genome than does the younger population. Genetics, environment, and life style interact and are related to the pathogenesis and progression of life style-related diseases. Among life style factors, food is especially important. The Ministry of Health formed a committee to study nutrition and foods for the twenty-first century. The committee reported the following in March 1997: (1) establishment of a general monitoring system for nutrition and food; (2) solid, basic investigation and research on nutrition and nutritional demand; (3) nutritional value of dishes in restaurants and foods in general; (4) education for people engaged in health-giving or nutrition-related work.

Presently, various treatment regimens, including drug therapy, have been applied to life style-related diseases. However, from the standpoint of prophylactic medicine, dietary therapy and drug therapy comprise only a minor part of treatment. In addition, these prophylactic treatments are started after a diagnosis as palliative therapy to prevent disease progression in most cases. My thoughts are focused on prophylaxis—before the appearance of disease symptoms and signs. These pathological conditions are derived from food after their absorption from the gastrointestinal tract and the appearance of metabolites. Therefore, the target of treatment should be restriction of absorption from the gastrointestinal tract.

Diet fiber and phytochemicals are especially important in foods.

1. *Dietary fiber*: Quantitation of diet fiber has been available since Prosky established the method.

2. *Physiological function*: Dietary fiber is not digested and not absorbed in the small intestine. In the colon, bacteria digest diet fiber and produce short-chain fatty acids. Vitamins, methane, and hydrogen lower the pH in the colon; and some of the short-chain fatty acids are absorbed. These absorbed materials correspond to approximately 10% of nutrients.

3. *Phytochemicals*: In addition to nutrients (i.e., carbohydrate, protein, lipid), plants produce polyphenol alleyl compounds, terpenoid compounds (β-carotene), vitamins

(α-tocopherol), and chlorophyll, which are secondary metabolites of photosynthesis. These secondary metabolites, called phytochemicals, have various biological functions and pharmacological actions, including: (1) prevention of cancer; (2) antioxidation; (3) biological protection; (4) immune potentiation; and (5) prevention of dental caries. Vegetables contain antioxidants that are not produced by animals. The typical antioxidant is phenol compound, which mainly binds to radicals and has a chelating effect on heavy metals.

Polyphenol extracted from red wine has a stronger effect on the peroxidation of LDL than does α-tocopherol. There have been few papers on absorption from the gastrointestinal tract and the tissue distribution, accumulation, and action of flavonoid. Recently a group at the National Institute of Nutrition and Health demonstrated that red wine stabilizes the oxidation of LDL. It was shown that red wine and green tea enhance the antioxidation effect in serum. After administration of 230–540 mg, green tea catechins the plasma concentration was increased in a dose-dependent manner up to 4500 pmol/ml. The absorption and metabolism of flavonoid await future study. Phytochemicals in daily foods are considered safe. Most catechins exist in a glucuronic acid-conjugated form. In general, foreign bodies are excreted by glucuronic acid conjugation. The safety of catechins should be reevaluated in case of megadose intake.

As described above, foods, exercise, relaxation, and antioxidation are highly effective for controling life style-related diseases. In 1970 it was thought that Japanese foods had an ideal balance of nutrients. Fat intake gradually increased, however, and now comprises more than 25% of total calories. In 1974 fat intake was 22.3%, in 1970 it was 25.3%, and in 1997 it was 26.6%; and it continues to increase. In 1988 the Ministry of Education Research Committee proposed a third function of foods: nutrition and taste.

We must recognize that nutrition and function are totally different concepts. The effect of functional foods must be evaluated qualitatively. It is difficult to demonstrate a dose-response effect, which contributes to own difficulty recognizing the problem. Gastroenterologists have an important role to play in resolving this issue. The following factors are important for this purpose.

1. Precise epidemiological investigation
2. Verification of the dose-response effect: quantitation of functional contents in foods, kinetics in the gastrointestinal tract, metabolism in the body, and the mechanism of action in the target organ
3. Interaction with other content in foods or metabolism in the body
4. Appropriateness of the food to supply enough nutrition and satisfy the taste, visual sense, and smell
5. Function and safety of foods made by DNA recombination

Physicians with expertise in cardiology, DM, and cancer have already played important roles in the prophylaxis and treatment of life style-related diseases. To go one step further, we must prevent life style-related diseases at the port of entry, that is, before digestion and absorption in the gastrointestinal tract. The role of researchers in gastroenterology is important, and they should be in forefront of our consideration.

Part 4
Apoptosis in Digestive Organs

Examination of Cytotoxic T Lymphocyte-Mediated Apoptosis Pathway in Peptic Ulcer Formation with or without *H. pylori* Infection

TADASHI OHARA[1,*], YUHSAKU KANOH[2], TAKAOMI MASHIKO[2], SHIGERU ASAKI[3], and SHINEI KUDOH[1]

Summary. Perforin/granzyme and Fas/Fas ligand (Fas L) pathways are two known major pathways of cytotoxic T lymphocyte (CTL)-mediated apoptosis. We clinically studied whether CTL-mediated apoptosis associated with peptic ulcer formation may occur via either or both of these two pathways. In all mucosal biopsy specimens obtained from the peptic ulcer marginal zone endoscopically with or without *Helicobacter pylori* infection, perforin/granzyme B and caspase 3 were expressed consistently, but FasL was not. Apoptotic changes of target cells by perforin/granzyme B were then observed via immunohistochemistry. These results suggested that the main pathway of CTL-mediated apoptosis in peptic ulcer formation was the perforin/granzyme pathway.

Key words. Cytotoxic T lymphocyte, Perforin, Granzyme B, Apoptosis, Peptic ulcer

Introduction

Attention has been focused on apoptosis in terms of its involvement in the pathogenesis of various diseases including hepatitis, graft-versus-host disease (GVHD), and multiple sclerosis [1–3]. It has also been reported that the inflammatory immune response may play a key role in peptic ulcer formation. Thus, there is a growing body of evidence suggesting that apoptosis may act as a trigger for the inflammatory response.

In a previous report, we investigated cytokine production in these patients and showed that the biological polarity of the mucosal immune response shifted to type-

[1] Department of Gastroenterology, Showa Northern Yokohama Hospital, School of Medicine, Showa University, 37-1 Chigasaki Chuo, Tsuzuki-ku, Yokohama 244-0032, Japan
[2] Department of Laboratory Medicine, Kitasato University School of Medicine, 1-15-1 Kitasato, Sagamihara, Kanagawa 228-8555, Japan
[3] Department of Gastroenterology, Tohoku University, School of Medicine, 1-1 Seiryo-machi, Aoba-ku, Sendai 980-8555, Japan
* e-mail: jlohara@sm.rim.or.jp

1 T-helper (Th1) lymphocytes dominant at the peptic ulcer marginal zone. We also showed the possibility that apoptosis induction by cytotoxic T lymphocytes (CTLs) derived from Th1 lymphocytes may be involved in the development of mucosal damage [4].

Some pathways are known to be implicated in CTL-mediated apoptotic induction: perforin/granzyme pathway (based on granules stored in cytoplasmic azurophile granules of CTLs), Fas/Fas ligand (FasL), tumor necrosis factor (TNF)/TNF receptor(TNFR), or TNF-related apoptosis-inducing ligand (TRAIL) pathways based on type II transmembrane proteins belonging to the TNF family expressed on the cell surface. Among them, the perforin/granzyme and Fas/FasL pathways are considered the two major routes of apoptosis. The aim of this study was to investigate whether apoptosis associated with peptic ulcer formation occurs via either or both of these two pathways.

Materials and Methods

Mucosal biopsy specimens were obtained endoscopically from the peptic ulcer marginal zone of patients who had active peptic ulcers at the A1-A2 stage, with or without *Helicobacter pylori* infection. *H. pylori* infection was diagnosed by an enzyme-linked immunosorbent assay (ELISA). These samples were examined for expression of perforin, Fas, FasL, and caspase 3, which is located upstream of a caspase group of interleukin-1b converting enzyme (ICE)/CD-3 family cystein protease, involved in transduction of apoptotic signals. Expressions of perforin, Fas, and FasL were determined by the reverse transcriptase-polymerase chain reaction (RT-PCR). Perforin and Fas primer were purchased from Ambion the RNA Company (USA), and a custom-made FasL primer was purchased from Japan Immuno-research Laboratories. Expression of caspase 3 was analyzed by immunoblot by means of anti-caspase 3 antibody obtained from Santa Cruz Biotechnology (USA). Molecular groups whose expression was detected and granzyme B were then examined for intramucosal localization by immunohistochemical staining using light microscopy. The anti-perforin antibody and anti-granzyme B antibody used for the experiments were purchased from Santa Cruz Biotechnology. As previously reported, immunohistochemical analysis was done by peroxidase staining based on the avidin biotin affinity cytochemistry (ABC) method.

Results

Expression of perforin and Fas was observed in all mucosal biopsy specimens obtained from the ulcer marginal zone irrespective of *H. pylori* infection by RT-PCR; expression of FasL was not observed consistently. Immunoblot analysis also showed constant expression of caspase 3 in all specimens regardless of *H. pylori* infection (Fig. 1).

Immunohistochemical analysis revealed that perforin and granzyme B were localized in the CTL cytoplasm, present between the proper mucous membrane and the epithelium, to the target cell. Moreover, caspase 3 was seen in granzyme B-expressing

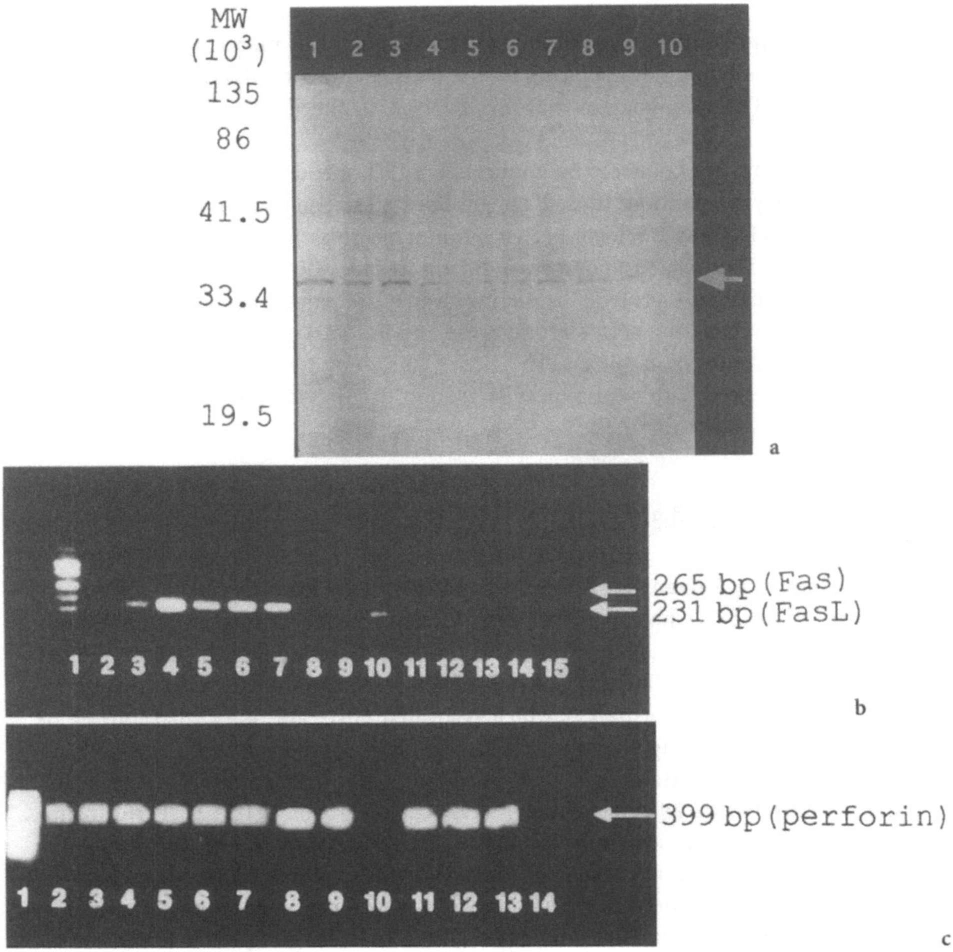

FIG. 1 **a.** Expression of caspase 3 by immunoblot in gastric mucosa infected with *Helicobacter pylori* (or not). *1*, gastric ulcer marginal zone (*H. pylori*$^+$); *2*, duodenal ulcer marginal zone (*H. pylori*$^+$); *3*, duodenal ulcer marginal zone (*H. pylori*$^+$); *4*, duodenal ulcer marginal zone (*H. pylori*$^-$); *5*, duodenal ulcer marginal zone (*H. pylori*$^+$); *6*, duodenal ulcer marginal zone (*H. pylori*$^-$); *7*, gastric ulcer marginal zone (*H. pylori*$^-$); *8*, gastric ulcer marginal zone (*H. pylori*$^+$); *9*, gastric ulcer marginal zone (*H. pylori*$^-$); *10*, gastric ulcer marginal zone (*H. pylori*$^+$). **b.** Expression of Fas. Fas L in gastric mucosa infected with *H. pylori* or not [by reverse transcriptase-polymerase chain reaction (RT-PCR)]. *1*, marker (pBR322/MSPI); *2*, normal mucosa (*H. pylori*$^+$); *3*, marginal zone (A2) (*H. pylori*$^+$); *4*, marginal zone (A2) (*H. pylori*$^+$); *5*, marginal zone (A2) (*H. pylori*$^+$); *6*, marginal zone (A2) (*H. pylori*$^-$); *7*, bleeding, erosion (*H. pylori*$^-$); *8*, normal mucosa (*H. pylori*$^+$); *9*, marginal zone (A2) (*H. pylori*$^+$); *10*, marginal zone (A2) (*H. pylori*$^+$); *11*, marginal zone (A2) (*H. pylori*$^+$); *12*, bleeding, erosion (*H. pylori*$^+$); *13*, bleeding, erosion (*H. pylori*$^-$); *14*, bleeding, erosion (*H. pylori*$^-$); *15*, normal mucosa (*H. pylori*$^-$). **c.** Expression of perforin in gastric mucosa infected with *H. pylori* (or not) (RT-PCR). *1*, marker (pBR322/MSPI); *2*, marginal zone (H1) (*H. pylori*$^+$); *3*, marginal zone (H1) (*H. pylori*$^+$); *4*, marginal zone (A2) (*H. pylori*$^+$); *5*, marginal zone (A2) (*H. pylori*$^+$); *6*, marginal zone (A2) (*H. pylori*$^+$); *7*, bleeding, erosion (*H. pylori*$^+$); *8*, marginal zone (A2) (*H. pylori*$^-$); *9*, marginal zone (A2) (*H. pylori*$^-$); *10*, normal mucosa (*H. pylori*$^+$); *11*, marginal zone (A2) (*H. pylori*$^-$); *12*, marginal zone (A2) (*H. pylori*$^-$); *13*, bleeding, erosion (*H. pylori*$^-$); *14*, normal mucosa (*H. pylori*$^-$)

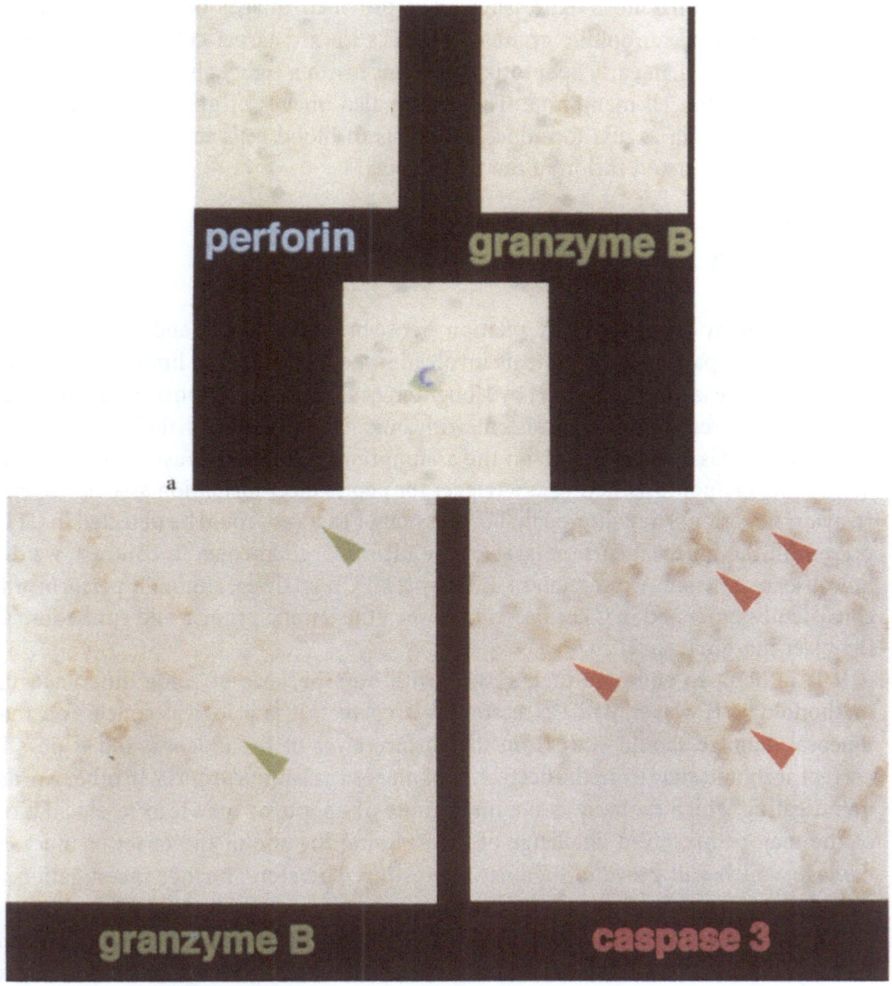

Fig. 2. **a** Expression of perforin granzyme B by immunohistochemistry in gastric ulcer marginal zone. Perforin and granzyme B are marked blue and green individually, by treatment of a computer graphic. The *lower picture* shows a composite photograph. **b** Expression of granzyme B caspase 3 by immunohistochemistry in a gastric ulcer marginal zone. *Arrowheads* indicate the expression of granzyme B caspase 3 individually

CTLs and their surrounding interstitium (Fig. 2). Immunoelectron microscopy of perforin- and granzyme B-expressing CTLs provided images of perforin released from cytoplasmic azurophilic granules of CTLs toward target cells; and images of target cells showed an early apoptotic appearance with a tight spherical body change and oscula in the cell membrane. There were also images of granzyme B invading target cells through oscula to induce apoptosis of blood cells in the tissue, in turn causing exfoliation and fusion of the tissue (Fig. 3).

Discussion

There are many reports on the relation between peptic ulcers and apoptosis, but reports on the pathway of apoptosis involved in peptic ulcers are limited. Except for our study, there is only one report by Houghton et al. on *H. pylori*-positive peptic ulcer [5], and their results are inconsistent with ours. They examined the expression of mRNA in mucosal tissue in situ on the assumption that the Fas/FasL pathway is the main route of apoptosis, acting as a trigger for peptic ulcer formation associated with *H. pylori* infection. They showed that expression of Fas/FasL could be detected in CTLs present in the mucosal surface layer of the ulcer marginal zone. In contrast, we did not observe constant expression of FasL by RT-PCR analysis, although perforin was consistently expressed in CTLs present between the lamina propria and epithelium of the ulcer marginal zone.

It is difficult to compare their results with ours because of some differences in methodology. However, if their reasoning is correct, it is a logical conclusion that mucosal damage should start from the surface layer of the mucosa; and if ours is correct, it should start from the deep layer of mucosa as lamina propria. In other words, investigating which pathway is the main route of apoptosis may lead to elucidation of the major unresolved challenge of determining the site of the onset of mucosal damage, which will prove to be most interesting. Therefore, further investigation is expected.

With regard to the mechanism of target cell destruction by perforin and granzyme B, it has been proposed that perforin released from azurophile granules of CTLs to target cells forms oscula on the target cell membrane in a calcium ion-dependent manner. Granzyme B, a serine protease (flagmentin), then invades the target cell through the oscula, which in turn attacks cells in the form of bystander lysis, leading to cleavage of a caspase group (including caspases 3, 6, 7, and 8) to cause cascade activation. At the same time it directly cleaves caspase substrates such as DNA-dependent protein kinase catalytic subunit and nuclear mitotic apparatus protein. Finally, apoptosis accompanied with DNA fragmentation and destruction of the cytoskeleton is induced (Fig. 4). In the present study, a series of phenomena occurring through the apoptotic process could be observed by means of immunohistochemistry, and we believe that the involvement of apoptosis in mucosal damage was verified morphologically.

By all means, the present clinical investigation alone cannot determine whether the observed phenomena means the onset of mucosal damage or the process of regeneration. Interestingly enough, it was suggested that CTLs might be effecter cells for mucosal damage irrespective of *H. pylori* infection. If it could be demonstrated that a

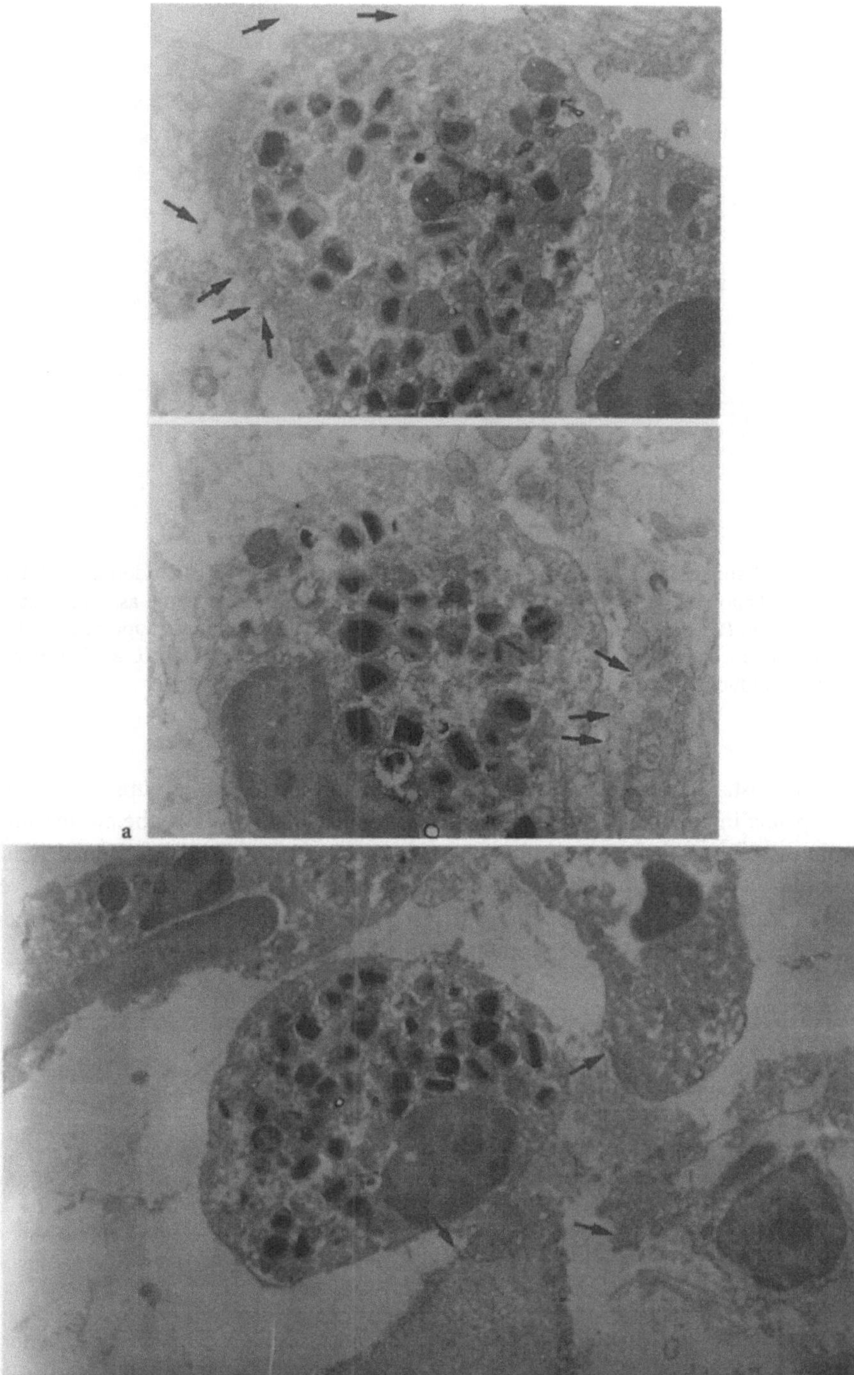

a

b

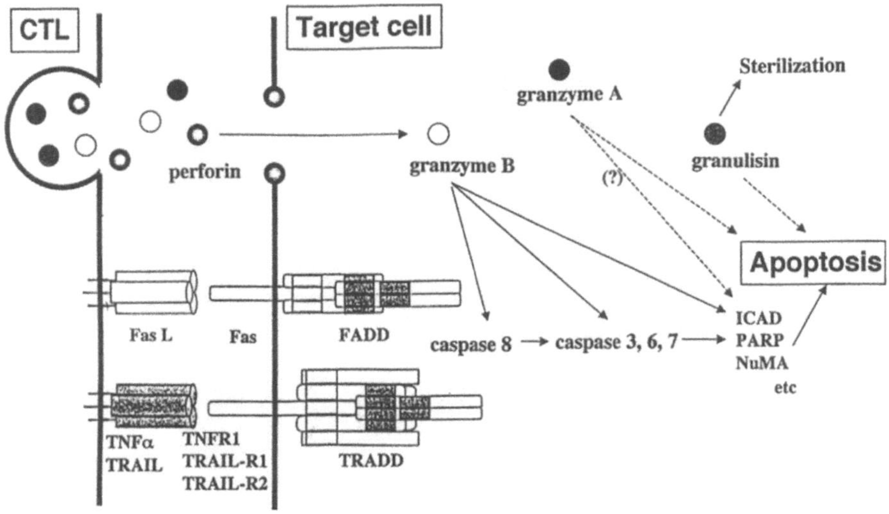

FIG. 4. Mechanism of CTL-mediated apoptosis. *FADD*, Fas-associated death domain; *TRADD*, TNF related apoptosis death domain; *ICAD*, interleukin-1b converting enzyme-associated apoptosis domain; *PARP*, poly(ADP-ribose) polymerase; *NuMA*, nuclear mitotic apparatus protein; *TNFR*, TNF receptor; *TRAIL*, TNF-related apoptosis-inducing ligand; *TRAIL-R*, TNF-related apoptosis-inducing ligand receptor

certain substance induces CTLs with a common epitope in both groups irrespective of *H. pylori* infection, it would signify the possibility that there may be an unknown antibody responsible for peptic ulcers. If such a substance could be determined, it may a significant discovery in terms of the investigation of peptic ulcers, and further development can be expected. Based on our results we are planning to investigate these various problems using an experimental animal model.

References

1. Ando K, Hiroishi K, Kaneko T, et al (1997) Perforin, Fas/Fas ligand, and TNF-alpha pathways as specific and bystander killing mechanisms of hepatitis C virsus-specific human CTL. J Immunol 158:5283–5291
2. Hattori K, Hirano T, Miyajima H, et al (1999) Differential effects of anti-Fas ligand and anti-tumor necrosis factor alpha antibodies on acute graft-versus-host disease pathologies. Blood 93:2738–2747

FIG. 3. **a** Examination of perforin by immunoelectron microscopy. *Top, arrows* indicate perforin released from azurophilic granules in cytotoxic T lymphocytes (CTLs) to the target cell. *Bottom, arrows* indicate a tight spherical body change of the target cell membrane. **b** Examination of granzyme B by immunoelectron microscopy. *Arrows* indicate granzyme B, which attacked various cells as bystander lysis

3. SabelkoDowners KA, Cross AH, Russell JH (1999) Dual role for Fas ligand in the initiation of and recovery from experimental allergic encephalomyelitis. J Exp Med 189: 1195–1205
4. Ohara T, Noguchi M, Yamaguchi M (1999) Role of perforin-granzyme pathway as a key effector for gastric mucosal injury (in Japanese). Proc Jpn Soc Gastric Secretion Res 31:55–59
5. Houghton JR, Korah RM, Condon M, Kim KH (1999) Apoptosis and *Helicobacter pylori*-associated gastric and duodenal ulcer disease is mediated via the Fas antigen pathway. Dig Dis Sci 44:465–478

Epidermal Growth Factor Inhibits *Helicobacter pylori* Lipopolysaccharide-Induced Apoptosis of Primary Cultures of Gastric Pit Cells

TSUKASA KAWAHARA*, SHIGETADA TESHIMA, KYOICHI KISHI, and KAZUHITO ROKUTAN

Summary. *Helicobacter pylori* (Hp) lipopolysaccharide (LPS) is generally considered to have low toxic virulence. However, when guinea pig pit cells were cultured under LPS-free conditions and treated with various concentrations of Hp LPS, low concentrations of Hp LPS (>2.1 endotoxin unit/ml) stimulated apoptosis of the cultured pit cells, and this apoptosis was induced by lipid A region of Hp LPS. Hp LPS caused activation of caspase 3, DNA fragmentation, and the appearance of nuclear condensation of the cells. Epidermal growth factor suppressed the Hp LPS-induced apoptosis. These results suggest that Hp LPS may play an important role in the pathogenesis of Hp infection.

Key words. *Helicobacter pylori*, Lipopolysaccharide, Apoptosis, Gastric pit cells

Introduction

Helicobacter pylori (Hp) infection causes type B chronic gastritis, peptic ulcer diseases, and mucosa-associated lymphoid tissue (MALT) lymphoma and is now considered to be a risk factor for the development of gastric adenocarcinoma. Chronic colonization of Hp also causes pathophysiological changes in gastric mucosa (e.g., gastrin secretion) and in the gastric epithelial cell cycle. In addition, increased alteration of gastric epithelial cell apoptosis is frequently observed in mucosal biopsy specimens obtained from patients with Hp-associated gastritis and duodenal ulcer; therefore, it is particularly important to reveal factor(s) that causes apoptosis of gastric epithelium.

Lipopolysaccharide (LPS) is a major component of the outer membranes of gram-negative bacteria. It is composed of the lipid A region, OS region, and polysaccharide chains that are also known as O antigen chains. Compared with other virulent factors, Hp LPS has been considered to be less toxic, as 1000 to 10,000 times higher concen-

Department of Nutritional Physiology, School of Medicine, The University of Tokushima, 3-18-15 Kuramoto-cho, Tokushima 770-8503, Japan
* e-mail: kawahara@nutr.med.tokushima-u.ac.jp

trations of Hp LPS are required for activation of host spleen cells or macrophages, compared with that from *Salmonella enterica* or *Escherichia coli.*

In this study, we examined the effects of Hp LPS on apoptosis. We found that Hp LPS at low concentrations could induce apoptosis of gastric pit cells.

Materials and Methods

Reagents

Epidermal growth factor (EGF) from mouse submaxillary glands (culture grade) was purchased from Becton Dickinson (Bedford, MA, USA); and RPMI 1640 liquid medium containing endotoxin [<0.01 endotoxin unit (EU)/ml] was purchased from GIBCO (Grand Island, NY, USA). Fetal bovine serum (FBS) containing endotoxin (<0.09 EU/ml), was purchased from ICN Biomedicals (Aurora, OH, USA).

Preparation and Culture of Gastric Mucosal Cells

Male guinea pigs weighing approximately 250 g were purchased from Shizuoka Laboratory Animal Center (Shizuoka, Japan). Gastric mucosal cells were isolated aseptically from guinea pig fundic glands as previously described [1]. In the present experiments, all reagents and media used were free from detectable amounts of LPS by the *Limulus amoebocyte* lysate assay (Endospecy; Seikagaku Kogyo, Tokyo, Japan). The isolated cells were cultured for 2 days in RPMI 1640 containing gentamicin 50 μg/ml, penicillin G 100 U/ml, and 10% FBS. This complete medium contained LPS at less than 0.01 EU/ml. Cell populations were determined by histochemical and immunohistochemical analyses, as described previously [1]. After culturing for 2 days, the growing cells consisted of pit cells (about 90%), pre-pit cells (about 5%), parietal cells (4%–5%), mucous neck cells (<1%), and fibroblasts (<1%).

Preparation of Hp LPS

NCTC11637 strain (kindly provided by Dr. Nakazawa, University of Yamaguchi, Yamaguchi, Japan) was cultured in *Brucella* broth (GIBCO), supplemented with 5% FBS and vancomycin 10 μg/ml, for 15 h at 37°C under microaerobic conditions (12% CO_2/5% O_2/83% N_2). Hp LPS was prepared by the hot-phenol water method of Westphal and Jann. The concentrations of prepared LPS were determined by the *Limulus amoebocyte* lysate assay (Endospecy).

Measurement of Apoptosis

Chromosomal condensation and fragmentation were assessed by staining with the fluorescent dye Hoechst 33342 (Sigma, St. Louis, MO, USA). After fixation with 2% paraformaldehyde, the preparation was washed with phosphate-buffered saline (PBS) and then exposed to Hoechst 33342 5 μg/ml. After washing, samples were mounted with glycerol/PBS (1:1, v/v) and subjected to fluorescence microscopic examination.

Caspase Assay

Measurement of caspase 3-like activity was performed as previously described [4]. After cells were lysed, the samples (100 μg protein) were mixed with reaction buffer containing the synthetic substrate *N*-acetyl-Asp-Glu-Val-Asp-*p*-nitroanilide (Ac-DEVD-pNa; BIOMOL Research Laboratories, Plymouth, PA, USA). Caspase 3-like activity was assayed by measuring the increase in absorbance at 405 nm.

Results

When gastric pit cells were treated with various concentrations of Hp LPS for 8 h, Hp LPS at 2.1 EU/ml or higher induced DNA ladder formation. The DNA ladder formation appeared within 5 h after treatment with Hp LPS. Consequently, the percentage of apoptotic cells after treatment with 2.1 EU/ml Hp LPS for 8 h significantly increased (Table 1). LPS was separated into free lipid A and polysaccharide fractions by boiling in 0.1 M acetate buffer. Lipid A, but not the polysaccharide fraction, caused apoptosis (data not shown). Apoptosis was mediated by activation of caspase 3 (Table 2). Furthermore, we found that EGF completely inhibited LPS-induced apoptosis and activation of caspase 3 (Table 2).

Discussion

Epidermal growth factor plays important role in the maintenance and repair of gastric glands by promoting cell migration, stimulating cell proliferation, and suppressing acid secretion. Furthermore, EGF promotes cell survival by the Ras-signaling pathway, the extracellular signal-regulated kinase-signaling pathway, and the pp90 ribosomal S6 kinase (p90 Rsks)-signaling pathway in neurons. Activation of p90 Rsks leads to phosphorylation of the Bad and cyclic adenosine-monophosphate response element-

Table 1. Inhibition of Hp LPS-induced apoptosis by EGF

	Apoptotic cells (%)	
Stimulus	EGF-negative	EGF-positive
None	3.8 ± 0.5	3.7 ± 1.8
Hp LPS	24.8 ± 0.7*	2.9 ± 1.3

Cells, maintained in RPMI 1640 containing 0.1% fetal bovine serum, were incubated with Hp LPS (21 endotoxin units (EU)/ml) for 8 h in the absence or presence of 20 nM EGF. Floating and attached cells were collected and stained with Hoechst 33342. Cells with a condensed nucleus were counted, and the percent of apoptotic cells are shown

Hp, *Helicobacter pylori*; LPS, lipopolysaccharide; EGF, epidermal growth factor

* $P < 0.05$ by ANOVA and Scheffè's test, compared with untreated cells

TABLE 2. Effects of Hp LPS on caspase activities in gastric pit cells

Stimulus	Caspase 3-like activities (absorbance at 450 nm/mg protein/h)
None	0.358 ± 0.029
EGF	0.203 ± 0.041*
Hp LPS	0.956 ± 0.106*
Hp LPS + EGF	0.300 ± 0.080

Gastric pit cells were incubated with Hp LPS (21 EU/ml) for 8 h in the absence or presence of 20 nM EGF. Caspase 3-like activities were measured

* $P < 0.05$ by ANOVA and Scheffè's test, compared with untreated cells

binding protein [2]. In this study, we found that EGF suppressed apoptosis. On the other hand, Hp LPS could up-regulate Mox1 oxidase components by the Toll-like receptor 4 (TLR4) signaling pathway [1,3] (data not shown). We also reported that Mox1-derived superoxide anion produced proliferation/survival signals through activation of nuclear factor κB [4]. Thus, TLR4-mediated signals may produced a number of diverse signals for both death and survival of gastric epithelium, and these signals may play an important role in the development of mucosal lesions caused by Hp infection.

References

1. Teshima S, Rokutan K, Nikawa T, et al (1998) Guinea pig gastric mucosal cells produce abundant superoxide anion through an NADPH oxidase-like system. Gastroenterology 115:1186–1196
2. Bonni A, Brunet A, West AE, et al (1999) Cell survival promoted by the Ras-MAPK signaling pathway by transcription-dependent and -independent mechanisms. Science 286:1358–1362
3. Teshima S, Tsunawaki S, Rokutan K (1999) *Helicobacter pylori* lipopolysaccharide enhances the expression of NADPH oxidase compornents in cultured guinea pig gastric mucosal cells. FEBS Lett 452:243–246
4. Teshima S, Kutsumi H, Kawahara T, et al (2000) Regulation of growth and apoptosis of primary cultured guinea pig gastric pit cells by Mox1 oxidase. Am J Physiol 279:G1169–G1176

Impaired Sensitivity to Fas-Induced Apoptosis of Lymphocytes in Ulcerative Colitis Lesions

HARUMI UEYAMA, TATSUYA KIYOHARA, YASUHISA SHINOMURA, and YUJI MATSUZAWA

Summary. We have previously reported that lamina propria lymphocytes (LPLs) in ulcerative colitis lesions express Fas ligand (FasL), suggesting that Fas/FasL-induced apoptosis participates in the mucosal damage of ulcerative colitis (UC). The aim of this study was to examine the sensitivity of Fas-mediated apoptosis in LPLs to analyze if down-regulation of LPL expansion is impaired. The sensitivity of Fas-mediated apoptosis of LPLs from UC, Crohn's disease (CD), and controls were examined by flow cytometry. Activation of NF-κB in LPLs was analyzed by immunohistochemistry and the electrophoretic mobility shift assay. The effect of NF-κB on the sensitivity of apoptosis in LPLs was examined with pyrrolidine dithiocarbamate and NF-κB decoy oligodeoxynucleotide. LPLs from UC and CD lesions, especially UC, showed decreased sensitivity of apoptosis. NF-κB was activated in LPLs from UC lesions. Inhibition of NF-κB activation increased apoptosis in UC LPLs. It is concluded that UC LPLs were resistant to Fas-mediated apoptosis, and activation of NF-κB was involved in the mechanism.

Key words. Ulcerative colitis, Lamina propria lymphocytes, Apoptosis, Fas ligand, Nuclear factor kappa B (NF-κB)

Introduction

Ulcerative colitis (UC) is characterized by chronic inflammation restricted to the colonic mucosa. We have previously reported that T lymphocytes infiltrating lesions of UC express Fas ligand (FasL), suggesting that Fas/FasL-induced apoptosis participates in the mucosal damage of UC [1].

Lymphocytes and colonic epithelia express Fas. At the end of inflammation, FasL expressed on the activated lymphocytes induces apoptosis in other lymphocytes to down-regulate the expansion of activated cells and suppress inflammation.

Department of Internal Medicine and Molecular Science, Graduate School of Medicine, Osaka University, 2-2 Yamadaoka, Suita, Osaka 565-0871, Japan

Despite the overexpression of FasL on T cells in UC lesions, inflammation is chronically observed. To prove the hypothesis that depletion of activated lymphocytes through the Fas/FasL system is impaired in UC, this paper reports an analysis of the sensitivity of Fas-mediated apoptosis in the lymphocytes of UC lesions. We also analyzed whether nuclear factor kappa B (NF-κB), which was recently reported to regulate Fas-mediated apoptosis of T cells [2], is important for apoptosis of UC lymphocytes.

Materials and Methods

Lamina Propria Lymphocytes and Detection of Apoptosis

Lamina propria lymphocytes (LPLs) were isolated from mucosal specimens of UC, Crohn's disease (CD), and controls by a density gradient method [1]. Isolated LPLs were incubated in RPMI medium supplemented with 5% fetal calf serum (FCS) at 37°C in a humid atmosphere of 5% CO_2/95% O_2. Apoptosis was induced by recombinant FasL peptide (kindly provided by Dr. S. Nagata). Cell viability was analyzed by the trypan blue exclusion method, and the cell cycle was analyzed by flow cytometry. Briefly, cells were fixed with ethanol and treated with RNAase and propidium iodide 50 μg/ml in 0.1% sodium citrate and 0.1% Triton X-100. The percentage of apoptotic cells was determined by evaluating hypodiploid nuclei.

Immunohistochemistry

Frozen sections were thawed, fixed in acetone, and treated with 3% H_2O_2 in cold methanol. The sections were irradiated with microwaves in 10 mM citrate buffer pH 6.0, washed in phosphate-buffered saline (PBS), and pretreated with goat serum, followed by treament with monoclonal mouse anti-human p65 antibody (Boehringer Mannheim Biochemica, Mannheim, Germany) overnight at 4°C. After washing, the sections were treated with biotinylated secondary antibody (Dako), incubated with the streptavidin-biotin peroxidase complex, washed again, and incubated in AEC.

Electrophoretic Mobility Shift Assay

Nuclear extracts from LPLs were prepared as described previously [3]. The electrophoretic mobility shift assay (EMSA) for NF-κB was performed by Gel Shift Assay Systems (Promega, Madison, WI, USA) according to the manufacturer's instructions. Double-stranded oligonucleotide probe for NF-κB was end-labeled with [γ-^{32}P]ATP. Nuclear extracts 10 μg were incubated with a radiolabeled DNA probe (5×10^4 cpm/reaction) and poly(dI-dC) 0.5 g/ml for 20 min at 20°C in 10 μl of binding buffer. Samples were run in 4% polyacrylamide gel with 0.5% Tris borate buffer.

NF-κB Decoy Oligodeoxynucleotides

The sequences of the double-stranded phosphorothioate oligodeoxynucleotides (ODNs) against the NF-κB binding site and scrambled ODNs were as follows (consensus sequences are underlined). Decoy ODNs have been reported to bind NF-κB [4].

NF-κB decoy ODNs: 5′-CCTTGAAGGGATTTCCCTCC-3′
3′-GGAACTTCCCTAAAGGGAGG-5′
Scrambled ODNs: 5′-TTGCCGTACCTGACTTAGCC-3′
3′-AACGGCATGGACTGAATCGG-5′

Transfection of ODNs

Cationic liposomes (Lipofectamine 2000 Reagent; Life Technologies, Gaithersburg, MD, USA) were used to transfect decoy ODNs into LPLs according to the manufacturer's instructions. Lipid–ODN complexes were formed by mixing 1 μl lipid and 1 μg ODN in 100 μl OPTI-MEN (Life Technologies). Cells were incubated in 24-well plates at 5×10^5 cells/ml, and the decoy was added at a final concentration of 2 μmol/l. We confirmed that this quantity of DNA and liposomes had no toxic effect on cell viability.

Results

We determined whether LPLs from inflammatory bowel disease (IBD) and control tissues differed in terms of susceptibility to undergo apoptosis when exposed to recombinant FasL peptide, which was previously shown to induce Fas-mediated apoptosis. As shown in Fig. 1, LPLs from IBD patients, especially those with UC, showed strikingly less Fas-mediated apoptosis; although the mean percent difference in celluler viability of normal colon LPLs was about 50% after exposure to recombinant FasL peptide, the cellular viability was about 80% in UC LPLs and 70% in CD LPLs. As UC, CD, and control LPLs were equivalent in their expression of Fas

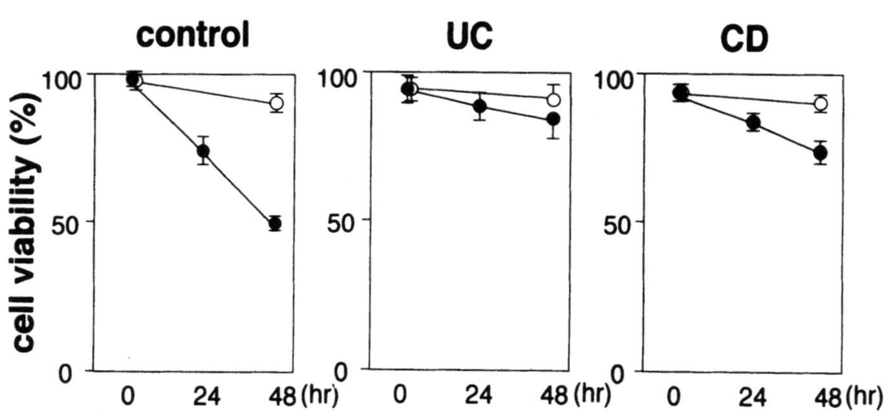

Fig. 1. Fas-mediated apoptosis of lamina propria lymphocytes (LPLs). LPLs isolated from lesions of ulcerative colitis (*UC*), Crohn's disease (*CD*), and controls were incubated in RPMI medium supplemented with 5% fetal calf serum (FCS) and antibiotics at 37°C in a humid atmosphere of 5% CO_2 and 95% O_2. LPLs were treated with (*open circles*) or without (*closed circles*) recombinant Fas ligand peptide at a concentration of 1 ng/ml. Cell viability was analyzed by trypan blue exclusion

(data not shown), the difference in the sensitivity of apoptosis was suggested to be caused by some deficiency in the signaling capacity of the intracellular Fas pathway.

Among the factors that could be defective during Fas signaling is NF-κB. Immunohistochemical study showed that activated NF-κB was detected in mononuclear cells in UC lesions (Fig. 2A). The EMSA analysis showed strong activation of NF-κB in UC LPLs (Fig. 2B). Pyrrolidine dithiocarbamate (PDTC), one of the inhibitors of NF-κB activation, strongly suppressed NF-κB activation in UC LPLs.

We next examined the effect of PDTC on Fas-mediated apoptosis (Fig. 3A). Compared with the controls, PDTC made LPLs more susceptible to Fas-mediated apoptosis. To examine the effect of NF-κB on Fas-mediated apoptosis more specifically, we analyzed the effect of NF-κB decoy ODNs (Fig. 3B). Transfection of decoy ODN significantly increased the susceptibility to Fas-mediated apoptosis in UC LPLs. In contrast, transfection of scrambled ODNs failed to influence Fas-mediated apoptosis.

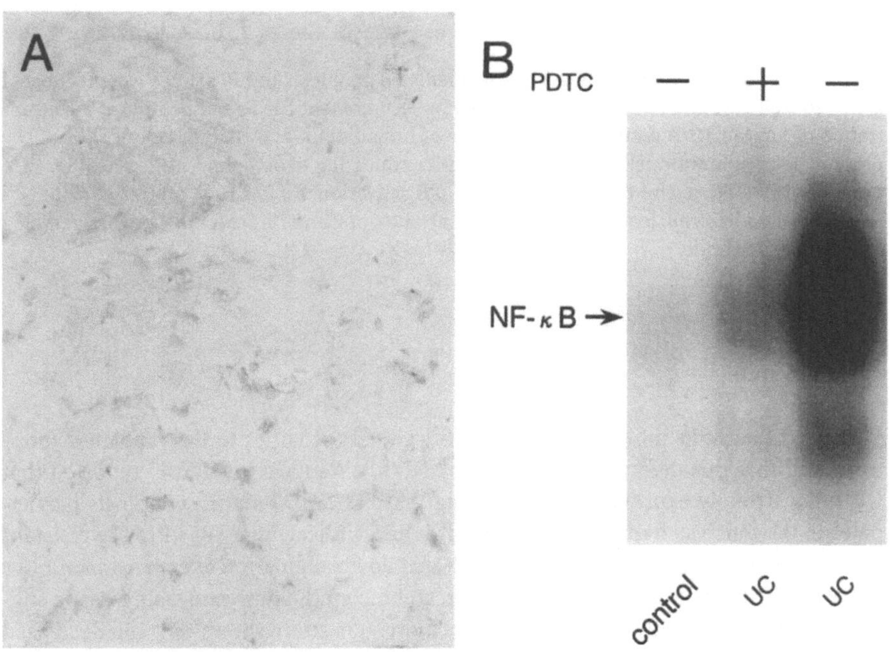

Fig. 2. Detection of activated nuclear factor kappa B (NF-κB) in LPLs infiltrating UC lesions. **A** Immunohistochemical detection of activated NF-κB in UC colonic mucosa. A section of a colonic specimen from active UC was stained with mouse monoclonal antibody against human p65. ×258. **B** Autoradiograph of an electrophoretic mobility shift assay using an NF-κB binding oligonucleotide. Nuclear extract were prepared from LPLs isolated from UC and normal colon. Pyrrolidine dithiocarbamate (*PDTC*) strongly suppressed NF-κB activation in UC LPLs. A representative blot is shown

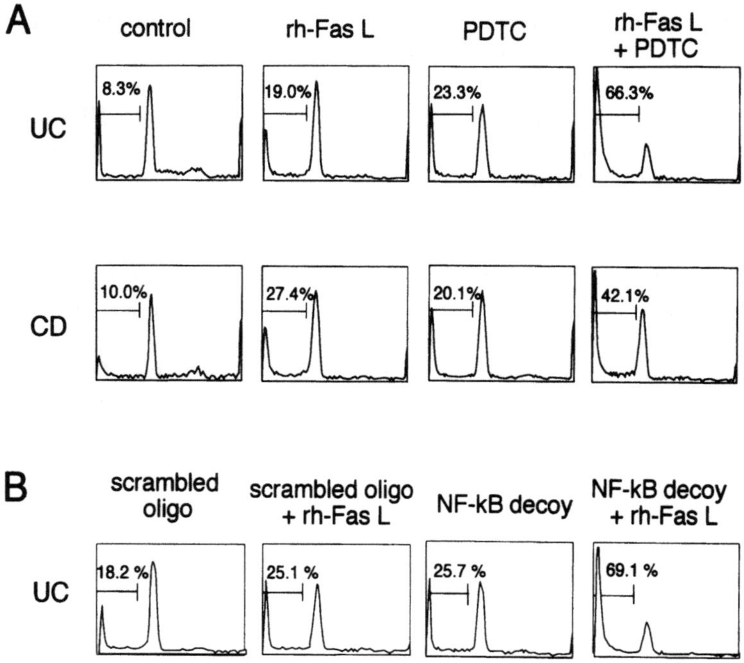

FIG. 3. Effect of inhibition of NF-κB on Fas-mediated apoptosis of LPLs. LPLs were incubated at 5×10^5 cells/ml, and apoptosis was induced by recombinant Fas ligand peptide at a concentration of 1 ng/ml. DNA fluorescence histogram of propidium iodide-stained cells is shown. The percentage of apoptotic cells were determined by evaluating hypodiploid nuclei. **A** LPLs were treated with PDTC, one of the inhibitors of NF-κB activation. **B** LPLs were pretreated with NF-κB decoy oligodeoxynucleotide at a final concentration of 2 μmol/l. Scrambled oligo, scrambled oligodeoxynucleotide

Discussion

We report that LPLs infiltrating UC lesions were less sensitive to Fas-mediated apoptosis, and that this defect was regulated by NF-κB. We have previously reported that UC LPLs strongly express FasL, suggesting that Fas/FasL-induced apoptosis participates in the mucosal damage of UC. Our data here indicate that UC LPLs are resistant to FasL-mediated apoptosis, with the result that down-regulation of expansion of LPLs expressing FasL is impaired. As the result, colonic epithelium expressing Fas is suggested to be chronically damaged. Furthermore, our study shows that the decreased sensitivity of apoptosis in UC LPLs is regulated by activation of NF-κB. Inhibition of NF-κB activation may decrease the defect in the mechanism to down-regulate expansion of activated LPLs and contribute to the treatment of UC.

References

1. Ueyama H, Kiyohara T, Sawada N, et al (1998) High Fas ligand expression on lymphocytes in lesions of ulcerative colitis. Gut 43:48–55

2. Dudly E, Hornung F, Zheng L, et al (1999) NF-κB regulates Fas/APO-1/CD95- and TCR-mediated apoptosis of T lymphocytes. Eur J Immunol 29:878–886
3. Brand K, Page S, Rogler G, et al (1996) Activated transcription factor nuclear factor kappa B is present in the atherosclerotic lesion. J Clin Invest 97:1715–1722
4. Morishita R, Sugimoto T, Aoki M, et al (1997) In vitro transfection of *cis* element "decoy" against nuclear factor-κB binding site prevents myocardial infarction. Nat Med 3:894–899

Tumor Necrosis Factor α-Induced Hepatic Apoptosis and Hepatocyte Sensitization

Masahito Nagaki*, Yosuke Osawa, Takafumi Naiki, and Hisataka Moriwaki

Summary. Tumor necrosis factor-α (TNFα) and Fas ligand are death factors that bind to their receptors, two TNF receptors (TNFR), TNFR1 and TNFR2, and Fas, respectively, and induce apoptosis in a variety of cell types. In galactosamine (GalN)-sensitized mice, hepatocyte apoptosis and liver failure were observed after injection of TNFα. On the contrary, neither apoptotic cell nor liver injury was shown in mice treated with TNFα alone. Histological analyses revealed that administration of GalN/TNF-α caused massive hemorrhagic liver damage and fragmented nuclei in hepatocytes, which were similar to those observed after the treatment with anti-Fas antibody. In contrast to hepatotoxicity by TNFα, however, GalN hardly sensitized the liver to injury by anti-Fas antibody. Compared with the GalN/TNFα model, most of the changes occurred earlier in the anti-Fas model. The expression of TNFR1 mRNA in the liver was up-regulated and reached a peak within 2h after GalN administration. However, the change of TNFR2 mRNA in the liver was less than that of TNFR1 mRNA. GalN treatment failed to affect TNFα-induced nuclear factor-κB activation. These results indicate that unlike apoptosis through Fas, TNFR-mediated liver cell apoptosis requires sensitization of the parenchymal cells. In the sensitization of hepatocytes to apoptosis, up-regulation of TNFR1 on hepatocytes could play an important role.

Key words. Tumor necrosis factor-α, Tumor necrosis factor receptor, Fas, Apoptosis, Liver failure

Three structurally related cell surface receptors have been identified, characterized, and implicated in the transduction of apoptotic death signals in a broad range of cell types. The three receptors belong to a family of cell surface glycoproteins, and include two distinct tumor necrosis factor receptor (TNFR) chains designated p55 [1,2] and p75 [3], as well as Fas antigen [4]. Administration of tumor necrosis factor-α (TNFα)

First Department of Internal Medicine, Gifu University School of Medicine, 40 Tsukasa-machi, Gifu 500-8705, Japan
* e-mail: mnagaki@cc.gifu-u.ac.jp

or the anti-Fas antibody to mice causes acute liver failure, which is lethal within hours owing to the induction of apoptosis in hepatocytes [5–7]. Increased susceptibility of rodents to TNF-induced death after pretreatment with D-galactosamine (GalN) is caused mainly by relatively selective liver failure [8,9]. The mechanisms responsible for the sensitization to TNF are largely unknown.

Although TNFRs and Fas are considered the two principal apoptosis-inducing receptors, whether they trigger cell death along the same or distinct pathways in liver injury is unclear. In the present study we investigated the differences between apoptotic liver cell death induced by TNFα and that induced by anti-Fas antibody, as well as the mechanism by which GalN sensitizes the hepatocyte to injury.

Lethal and Hepatotoxic Effects in GalN-Sensitized Mice Induced by TNFα or Anti-Fas Antibody

Either TNFα or anti-mouse Fas antibody was injected intraperitoneally into BALB/c mice with or without prior sensitization by GalN. Liver injury was assessed biochemically and histologically. Microscopically, GalN preceding TNFα caused massive hemorrhagic liver damage with fragmented hepatocyte nuclei resembling effects of anti-Fas antibody, but GalN largely failed to sensitize the liver to injury by the antibody. We quantitated hepatotoxicity by measuring serum alanine aminotransferase (ALT) activity and by counting apoptotic cells detected by terminal deoxynucleotidyl transferase (TdT) nick end-labeling (TUNEL) (Fig. 1). Neither liver injury nor apoptotic cells were found in mice treated with GalN or TNFα alone within 8h after administration (Fig. 1A). In GalN-sensitized mice, TUNEL-positive hepatocyte nuclei were observed 3h after TNFα injection when liver injury was not yet apparent (Fig. 1B). Increased numbers of TUNEL-positive apoptotic hepatocytes were observed, and hepatotoxicity became evident within 5h after administration. At 8h after administration the numbers of dead hepatocytes had increased further, and liver failure had fully developed. In mice treated with anti-Fas antibody, hepatotoxicity appeared soon (2h) after administration manifested as a high elevation of serum ALT activity and increased numbers of TUNEL-positive hepatocyte nuclei (Fig. 1C). Both hepatocyte apoptosis and liver injury occurred earlier in the anti-Fas model than in the GalN/TNFα model. Passive immunization against mouse TNFR1 conferred protection against the hepatotoxic effect of TNFα on GalN-sensitized mice. On the other hand, passive immunization with either hamster immunoglobulin G or monoclonal TNFR2 antibody failed to prevent hepatotoxicity.

Fig. 1. Liver injury and apoptotic cells over time in mice treated with tumor necrosis factor α (TNFα) (**A**), GalN/TNFα (**B**), and anti-Fas antibody (**C**). Liver sections were prepared 3, 5, and 8h after injection of TNFα or GalN/TNFα, and 1, 2, and 3h after injection of anti-Fas. *ALT*, alanine aminotransferase. (×180)

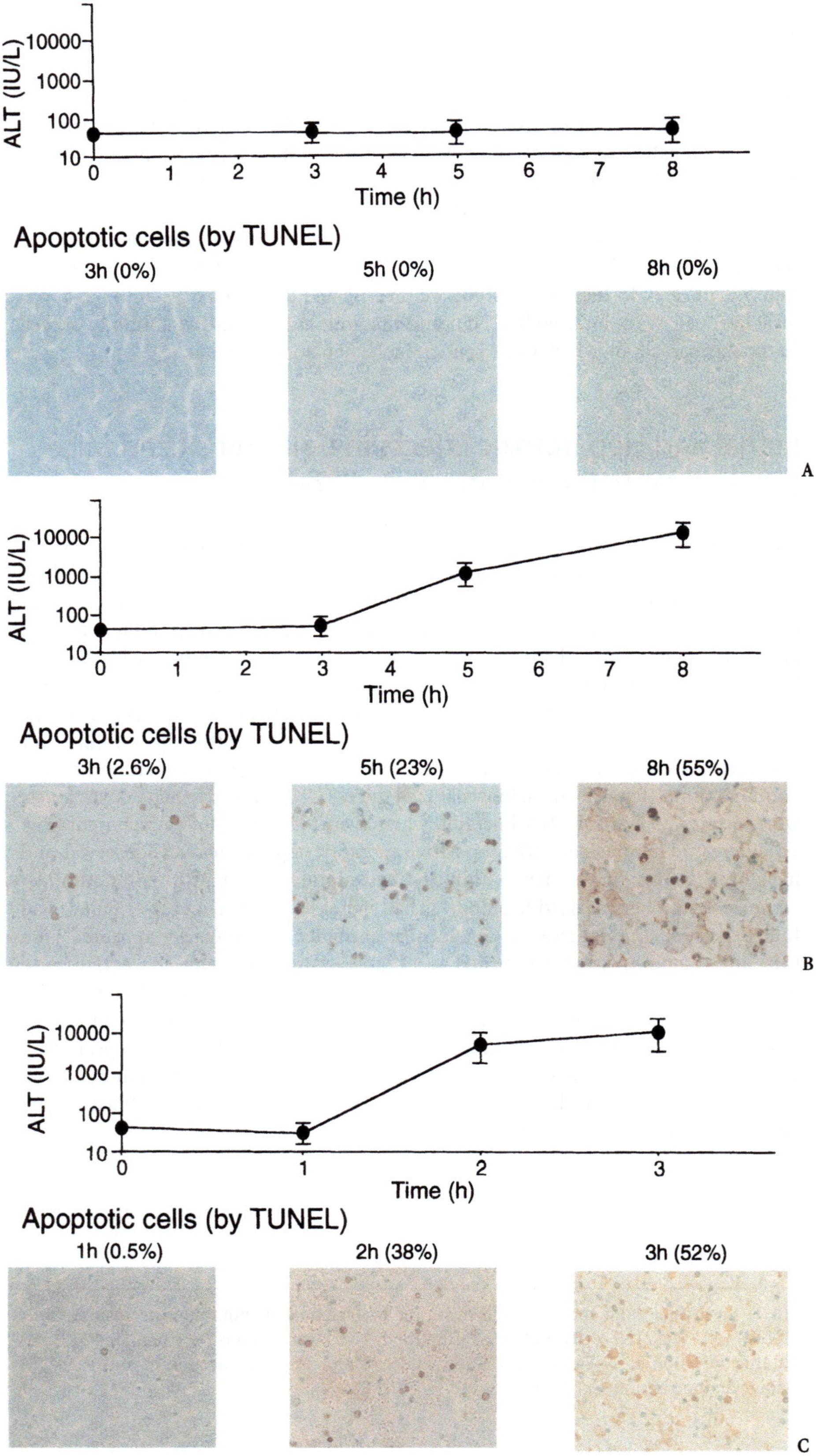

ALT (IU/L)
10000
1000
100
10
0
1
2
3
4
5
6
7
8
Time (h)
Apoptotic cells (by TUNEL)
3h (0%)
5h (0%)
8h (0%)
A
ALT (IU/L)
10000
1000
100
10
0
1
2
3
4
5
6
7
8
Time (h)
Apoptotic cells (by TUNEL)
3h (2.6%)
5h (23%)
8h (55%)
B
ALT (IU/L)
10000
1000
100
10
0
1
2
3
Time (h)
Apoptotic cells (by TUNEL)
1h (0.5%)
2h (38%)
3h (52%)
C

Activation of Caspase Proteases in Liver Damage Induced by GalN/TNFα

Studies suggest two major caspase cascades during apoptosis [10]. Cell surface receptors trigger activation of caspase-8 via Fas-associated death-domain protein (FADD) [and TNFR-1-associated death-domain protein (TRADD)], resulting in the processing of effector caspases such as caspases 3, 6, and 7. The other cascade is triggered by cytochrome c release from mitochondria, and consequently procaspase-9 is converted to the active caspase 9, which activates the effector caspases. Activation of caspases 9 and 3 and cytochrome c release into the cytosol were observed 5h after GalN/TNFα administration. These changes were not observed in mice treated with either GalN or TNFα alone.

Induction of TNFR1 Expression by GalN

Changes in expression of TNFR1 and TNFR2 mRNA in the liver were assessed in mice treated after administration of GalN or anti-Fas antibody. Expression of TNFR1 mRNA in the liver was up-regulated, reaching a peak within 2h after GalN administration and remaining present in small amounts 5h after administration. In contrast, TNFR2 mRNA showed little change. Neither TNFR1 nor TNFR2 mRNA were induced by anti-Fas antibody. We studied the in vivo expressions of TNFR1 or TNFR2 antigen in livers by immunohistochemistry. In normal livers neither TNFR1 nor TNFR2 antigen was observed. However, 60 min after GalN administration, moderate expression of TNFR1 antigen was found on the membrane of hepatocytes but not that of TNFR2 antigen [7].

Effects of GalN on the Inhibitory Signaling Pathway for TNFR-Mediated Apoptosis

Another possible mechanism for GalN sensitization effects on the signaling pathway for TNFR-mediated apoptosis should be considered. In addition to apoptosis-promoting pathways, cells have apoptosis-prevention mechanisms such as those related to nuclear factor kappa B (NF-κB) activation [11] and the Bcl-2 family proteins [12]. DNA gel shifts demonstrated that protein binding to an NF-κB consensus oligonucleotide was equivalent in livers treated with either TNFα alone or GalN/TNFα. The levels of Bax, Bad, and Bcl-X showed no significant changes after administration of TNFα, GalN, or GalN/TNFα.

Conclusions

Our data demonstrated that hepatocyte apoptosis is a critical event preceding hepatoxicity induced by either GalN/TNF-α or anti-Fas antibody. They also indicated that, unlike apoptosis involving Fas, TNFR-induced apoptosis requires sensitization of the parenchymal cells. Histologic changes in the liver observed in the two models appeared similar, but we and Leist et al. [6] found that Fas-mediated hepatocyte apoptosis was faster than TNFα-induced apoptosis and that the induction of anti-Fas-induced hepatotoxicity did not require pretreatment of mice with GalN or actinomycin D; sensitization was a necessary metabolic condition for TNF-induced hepatocyte apoptosis. These findings suggest that TNF receptors and Fas transduce similar and distinct signals resulting in apoptosis.

Apoptosis is a controlled process by which unwanted cells are selectively eliminated. In the various forms of hepatitis, the unwanted cells must be hepatocytes infected by hepatitis viruses or injured by drugs. The target cells may be susceptible or predisposed to apoptosis induced by TNFα or Fas ligand in such conditions. To gain insight into the mechanism by which TNFα-induced hepatocyte apoptosis requires sensitization in mice, we assessed the expression of TNF receptors in the liver. Expression of TNFR1, but not that of TNFR2, was up-regulated after GalN administration. GalN treatment failed to affect TNFα-induced NF-κB activation and expression of Bcl-2 family proteins, each preventing a signaling pathway for apoptosis. These findings demonstrate that up-regulation of TNFR1 on hepatocytes is important for the sensitization of these cells to subsequently triggered apoptosis.

Constitutive expression levels of Fas receptor have been shown to be functionally sufficient to mediate Fas-mediated apoptosis in mouse [13] and human [14] tissue. That observation supports our result that GalN only minimally sensitized the liver to injury by anti-Fas antibody. Fas expression was significantly elevated in hepatocytes in patients with acute liver failure [14] and chronic hepatitis C [15]. These findings are consistent with significant overexpression of cytokine receptors on target cells including TNFR1 and Fas. This process may occur beneficially during removal of virus-infected cells, but if exaggerated it can lead to fulminant hepatitis.

References

1. Loetscher H, Pan Y-CE, Lahm H-W, et al (1990) Molecular cloning and expression of the human 55kd tumor necrosis factor receptor. Cell 61:351–359
2. Schall TJ, Lewis M, Koller KJ, et al (1990) Molecular cloning and expression of a receptor human tumor necrosis factor. Cell 61:361–370
3. Heller RA, Song K, Onasch MA, et al (1990) Complementary DNA cloning of a receptor for tumor necrosis factor and demonstration of a shed form of the receptor. Proc Natl Acad Sci USA 87:6151–6155
4. Itoh N, Yonehara S, Ishii A, et al (1991) The polypeptide encoded by the cDNA for human cell surface antigen Fas can mediate apoptosis. Cell 66:233–243
5. Ogasawara J, Watanabe-Fukunaga R, Adachi M, et al (1993) Lethal effect of the anti-Fas antibody in mice. Nature 364:806–809
6. Leist M, Gantner F, Künstle G (1996) The 55-kD tumor necrosis factor receptor and CD95 independently signal murine hepatocyte apoptosis and subsequent liver failure. Mol Med 2:109–124
7. Nagaki M, Sugiyama A, Osawa Y, et al (1999) Lethal hepatic apoptosis mediated by tumor necrosis factor receptor, unlike Fas-mediated apoptosis, requires hepatocyte sensitization in mice. J Hepatol 31:997–1005
8. Galanos C, Freudenberg MA, Reutter W (1979) Galactosamine-induced sensitization to the lethal effects of endotoxin. Proc Natl Acad Sci USA 76:5939–5943
9. Nagaki M, Muto Y, Ohnishi H, et al (1994) Hepatic injury and lethal shock in galactosamine-sensitized mice induced by the superantigen staphylococcal enterotoxin B. Gastroenterology 106:450–458

10. Scaffidi C, Fulda S, Srinivasan A, et al (1998) Two CD95 (APO-1/Fas) signaling pathways. EMBO J 17:1675–1687
11. Beg AA, Baltimore D (1996) An essential role of NF-κB in preventing TNF-α-induced cell death. Science 274:782–784
12. Reed JC (1994) Bcl-2 and regulation of programmed cell death. J Cell Biol 124:1–6
13. Watanabe-Fukunaga R, Brannan CI, Itoh N, et al (1992) The cDNA structure, expression, and chromosomal assignment of the mouse Fas antigen. J Immunol 148: 1274–1279
14. Galle PR, Hofmann WJ, Walczak H, et al (1995) Involvement of the CD95 (APO-1/Fas) receptor and ligand in liver damage. J Exp Med 182:1223–1230
15. Hiramatsu N, Hayashi N, Katayama K, et al (1994) Immunohistochemical detection of Fas antigen in liver tissue of patients with chronic hepatitis C. Hepatology 19: 1354–1359

Molecular Mechanisms of D-Galactosamine/Lipopolysaccharide-Induced Fulminant Hepatic Failure in Mice and the Effects of Therapeutic Agents

Shuichi Hirono*, Tetsufumi Nakama, and Hirohito Tsubouchi

Summary. Treatment of experimental animals with D-galactosamine (GalN)/lipopolysaccharide (LPS) causes lethal liver injury that is characterized by apoptosis of the hepatocyte. We analyzed the molecular mechanism of GalN/LPS-induced apoptosis of hepatocytes and examined the therapeutic effects of etoposide on GalN/LPS-induced lethal liver injury. Serum tumor necrosis factor-α (TNF-α) levels were markedly increased in GalN/LPS-treated mice, and treatment with anti-TNF-α antibody of GalN/LPS-injected mice improved survival. The expression of tumor necrosis factor receptor-1 (TNFR1) mRNA, caspase 8 mRNA, and caspase 3 activity were enhanced in the liver of GalN/LPS-treated mice. Treatment of GalN/LPS-treated mice with etoposide markedly reduced lethality by preventing apoptosis of hepatocytes. The therapeutic effects of etoposide are thought to be caused by the enhancement of bcl-xL mRNA expression as etoposide did not alter serum TNF-α levels and TNFR1 mRNA expression. These findings suggest that antiapoptotic therapy is useful for the treatment of TNF-α-mediated liver diseases.

Key words. Etoposide, Acute hepatic failure, Apoptosis, GalN/LPS, TNF-α

Introduction

Liver transplantation is widely accepted as the treatment of choice for patients with fulminant hepatic failure. Unfortunately, however, the rapid progression of fulminant hepatic failure often precludes the possibility of transplantation. Plasma exchange is the only alternative in cases where transplantation is not possible, even though its efficacy is low. This study suggests that etoposide may be more effective than plasma exchange in improving the prognosis of patients with fulminant hepatic failure.

Administration of D-galactosamine (GalN)/lipopolysaccharide (LPS) causes lethal liver injury similar to fulminant hepatic failure. In this experimental model, tumor

Department of Internal Medicine II, Miyazaki Medical College, Kiyotake, Miyazaki 889-1692, Japan
*e-mail: hshuic@post.miyazaki-med.ac.jp

necrosis factor-α (TNF-α) is thought to be a key cytokine causing apoptosis of hepatocytes and resulting in lethal liver injury. The production of TNF-α in mononuclear cells of patients with fulminant hepatic failure is increased, and serum TNF-α levels of the patients are also reported to be increased. Whereas the molecular mechanism of TNF-α-mediated apoptosis has been clarified, the signal transduction system in TNF-α-mediated apoptosis in GalN/LPS-treated animals remains unclear. The animal model for fulminant hepatic failure induced by GalN/LPS treatment is useful for testing the effects of therapeutic agents. Therefore, we examined the molecular mechanism of TNF-α-mediated apoptosis in mice with GalN/LPS-induced lethal liver injury and the therapeutic effects of etoposide on GalN/LPS-induced lethal liver injury.

D-Galactosamine/Lipopolysaccharide-Induced Lethal Liver Injury as an Animal Model for Fulminant Hepatic Failure

The maximum serum alanine aminotransferase (AST) level of rats injected intraperitoneally with a high dose of GalN (up to 1.5 g/kg body weight) reaches less than 100 IU/L and does not induce lethal injury. However, administration of a subtoxic dose of D-galactosamine together with or followed by lipopolysaccharide (LPS) causes lethal liver injury consistent with fulminant hepatic failure [1]. In contrast, when LPS is injected into rats intravenously 7 days after intravenous injection of *Corynebacterium parvum*, lethal liver injury with extensive hepatocyte necrosis occurs within 12 h after LPS injection [2]. Administration of *C. parvum* induces infiltration of a large number of macrophages into the liver, and the activated macrophages are thought to increase the production of active oxygen and inflammatory cytokines such as TNF-α. In contrast, GalN inhibits RNA metabolism by depleting hepatic uridine trephosphate (UTP) content and is thought to cause cell membrane damage. The hepatocyte condition of rats treated with GalN is similar to those treated with *C. parvum*.

Molecular Mechanism of GalN/LPS-Induced Fulminant Hepatic Failure

Activated liver macrophages play an important role in the extensive hepatic necrosis seen after treatment with GalN/LPS. The serum TNF-α levels are markedly increased in Balb/c mice 1 h after GalN/LPS injection. TUNEL-positive hepatocytes indicating apoptosis of the hepatocytes in the livers of mice are first seen 3 h after GalN/LPS administration. After GalN/LPS injection into mice, serum levels of alanine aminotransferase are increased at 6 h, and massive hepatic necrosis is seen at 8 h. Most mice die from acute hepatic failure within 12 h after GalN/LPS administration. The key cytokine of this lethal liver injury is TNF-α as GalN/LPS-induced liver injury is completely prevented by treatment with anti-TNFα antibody. We confirmed the pivotal role of TNF-α in GalN/LPS-induced lethal liver injury and analyzed the mechanism of TNFα-mediated apoptosis of the hepatocytes.

The mRNA levels of TNF receptor 1 (TNFR1) and caspase 8 in the liver of mice treated with GalN/LPS injection were increased. The caspase 3 activity in the liver of mice 8 h after GalN/LPS administration was also increased approximately fivefold that

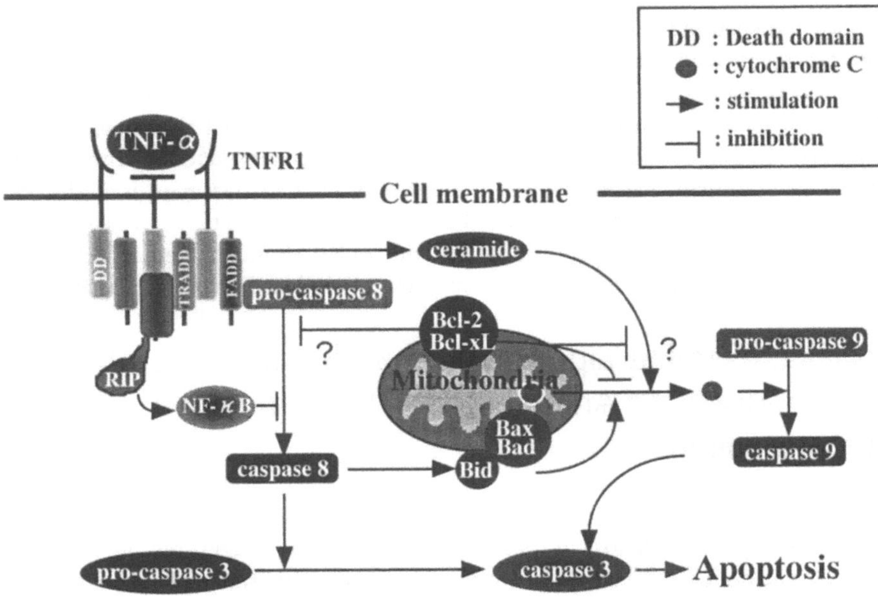

FIG. 1. Regulatory mechanism of apoptosis induced by tumor necrosis factor-α (TNF-α). TNF receptor 1 (TNFR1) has a death domain similar to Fas. TNF-α activates the caspase cascade by binding with TNFR1 and induces apoptosis. TNF-α also activates Nf-κB, which is one antiapoptotic molecule; however, the apoptotic change is dominant in the liver from GalN/LPS-treated mice. Apoptosis is also regulated by mitochondrial proteins, such as Bcl-2 family proteins. *DD*, death domain; *TRADD*, TNFR1-associated death domain protein; *FADD*, Fas-associating protein with a novel death domain; *RIP*, receptor-interacting protein; *Bax*, bcl-2-associated X ptotein; *Bad*, bcl-xL/bcl-2-associated death promotor; *Bid*, BH_3 interacting domain death agonist

of the control mice (without GalN/LPS treatment). Thus, the TNF-α-induced apoptotic signal transduction in GalN/LPS-treated mice livers seems to be mediated through the activation of the caspase 8/caspase 3 cascade via TNFR1-associated death domain protein/Fas-associating protein with a novel death domain (TRADD/FADD). A caspase-independent, ceramide-mediated signal transduction has been reported in TNFα-induced apoptosis [3,4]. The Bcl-2 family proteins, membrane proteins of the mitochondria, inhibit apoptosis by affecting these two systems. The molecular mechanisms of TNF-α-induced apoptosis are summarized in Fig. 1.

Preventive Agents for GalN/LPS-Induced Fulminant Hepatic Failure

Until now several preventive agents for GalN/LPS-induced fulminant hepatic failure have been reported. Gadolinium chloride inhibits the phagocytic activity of the Kupffer cells and decreases the production of TNF-α in GalN/LPS-treated mice, resulting in reduction of the lethal liver injury. Tetrahydroswertianolin, a hepatoprotective agent isolated from *Swertia japonica*, inhibits TNF-α production and decreases lethality in GalN/LPS-treated mice. Hepatocyte growth factor has also been reported to prevent the lethality of GalN/LPS-treated mice by up-regulation of Bcl-xL expression in the liver.

Etoposide, a topoisomerase II inhibitor, is well known to be an antineoplastic agent and causes antitumor effects by inducing apoptosis of malignant tumor cells. Etoposide is effective for treating patients with hemophagocytic syndrome whose serum cytokine levels including TNF-α are markedly high and whose prognosis is poor. The effectiveness of etoposide for patients with hemophagocytic syndrome is thought to be caused by suppression of inflammatory cytokine production. Therefore, we examined the effects of etoposide on mice with GalN/LPS-induced fulminant hepatic failure. We demonstrated that etoposide prevented lethality in mice with GalN/LPS- and GalN/TNF-α-induced fulminant hepatic failure. ICRF-193, another topoisomerase II inhibitor, showed no antilethal effects on the GalN/LPS-treated mice. Etoposide inhibited apoptosis of the hepatocytes without reducing the serum TNF-α levels in GalN/LPS-treated mice. Treatment of GalN/LPS-treated mice with etoposide increased bcl-xL mRNA expression in the liver and reduced caspase 3 activity in the liver. It is likely that increased Bcl-xL plays an important role in the antiapoptotic effect of etoposide on the GalN/LPS-induced liver injury.

Conclusions

The TNF-α induced by GalN/LPS treatment causes apoptosis of hepatocytes through a caspase 8/caspase 3 cascade followed by binding with TNFR1. Etoposide completely prevents lethal liver injury of GalN/LPS-treated mice by up-regulation of antiapoptotic bcl-xL without affecting TNF-α-mediated signal transduction.

References

1. Galanos C, Freudenberg MA, Reutter W (1979) Galactosamine-induced sensitization to the lethal effects of endotoxin. Proc Natl Acad Sci USA 76:5939–5943
2. Ferluga J, Allison AC (1978) Role of mononuclear infiltrating cells in pathogenesis of hepatitis. Lancet 2:610–611
3. Obeid LM, Linardic CM, Karolak LA, et al (1993) Programmed cell death induced by ceramide. Science 259:1769–1771
4. Jones BE, Lo CR, Srinivasan A, et al (1999) Ceramide induces caspase-independent apoptosis in rat hepatocytes sensitized by inhibition of RNA synthesis. Hepatology 30:215–222

Ethanol-Induced Apoptosis Mediated by Mitochondrial Permeability Transition in Primary Cultured Sinusoidal Endothelial Cells

Tsuneo Kitamura*, Liang Xiu Li, Miyoko Hirose, Kenichi Iejima, Nobuyuki Enomoto, Syujiro Matsuyama, Yoshiyuki Takei, and Nobuhiro Sato

Summary. Accumulating evidence suggests that ethanol delays liver regeneration in response to liver injury. The responsible mechanisms have been less well understood in sinusoidal endothelial cells (SECs) than in hepatocytes. To test this theory in vitro we prepared primary cultured SECs in rats and investigated the effect of ethanol on apoptosis and mitochondrial permeability transition (MPT), which is involved in the process of apoptosis. SECs were isolated based on a modification of the method of Wisse et al. SECs were cultured in EBM-2 containing vascular endothelial growth factor (20 ng/ml) at 37°C for 5 days. SECs displayed a confluent cell sheet at day 5 in culture. The bromodeoxyuridine labeling index was decreased whereas the apoptotic cells increased during the time in culture. Addition of 100 mM ethanol to the medium for 6 h induced two- and four-fold increases in apoptosis at days 2 and 5, respectively. This apoptotic effect was augmented in a dose-dependent manner by ethanol (50–150 mM). When SECs were exposed to ethanol for 3 h, MPT was observed, but there was no significant increase in apoptotic cells. Furthermore, cyclosporin A, an MPT inhibitor, suppressed apoptosis in SECs exposed to ethanol for 6 h. These results indicate that ethanol induces apoptosis in SECs, a process is mediated by MPT. It may therefore be hypothesized that ethanol-induced apoptosis in SECs causes impaired angiogenesis in liver, contributing to the delay in liver regeneration.

Key words. Ethanol, Liver sinusoidal endothelial cells, Mitochondrial permeability transition

Introduction

Based on experimental studies, evidence suggests that ethanol delays liver regeneration in response to liver injury [1–4]. The responsible mechanisms have been less well understood in sinusoidal endothelial cells (SECs) than in hepatocytes. Because SECs

Department of Gastroenterology, Juntendo University School of Medicine, 2-1-1 Hongo, Bunkyo-ku, Tokyo 113-8421, Japan
* e-mail: kitamura@med.juntendo.ac.jp

are initially exposed to ethanol in animals receiving ethanol administration, it is possible to assume that death of SECs plays an important role in delaying liver regeneration.

To test this idea in vitro, we prepared primary cultured SECs in rats and investigated the effect of ethanol on apoptosis and mitochondrial permeability transition (MPT), which is involved in the process of apoptosis [5,6].

The SECs were isolated based on a modification of the method of Wisse et al. [7]. Briefly, Wistar female rat liver was perfused with collagenase A, and cells were purified by isopyknic sedimentation in a two-step Percoll gradient. Cell viability, determined by trypan blue exclusion, was typically 90%. After isolation, cells were plated on a 60-mm collagen-coated dish at a concentration of 3×10^6 cells per dish. After 2h of incubation in 5% CO_2/air at 37°C, the cells were washed with RPMI 1640 to remove dead cells, and the medium was changed to EBM-2. After 24h of incubation, the medium was again changed to EBM-2 containing vascular endothelial growth factor (VEGF) (20ng/ml) and subsequently at 48-h intervals. SECs were used after 2 and 5 days of culture.

The DNA synthesis of cells was determined by bromodeoxyuridine (BrdU) incorporation. The percent of apoptotic cells was assessed by the TUNEL assay. After loading cells with tetramethylrhodamine methylester (TMRM), a cationic fluorescence dye, the MPT was monitored in SECs using fluorescence microscopy. It was defined by detecting the release of TMRM from mitochondria into the cytoplasm of SECs.

The SECs displayed a confluent cell sheet at day 5 in culture. The BrdU labeling index was decreased whereas apoptotic cells increased during the time in culture. Addition of 100mM ethanol to the medium for 6h induced two- and four-fold increases in apoptosis of cells at days 2 and 5 in culture, respectively. This apoptotic effect was augmented in a dose-dependent manner by ethanol (50–150mM) at both days 2 and 5 in culture.

To test whether MPT is involved in ethanol-induced apoptosis, the intracellular distribution of TMRM was investigated in SECs at day 2 in culture. In the absence of ethanol, TMRM accumulated in the mitochondria of SECs presumably in response to the negative mitochondrial membrane potential. However, when SECs were exposed to ethanol for 3h on culture day 2, the accumulation of TMRM fluorescence in mitochondria was lost, indicating that mitochondrial depolarization caused TMRM to be released from the mitochondria into the cytoplasm.

This phenomenon was inhibited by cyclosporin A, an MPT transition inhibitor, strongly suggesting that incubation of cells with ethanol for 3h induced MPT [8]. Furthermore, there was no significant increase in apoptotic cells in the presence of ethanol for 3h, and cyclosporin A suppressed apoptosis in SECs incubated with ethanol for 6h.

Conclusions

These results indicate that ethanol induces apoptosis in SECs, the process of which is mediated by MPT. Although endothelial cells, rather than other cell types, are generally susceptible to apoptosis, the present findings reveal that apoptosis could be induced by ethanol in SECs, which are highly proliferating (day 2 in culture) as well.

In the normal liver, hepatocytes are in direct contact with hepatic sinusoids, which are formed by SECs. During liver regeneration, hepatocyte mitotic activity at first leads to the formation of hepatocyte clusters without sinusoids. Following hepatocyte regeneration, SECs proliferate, sinusoids insinuate themselves into hepatocyte clusters, and normal hepatic size and architecture are achieved [9]. Therefore, during liver regeneration not only hepatocyte regeneration but also SEC regeneration and sinusoidal formation appear to be important.

Based on these findings, it seems that apoptosis of SECs plays a crucial role in liver regeneration. It is therefore possible to offer a novel hypothesis that ethanol-induced apoptosis in SECs causes impaired sinusoidal formation in the liver, thereby contributing to delayed liver regeneration.

References

1. Wands JR, Carter EA, Bucher NL, et al (1979) Inhibition of hepatic regeneration in rats by acute and chronic ethanol intoxication. Gastroenterology 77:528–531
2. Diehl AM, Thorgeirsson SS, Steer CJ (1990) Ethanol inhibits liver regeneration in rats without reducing transcripts of key protooncogenes. Gastroenterology 99:1105–1112
3. Lumpkin CK Jr, Moore TL, Tarpley MD, et al (1995) Acute ethanol and selected growth suppressor transcripts in regenerating rat liver. Alcohol 12:357–362
4. Zhang MN, Gong Y, Minuk GY (2000) The effects of acute ethanol exposure on inhibitors of hepatic regenerative activity in the rat. Mol Cell Biochem 207:109–114
5. Marchetti P, Castedo M, Susin SA, et al (1996) Mitochondrial permeability transition is a central coordinating event of apoptosis. J Exp Med 184:1155–1160
6. Green DR, Reed JC (1998) Mitochondria and apoptosis. Science 281:1309–1312
7. Braet F, De Zanger R, Sasaoki T, et al (1994) Assessment of a method of isolation, purification, and cultivation of rat liver sinusoidal endothelial cells. Lab Invest 70:944–952
8. Pastorino JG, Snyder JW, Serroni A, et al (1993) Cyclosporin and carnitine prevent the anoxic death of cultured hepatocytes by inhibiting the mitochondrial permeability transition. J Biol Chem 268:13791–13798
9. Martinez-Hernandez A, Delgado FM, Amenta PS (1991) The extracellular matrix in hepatic regeneration: localization of collagen types I, III, IV, laminin, and fibronectin. Lab Invest 64:157–166

Therapeutic Strategies for Hepatocellular Carcinoma Based on Analyses for Resistance to Apoptosis Mediated by Activation of Intracellular Signal Pathways

Toshifumi Ito[1,*], Yutaka Sasaki[2], Harumasa Yoshihara[1], Kunio Suzuki[1], Eiji Masuda[1], Yukinori Yamada[1], Keiichi Arai[1], Takenobu Kamada[1], Norio Hayashi[2], and Jack R. Wands[3]

Summary. Evidence clearly demonstrates that transforming hepatocytes are gaining phenotypes, either accelerating cell cycles or resisting apoptosis, during hepatocarcinogenesis. Disorder of intracellular signaling seems to be closely related to the acquisition of such malignant phenotypes. Thus it is important to understand how the intracellular signaling is constitutively activated or improperly regulated. It is beneficial to clarify these pathways for the sake of preparing new therapeutic strategies against human hepatocellular carcinoma (HCC). On the other hand, insulin is a hepatotrophic factor that stimulates growth of normal hepatocytes and HCC-derived cell lines. The insulin receptor substrate-1 protein (IRS-1) is a specific substrate for insulin receptor tyrosine kinase. Expression and tyrosyl phosphorylation of IRS-1 plays an important role during normal hepatocyte growth, and the gene is overexpressed in HCC tissue. Previously, we reported that IRS-1 could induce cellular transformation similar to a dominant oncogene. Interestingly, it has been reported that several cytokines, such as insulin and insulin-like growth factors, could inhibit apoptotic phenomena. Here we reviewed the role of IRS-1 overexpression in hepatic carcinogenesis from the viewpoint of transforming activities and acquisition of resistance to apoptosis. These analyses may permit a new understanding of oncogenes, by which overexpression cells could acquire not only the transforming phenotype but also the ability to escape from programmed cell death, thereby becoming resistant to therapy. Moreover, they may lead to new therapeutic strategies for HCC, targeting the intracellular signaling molecules.

[1]Department of Gastroenterology, Osaka Rosai Hospital, 1179-3 Nagasone-cho, Sakai, Osaka 591-8025, Japan
[2]Department of Molecular Therapeutics, Osaka University Postgraduate School of Medicine, 2-2 Yamadaoka, Suita, Osaka 565-0871, Japan
[3]The Liver Research Center, Rhode Island Hospital and Brown University School of Medicine, 55 Claverick Street, 4th Floor, Providence, RI 02903, USA
* e-mail: tito@orh.go.jp

Key words. Apoptosis, Signal transduction, Insulin receptor substrate-1, Mitogen-activated protein kinase, Hepatocellular carcinoma

Introduction

Insulin is a pleiotrophic factor with both mitogenic and metabolic effects on cells. Insulin receptor substrate-1 (IRS-1) protein is the principal intracellular substrate of the insulin receptor tyrosine kinase activity and is the most upstream molecule in the signal transduction cascade mediated by insulin, interleukin-4 (IL-4), and insulin-like growth-I factor stimulation [1,2]. Our previous preport showed the cloning of the human IRS-1 (hIRS-1) gene and overexpression in human hepatocellular carcinoma (HCC) tissue compared to adjacent noninvolved normal liver. We also showed that expression and phosphorylation of IRS-1 was important during normal liver growth induced by partial hepatectomy [3].

It has been simply demonstrated that IRS-1 has multiple tyrosine phosphorylation residues that allow it to associate with other signal molecules containing *src* homology 2 (SH2) domains, such as the p85 subunit of the phosphatidylinositol 3′-kinase (PI3-K), growth factor receptor-bound protein 2 (Grb2) [which interacts with *son of sevenless* (SOS) and induces *ras* activation], and Syp. These protein–protein interactions play essential roles in the intracellular signaling process.

The insulin signal transduction pathway activates the mitogen-activated protein kinase (MAPK, or extracellular signal-regulated kinase, Erk) cascade. This MAPK cascade is comprised of MAPKs, MAPKK [Erk kinase, *M*APK/*E*rk *K*inase (MEK)] and Raf or MEK kinase. In addition, *ras* functions as an activator of *raf* and leads to activation of the cascade. It has also been established that *ras*-dependent signal transduction converges to activate the MAPK cascade, and this event appears necessary for cell proliferation to occur (Fig. 1).

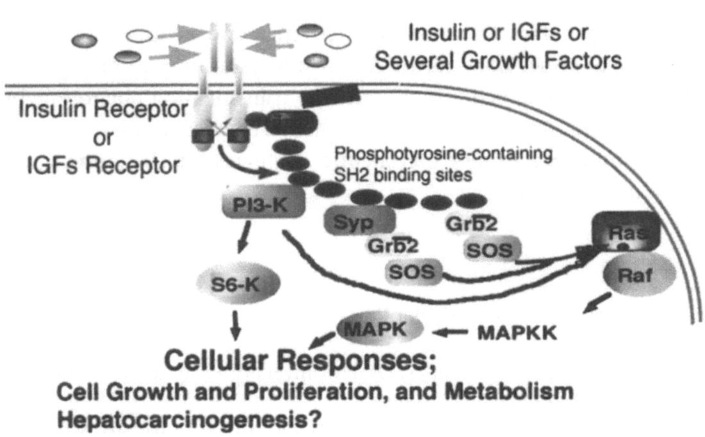

FIG. 1. Insulin receptor substrate-1 (IRS-1) signaling system. *IGFs*, insulin-like growth factors

IRS-1: A Dominant Oncogene?

It has been proposed that IRS-1 is essential for insulin-induced mitogenic effects. Thus, the components of this cascade, including IRS-1, may be required for hepatocyte proliferation and even contribute to hepatic carcinogenesis. Therefore, we tested the hypothesis that constitutive overexpression of this molecule may result in generation of the malignant phenotype. In the previous investigation [4] we determined if up-regulation of the IRS-1 gene activates the downstream MAPK cascade and is associated with malignant transformation of NIH 3T3 cells.

The IRS-1 protein is the most upstream molecule in the signal transduction cascade as one of the principal intracellular substrates for receptor tyrosine kinase of insulin, IGFs, and several cytokines, such as IL-4, as shown in Fig. 1. We previously reported that the IRS-1 gene could act like a dominant oncogene [4,5]. Overexpression of this gene in NIH 3T3 fibroblasts could lead these cells to acquire the transforming phenotype. NIH 3T3 cells overexpressing the IRS-1 gene could form transforming foci, make up colonies in soft agar, proliferate under low serum conditions, and grow up in nude mice. In other words, these cells could grow up anchorage-independently without contact inhibition and under low growth stimulation. Finally, to further investigate the phenotype of the three cell lines overexpressing IRS-1 and associated activation of downstream MAPKs, the ability of such cell lines to form solid tumors in nude mice was assessed. It is noteworthy that cells overexpressing IRS-1 produced tumors in most mice, but *v-src*-transformed NIH 3T3 cells were the most. It was of interest that there may be a correlation of tumor growth rate with the degree of MAPKs activation in these hIRS-1-transfected NIH 3T3 cell lines. In addition, we showed that simple overexpression of IRS-1 could be followed by increased tyrosine phosphorylation of IRS-1 molecules with MAPKs. IRS-1 overexpression could be induced to activate the cascade Ras to MAPKs through MAPKK with dominantly increased protein–protein interaction between IRS-1 and Grb-2.

These findings were interesting in that simple overexpression of the most upstream signal molecule without catalytic activity like IRS-1 could make cells acquire the transforming phenotype with activation of the MAPK cascade (Fig. 2).

IRS-1 Overexpression: Induction of Resistance to Apoptosis

Evidence suggests that several growth factors, including insulin and IGFs, may protect cells from apoptosis; that is, they function as survival factors. This implies the possibility that intracellular signaling evoked by the IGF family plays an important role in protecting cells from apoptosis. Moreover, insulin and IGFs are pleiotrophic factors with both mitogenic and metabolic effects on cells. Altered regulation of apoptosis may be important in tumorigenesis. However, little is known which signal transduction pathways are involved in this escape from programmed cell death. Previous studies have shown that overexpression of IRS-1 promotes resistance to apoptosis. Our hypothesis—*ras* activation following IRS-1 overexpression—seemed pivotal in

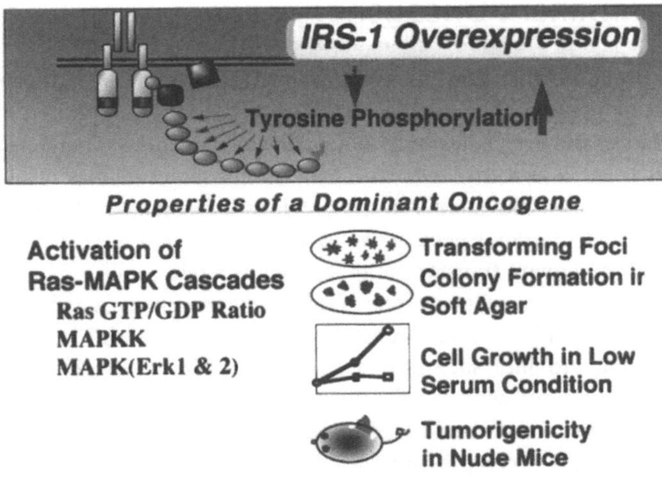

FIG. 2. IRS-1 has properties of a dominant oncogene

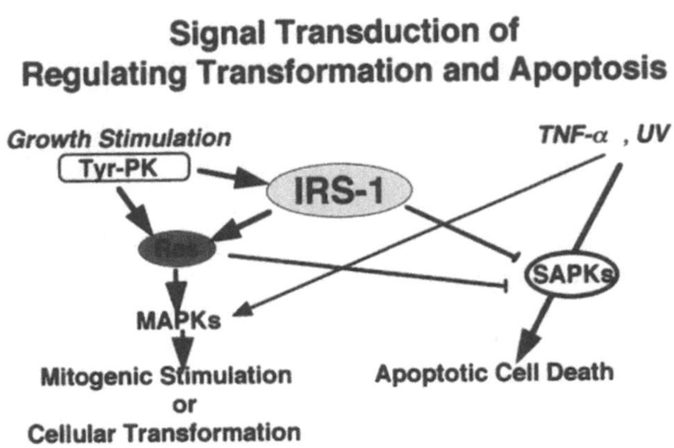

FIG. 3. Our hypothesis. Signaling from IRS-1 to *ras* may have a close relation to cellular transformation and resistance to apoptosis

preventing programmed cell death. On the other hand, there should be a close relationship between apoptosis and the function of the stress-activated protein kinase (SAPK) cascade (Fig. 3). Unfortunately, little is known about the relation of SAPK activation and apoptosis induced by IRS-1 overexpression with *ras* activation. In future, the downstream signaling that contributes to the acquisition of such a malignant phenotype should be addressed.

References

1. Myers MG Jr, Sun XJ, White MF (1994) The IRS-1 signaling system. Trends Biochem Sci 19:289–293
2. White MF, Kahn CR (1994) The insulin signaling system. J Biol Chem 269:1–4
3. Sasaki Y, Zhang XF, Nishiyama M, et al (1993) Expression and phosphorylation of insulin receptor substrate 1 during rat liver regeneration. J Biol Chem 268:3805–3808
4. Ito T, Sasaki Y, Wands JR (1996) Overexpression of human insulin receptor substrate 1 induced cellular transformation with activation of mitogen-activated protein kinases. Mol Cell Biol 16:943–951
5. Tanaka S, Ito T, Wands JR (1996) Neoplastic transformation induced by insulin receptor substrate-1 overexpression requires an interaction with both Grb2 and Syp. J Biol Chem 271:14610–14616

Expression of Apoptosis-Related Factors in Human Pancreatic Duct Cell Carcinoma and Intraductal Papillary-Mucinous Tumor

KENICHI SATOH*, ATSUSHI MASAMUNE, KENZO KANEKO, MORIHISA HIROTA, AKIHIKO SATOH, and TOORU SHIMOSEGAWA

Summary. Pancreatic duct cell carcinoma (PDC) is one of the most malignant of the gastrointestinal tumors. Expression of the apoptosis-related factors Fas ligand (FasL) and caspase-3 and the antiapoptotic factor survivin was examined in PDC and in intraductal papillary-mucinous tumor (IPMT) by reverse transcriptase-polymerase chain reaction (RT-PCR), immunoblot analysis, and immunohistochemistry. Frequent expression of FasL was observed in PDC. The co-culture experiments showed that PANC-1 cells induced apoptosis of Jurkat cells, whereas the PANC-1 cells themselves and Jurkat cells cultured without the presence of PANC-1 showed few apoptotic changes. The immunoreactivity of caspase-3 was predominantly found in the cytoplasm of invasive tumors (PDC and invasive IPMT). There was a significant correlation between the cytoplasmic staining and malignant grade of the tumors. In contrast, the nuclear expression of this enzyme was significantly higher in noninvasive tumors than in invasive tumors. Survivin was more frequently expressed in malignant tumors than in benign tumors. In PDC, high levels of survivin expression were significantly associated with a reduction in the apoptotic index of the tumor cells. These findings suggest that: (1) Fas-L may play an important role in the ability of PDC to escape from immune surveillance through the induction of apoptosis in tumor-attacking lymphocytes; (2) cytoplasmic expression of caspase-3 may be related to the invasiveness of pancreatic tumors; and (3) the expression of survivin may be up-regulated during the development of cancer by reducing the cancer cell apoptosis.

Key words. Pancreatic tumor, Fas ligand, Caspase-3, Survivin, Apoptosis

Introduction

Pancreatic duct cell carcinoma (PDC) is one of the most malignant of the gastrointestinal tumors. Once PDC is clinically evident, it progresses rapidly to develop metastatic lesions, frequently by the time of diagnosis. Furthermore, these tumors are

---

Department of Gastroenterology, Division of Internal Medicine, Tohoku University Graduate School of Medicine, 1-1 Seiryo-machi, Aoba-ku, Sendai 980-8574, Japan
* e-mail: ksatoh@int3.med.tohoku.ac.jp

usually resistant to conventional chemotherapy and radiation therapy. The pathogenic mechanisms that regulate this aggressive growth behavior in PDC remain to be clarified. On the other hand, intraductal papillary-mucinous tumor (IPMT) of the pancreas is a unique neoplasm that is considered a precancerous lesion analogous to adenomatous polyps of the colon [1]. The basically favorable prognosis of the patients with IPMT suggests that the dysplastic component may remain in situ for a long time [1]. We previously demonstrated, however, the activation of oncogenes such as K-*ras* [2] and c-*erb* B-2 [3], the accumulation of p53 [2], and the loss of chromosome 18q [4] in IPMT, suggesting the malignant potential of this neoplasm. In addition, stromal infiltration and distal metastasis have been reported even in this type of tumor [5,6].

Apoptosis, or programmed cell death, plays a critical role in normal morphogenesis and homeostatic mechanisms in both normal and neoplastic cells [7]. Fas ligand (Fas-L) and its receptor Fas (also known as APO-1 and CD 95) play a key role in the regulation of apoptosis in the immune system [8]. Ligation of Fas with either activating antibodies or Fas-L transmits a "death signal" to the target cell, resulting in the triggering of apoptosis [9,10]. The interaction between Fas-L and Fas has been shown to play a pivotal role in the maintenance of immunological homeostasis and peripheral tolerance by the deletion of activated T lymphocytes [11,12].

It has been demonstrated that Fas-L is expressed in human melanoma [13], hepatocellular carcinoma [14], colon cancer [15,16], lung carcinoma [17], and pancreatic cancer cell lines [18]. These studies suggested that the expression of Fas-L may play an important role in establishing immunologically privileged environments that allow tumors or metastatic cancer cells to escape from the host's immune surveillance.

To date, at least 14 members of the ICE/ced-3 family (caspases) have been identified, and most can induce apoptosis when overexpressed in mammalian cells [19]. One of these cystein proteases, caspase-3 (CPP32, Yama, apopain), is believed to be most commonly involved in the execution of apoptosis in various cell types [20]. Activation of caspase-3 has been described in a number of cell types undergoing apoptosis in response to a variety of stimuli including CD95 (Fas/Apo-1) signaling [20]. Caspase-3 expression has been demonstrated in neoplastic cells such as gastric cancer [21], Hodgkin's lymphoma [22], and neuroblastomas [23]. In neuroblastoma [23] and gastric cancer [21], high levels of caspase-3 may be involved in the development or regulation of apoptotic cell death.

Suppression of apoptosis by aberrantly prolonging cell viability is considered to contribute to carcinogenesis and carcinoma progression by facilitating gene mutations and promoting resistance to immune-based cytotoxicity [7]. Survivin is a new member of the inhibitor of apoptosis (IAP) family of antiapoptotic proteins [24]. Unlike other IAP proteins, survivin contains a single baculovirus IAP repeat but no RING finger. Survivin was expressed selectively during development and in all the most common human cancers but not in normal adult tissues [24]. Overexpression of survivin has been shown to be associated with aggressive forms of neuroblastoma [25] and is correlated with a reduction of apoptosis in colorectal [26] and stomach [27] cancer. In addition, survivin expression was frequently observed in skin cancer and in premalignant lesions of Bowen's disease, suggesting that its expression occurs early during skin carcinogenesis [28]. To our knowledge, the relation between survivin expression and apoptosis or tumorigenesis has not yet been studied in pancreatic neoplasms. In this study we investigated the expression of survivin in PDC and IPMT including premalignant lesions, and we examined the association of its expression with tumor cell apoptosis or tumorigenesis.

FasL Expression in Pancreatic Tumors

The mRNA and protein expression of Fas-L [29] was investigated in four pancreatic cancer cell lines and 19 human pancreatic duct cell carcinomas (PDCs) by the reverse transcriptase-polymerase chain reaction (RT-PCR) and immunohistochemistry, respectively. In addition, a co-culture assay of Fas-L and Fas-expressing PANC-1 cells and Fas-sensitive Jurkat cells was performed. Fas-L mRNA expression was observed in all four cell lines and in 10 PDC tissues; and the protein expression was frequently detected in the PDC tissues (16 of 19 cases). The co-culture experiments showed that PANC-1 cells induced apoptosis of Jurkat cells, whereas the PANC-1 cells themselves and Jurkat cells cultured without the presence of PANC-1 showed few apoptotic changes.

Caspase-3 Expression in Pancreatic Tumors

To determine whether caspase-3 expression [30] reflects the biological behavior of pancreatic tumors, we investigated this enzyme expression by RT-PCR and immunohistochemistry in 22 PDCs and 13 IPMTs. Caspase-3 mRNA was overexpressed in PDCs and IPMTs with carcinoma when compared with normal pancreatic tissues or IPMT with adenoma. The immunoreactivity of this enzyme was found predominantly in the cytoplasm of invasive tumors (PDCs and invasive IPMTs). There was a significant correlation between cytoplasmic staining and the malignant grade of the tumor. In contrast, the nuclear expression of this enzyme was significantly higher in noninvasive tumors than in invasive tumors.

Survivin Expression in Pancreatic Tumors

We investigated the expression of survivin in 4 pancreatic carcinoma cell lines and 56 human pancreatic tissues [5 normals, 12 cases of chronic pancreatitis (CP), 26 PDCs, 13 IPMTs (9 adenomas, 4 carcinomas including 2 invasive lesions)] by immunohistochemistry, immunoblotting, and RT-PCR to examine the association of its expression with tumor apoptosis and tumorigenesis. By immunohistochemistry, immunoblotting, and RT-PCR, survivin expression was found in the tumor cells but not in the nonneoplastic pancreatic tissues (normal and CP tissues). Survivin expression was observed in 20 of 26 PDCs (76.9%) and in 9 of 16 IPMTs, which ranged from adenoma to invasive lesions (56.3%) by immunohistochemistry. Survivin was expressed more frequently in malignant tumors than in benign tumors. In PDCs high levels of survivin expression were significantly associated with a reduction in the apoptotic index of the tumor cells. In addition, cells expressing this protein appeared to increase in the transition from adenoma to cancer in situ (CIS) and in that from CIS to invasive IPMT.

Conclusions

Fas-L may play an important role in the ability of PDCs to escape from immune surveillance. It does it through the induction of apoptosis in tumor-attacking lymphocytes [29].

Cytoplasmic expression of caspase-3 may be related to the invasiveness of pancreatic tumors. In contrast, nuclear expression of this enzyme may reflect the benign biological behavior of IPMTs [30].

Expression of survivin may be up-regulated during an early step of tumorigenesis and during the development of cancer by reducing cancer cell apoptosis.

References

1. Loftus EV Jr, Olivares-Pakzad BA, Batts KP, et al (1996) Intraductal papillary-mucinous tumors of the pancreas: clinicopathologic features, outcome, and nomenclature. Gastroenterology 110:1909–1918
2. Satoh K, Shimosegawa T, Moriizumi S, et al (1996) K-*ras* mutation and p53 protein accumulation in intraductal mucin-hypersecreting neoplasms of the pancreas. Pancreas 12:362–368
3. Satoh K, Sasano H, Shimosegawa T, et al (1993) An immunohistochemical study of the c-*erb* B-2 oncogene product in intraductal mucin-hypersecreting neoplasms and in ductal cell carcinomas of the pancreas. Cancer 72:51–56
4. Fukushige S, Furukawa T, Satoh K, et al (1998) Loss of chromosome 18q is an early event in pancreatic ductal tumorigenesis. Cancer Res 58:4222–4226
5. Sugiyama M, Atomi Y (1998) Intraductal papillary-mucionus tumors of the pancreas: imaging studies and treatment strategies. Ann Surg 228:685–691
6. Yasuda H, Takada T, Amano H, et al (1998) Surgery for mucin-producing pancreatic tumor. Hepatogastroenterology 45:2009–2015
7. Thompson CB (1995) Apoptosis in the pathogenesis and treatment of disease. Science 267:1456–1462
8. Nagata S, Golstein P (1995) The Fas death factor. Science 267:1449–1456
9. Yonehara S, Ishii A, Yonehara M (1989) A cell-killing monoclonal antibody (anti-Fas) to cell surface antigen co-downregulated with the receptor of tumor necrosis factor. J Exp Med 169:1747–1756
10. Oehn A, Behrman I, Falk W, et al (1992) Purification and molecular cloning of the APO-1 cell surface antigen, a member of the tumor necrosis factor/nerve growth factor receptor family: sequence identity with the Fas antigen. J Biol Chem 267:10709–10715
11. Singer GG, Abbas AK (1994) The Fas antigen is involved in peripheral but not thymic deletion of T lymphocytes in T cell receptor transgenic mice. Immunity 1:365–371
12. Alderson MR, Tough TW, Davis-Smith T, et al (1995) Fas ligand mediates activation-induced cell death in human T lymphocytes. J Exp Med 181:71–77
13. Hahne D, Rimoldi M, Schröter P, et al (1996) Melanoma cell expression of Fas (Apo-1/CD95) ligand: implications for tumor immune escape. Science 274:1363–1366
14. Strand S, Hofmann WJ, Hug H, et al (1996) Lymphocyte apoptosis induced by CD95 (APO-1/Fas) ligand-expressing tumor cells: a mechanism of immune evasion? Nat Med 2:1361–1366
15. O'Connell BJ, O'Sullivan GC, Collins JK, et al (1996) The Fas counterattack: Fas-mediated T cell killing by colon cancer cells expressing Fas ligand. J Exp Med 184:1075–1082
16. Shiraki K, Tsuji N, Shioda T, et al (1997) Expression of Fas ligand in liver metastases of human colonic adenocarcinomas. Proc Natl Acad Sci USA 94:6420–6425

17. Niehans GA, Brunner T, Frizelle SP, et al (1997) Human lung carcinomas express Fas ligand. Cancer Res 57:1007–1012
18. Ungefroren H, Voss M, Jansen M, et al (1998) Human adenocarcinomas express Fas and Fas ligand yet are resistant to Fas-mediated apoptosis. Cancer Res 58:1741–1749
19. Nuñez G, Benedict MA, Hu Y, et al (1998) Caspases: the proteases of the apoptotic pathway. Oncogene 17:3237–3245
20. Tewari M, Quan LT, O'Rouke K, et al (1995) Yama/CPP32β, a mammalian homologue of CED-3, is a crmA-inhibitable protease that cleaves the death substrate poly ADP-ribose polymerase. Cell 81:801–809
21. Hoshi T, Sasano H, Kato K, et al (1998) Immunohistochemistry of Caspase3/CPP32 in human stomach and its correlation with cell proliferation and apoptosis. Anticancer Res 18:4347–4353
22. Krajewski S, Gascoyne RD, Zapata JM, et al (1997) Immunolocalization of ICE/ced-3-family protease, CPP-32 (caspase-3), in non-Hodgkin's lymphomas, chronic leukemias, and reactive lymph nodes. Blood 89:3817–3825
23. Nakagawara A, Nakamura Y, Ikeda H, et al (1997) High levels of expression and nuclear localization of interleukin-1β converting enzyme (ICE) and CPP32 in favorable human neuroblastomas. Cancer Res 57:4578–4584
24. Ambrosini G, Adida C, Altieri DC (1997) A novel anti-apoptosis gene, survivin, expressed in cancer and lymphoma. Nat Med 3:917–921
25. Adida C, Berrebi D, Peuchmaur M, et al (1998) Anti-apoptosis gene, survivin, and prognosis of neuroblastoma. Lancet 351:882–883
26. Kawasaki H, Altieri DC, Lu C-D, et al (1998) Inhibition of apoptosis by survivin predicts shorter survival rates in colorectal cancer. Cancer Res 58:5071–5074
27. Lu CD, Altieri DC, Tanigawa N (1998) Expression of a novel antiapoptosis gene, survivin, correlated with tumor cell apoptosis and p53 accumulation in gastric carcinomas. Cancer Res 58:1808–1812
28. Grossman D, McNiff JM, Li F, et al (1999) Expression of the apoptosis inhibitor, survivin, in nonmelanoma skin cancer and gene targeting in a keratinocyte cell line. Lab Invest 79:1121–1126
29. Satoh K, Shimosegawa T, Masamune A, et al (1999) Fas ligand is frequently expressed in human pancreatic duct cell carcinoma. Pancreas 19:339–345
30. Satoh K, Kaneko K, Hirota M, et al (2000) The pattern of CPP 32/Caspase-3 expression reflects the biological behavior of the human pancreatic duct cell tumors. Pancreas (in press)

Part 5
Is Nitric Oxide Friend or Foe?

Effect of Exogenous and Endogenous Nitric Oxide on Endothelial Permeability Induced by Oxidants In Vitro

NAOTSUKA OKAYAMA[1,*], MAKOTO ITOH[1], and J. STEVEN ALEXANDER[2]

Summary. Nitric oxide (NO) can be divided into two types: exogenous and endogenous. In this study we examined the effects of exogenous and endogenous NO on endothelial permeability induced by oxidants, such as hydrogen peroxide and superoxide, using bovine pulmonary artery endothelial cells and a chromatographic cell column technique. An NO donor, supermine-NONOate (SNO), at a concentration of 1 mM significantly exacerbated endothelial permeability induced by 0.1 mM peroxide by activating the Fenton reaction and reducing the intracellular glutathione level. Conversely, an NO synthase (NOS) inhibitor, L-N^5-(1-iminoethyl)-ornithine (L-NIO, 10 μM) completely inhibited peroxide-mediated permeability, suggesting that both exogenous and endogenous NO have aggressive effects on this event. On the other hand, SNO completely inhibited superoxide-mediated endothelial permeability by consuming the oxidant when flux of NO from an NO donor was similar to that of superoxide from its generating system (xanthine plus xanthine oxidase). An NOS inhibitor, L-NIO (10 μM), did not affect this system. These results suggest that NO is a controversial chemical agent because it depends on the type of oxidant as to whether NO has defensive or aggressive effects on endothelial permeability induced by oxidants.

Key words. Nitric oxide, Endothelial permeability, Hydrogen peroxide, Superoxide, Peroxynitrite

Introduction

Nitric oxide (NO) can be divided into two types: endogenous (generated from endothelial cells) and exogenous (generated from smoking, air pollution, medicines, among other sources). Oxidants such as hydrogen peroxide and superoxide are also

[1] First Department of Internal Medicine, Nagoya City University Medical School, 1 Kawasumi, Mizuho-cho, Mizuho-ku, Nagoya 467-8601, Japan
[2] Department of Molecular and Cellular Physiology, Louisiana State University Medical Center, 1501 Kings Highway, Shreveport, LA 71130, USA
* e-mail: nokaya@med.nagoya-cu.ac.jp

generated from endothelial cells in such stress conditions as produced by gastroenterological diseases, resulting in increasing endothelial permeability [1,2]. It is still not known whether NO has a defensive or aggressive effect on these events. In this study we examined the effects of exogenous and endogenous NO on endothelial permeability induced by oxidants in vitro to define whether NO is a good or bad influence.

Materials and Methods

After bovine pulmonary artery endothelial cells were cultured on Cytodex-3 microcarrier beads (Sigma, St. Louis, MO, USA), chromatographic cell columns were filled with the cell-covered beads and perfused with Hank's balanced salt solution containing 15 mM HEPES (pH 7.4) and 0.5% bovine serum albumin. The endothelial permeability was determined by comparing the elution curves of three tracers (2000 kDa blue dextran as a flow tracer and 1355-Da cyanocobalamin and 376-Da sodium fluorescein as membrane-permeable tracers) injected into the flow at the top of the column as previously reported [3,4].

Results and Discussion

Hydrogen peroxide at a concentration of 0.1 mM significantly increased endothelial permeability after 70 min. An NO donor, supermine-NONOate (SNO), at a concentration of 1 mM significantly exacerbated an increase in permeability induced by peroxide. Interestingly, an NO synthase (NOS) inhibitor, L-N^5-(1-iminoethyl)-ornithine (L-NIO, 10 μM; Calbiochem, La Jolla, CA, USA) completely inhibited 0.1 mM peroxide-mediated permeability. These data suggest that exogenous and endogenous NO have aggressive effects on endothelial permeability induced by peroxide.

To define the mechanisms of these events, we first measured intracellular glutathione concentrations after exposure to peroxide and SNO and found that SNO (1 mM) but not peroxide (0.1 mM) significantly reduced the glutathione level after 60 min. We also found that desferrioxamine (0.1 mM), an iron chelator, and methionine (1 mM), a hydroxyl radical scavenger, completely blocked peroxide/SNO-mediated permeability.

Based on these results we speculated that NO stimulates the Fenton reaction, in which oxidation of iron from the ferrous (Fe^{2+}) state to the ferric (Fe^{3+}) state generates hydroxyl radicals from hydrogen peroxide, which results in an increase in endothelial permeability due to peroxide. NO also makes cells more sensitive to oxidants by reducing the intracellular glutathione level.

A superoxide-generating system, xanthine (X; 0.1 mM) plus xanthine oxidase (XO; 25 mU/ml), also significantly increased endothelial permeability 60 min earlier than 0.1 mM peroxide. The early increase in permeability due to X/XO was likely mediated by superoxide because this system generates both superoxide and peroxide. Because this event was completely inhibited by superoxide dismutase (100 U/ml), catalase (1000 U/ml), desferrioxamine (0.1 mM), and methionone (1 mM), superoxide is thought to stimulate the Fenton reaction and increase permeability in this system. Supermine-NONOate at a concentration of 0.1 mM completely blocked X/XO-mediated permeability, but 0.01 and 1 mM SNO partially attenuated it. We also found that the flux of NO generated from 0.1 mM SNO was similar to that of superoxide from the X/XO system. These results suggest that equal flux of exogenous NO inhibits superoxide-mediated endothelial permeability by consuming the oxidant.

To evaluate the effects of peroxynitrite produced by the reaction between NO and superoxide on permeability, we used 3-morphosyndiomine (SIN-1 1 mM; Alexis, San Diego, CA, USA) plus catalase (1000 U/ml), a peroxynitrite generating system. This system did not affect permeability in this study. Conversely, an NOS inhibitor, L-NIO (10 μM), did not affect the early increase in X/XO-mediated permeability due to superoxide, suggesting that endogenous NO has no effect on superoxide-mediated permeability.

Conclusions

We found that exogenous and endogenous NO caused an increase in endothelial permeability induced by hydrogen peroxide. However, exogenous, but not endogenous, NO had defensive effects on superoxide-mediated permeability in this study. These findings suggest that NO is a controversial chemical agent: Whether NO has a defensive or an aggressive effect on endothelial permeability induced by oxidants depends on the oxidant.

References

1. Kevil CG, Ohno N, Gute D, et al (1998) Role of cadherin internalization in hydrogen peroxide-mediated endothelial permeability. Free Radic Biol Med 24:1015–1022
2. Berman RS, Martin W (1993) Arterial endothelial barrier dysfunction: actions of homocysteine and the hypoxanthine-xanthine oxidase free radical generating system. Br J Pharmacol 108:920–926
3. Okayama N, Kevil CG, Correia L, et al (1997) Nitric oxide enhances hydrogen peroxide-mediated endothelial permeability in vitro. Am J Physiol 273(Cell Physiol 42):C1581–C1587
4. Okayama N, Grisham MB, Kevil CG, et al (1999) Effect of reactive oxygen metabolites on endothelial permeability: role of nitric oxide and iron. Microcirculation 6:107–116

Gastric Carcinoma and *Helicobacter pylori* Infection: Role of Nitric Oxide and Inflammatory Cytokines in Gastric Carcinogenesis

Yasuhiko Kitadai*, Ken Haruma, Toyoko Goto, Kunihiko Komoto, Shinji Tanaka, Masaharu Yoshihara, Koji Sumii, and Kazuaki Chayama

Summary. Recent studies have shown that *Helicobacter pylori* infection is etiologically and experimentally associated with gastric carcinoma. However, the role of *H. pylori* in carcinogenesis has not been clarified. *H. pylori* infection leads to sustained production of the reactive nitrogen species that cause DNA damage. We discuss hypotheses related to possible mechanisms of action of *H. pylori* in human gastric carcinogenesis and tumor progression, especially the role of reactive nitrogen species and inflammatory cytokines. Immunohistochemical analysis revealed that the expression of inducible nitric oxide synthase (iNOS) and nitrotyrosine in the gastric mucosa was significantly higher in *H. pylori*-positive subjects than in *H. pylori*-negative subjects. Among the *H. pylori*-positive patients, the expression of iNOS and nitrotyrosine in the gastric mucosa was significantly higher in those who developed gastric carcinoma than in the controls. *H. pylori* with *cagA* gene induces inflammatory cytokines, including interleukin (IL)-1, IL-6, IL-8, and tumor necrosis factor (TNF). IL-1 and TNF may cause overexpression of iNOS and nitrotyrosine in gastric mucosa, and IL-8 may promote tumor growth through its angiogenic activity.

Key words. iNOS, Nitrotyrosine, Interleukin-8, *Helicobacter pylori*, Gastric carcinoma

Introduction

Gastric carcinoma is one of the most common malignancies in the world. Advances in molecular analyses are uncovering a large number of genetic and epigenetic alterations that determine a multistep process of stomach carcinogenesis [1]. *Helicobacter pylori* infection has been considered to be greatly responsible for the pathogenesis of atrophic gastritis and intestinal metaplasia. Epidemiologic studies have indicated that infection with *H. pylori* is considered a risk factor for gastric carcinoma, and the WHO IARC classified this bacterium as a definite biological carcinogen in 1994. In addition, the model of Mongolian gerbils with *H. pylori* inoculated into the stomach is closely

First Department of Internal Medicine, Hiroshima University School of Medicine, 1-2-3 Kasumi, Minami-ku, Hiroshima 734-8551, Japan
* e-mail: ykitadai@mcai.med.hiroshima-u.ac.jp

TABLE 1. Comparison of the measured parameters among patients with gastric carcinoma and control subjects

Parameter	Carcinoma	Control
No.	105	105
M/F	82/23	82/23
Age (years), mean	64.9 ± 1.2	62.4 ± 1.1
Hp-antibody-positive rate (%)	93.3*	71.4
Odds ratio	5.6	1.00
95% CI	2.33–13.45	
Hp-Giemsa stain-positive rate (%)	96.2*	73.3

* $P < 0.05$ compared with control subjects
Hp, *Helicobacter pylori*; CI, confidence interval

associated with the occurrence of chronic gastritis, intestinal metaplasia, and adenocarcinoma. The mechanisms linking *H. pylori* infection and carcinogenesis remain unclear. Here we describe our recent data indicating the possible contribution of nitric oxide and inflammatory cytokines to human stomach carcinogenesis and tumor progression.

H. pylori Infection and Gastric Carcinoma

To clarify the relation between *H. pylori* infection and gastric carcinoma, we investigated the prevalence of *H. pylori* infection of 105 patients with gastric carcinoma and 105 age- and gender-matched control subjects [2]. As shown in Table 1, the prevalence of *H. pylori* seropositivity in patients with gastric carcinoma (93%) was significantly increased compared to that in control subjects (71%), with an odds ratio of 5.60. *H. pylori* was identified by Giemsa stain in 96% of the patients with gastric carcinoma and 73% of the control subjects.

NO and Carcinogenesis

Although *H. pylori* has been reported to be associated with an increased risk of gastric carcinoma, most persons infected with *H. pylori* never have gastric carcinoma. Therefore, other factors that increase the risk of gastric carcinoma among those infected with *H. pylori* may exist. It has been proposed that reactive oxygen and nitrogen species play a role in human carcinogenesis. The reactive nitrogen species are derived from the synthesis of nitric oxide (NO) stimulated by inducible nitric oxide (iNOS). Mannick et al. reported that increased iNOS activity has been observed in patients with chronic gastritis and gastric carcinoma [3]. Furthermore, studies have revealed that *H. pylori* infection leads to the formation of nitrotyrosine, which may contribute to DNA damage and apoptosis in gastric mucosa.

We hypothesized that *H. pylori*-positive subjects with high levels of reactive nitrogen species in gastric mucosa may be at high-risk for gastric carcinoma. To prove this hypothesis, we prospectively examined the relation of reactive nitrogen species in gastric mucosa and patients' outcome [4]. We selected 34 subjects who developed

TABLE 2. Expression of iNOS and nitrotyrosine in the gastric mucosa

Parameter	Hp-positive Cancer group (group A)	Hp-positive Controls (group B)	Hp-negative controls (group C)
iNOS			
Antrum	2.24 ± 0.14*	1.00 ± 0.11**	0.57 ± 0.30
Corpus	2.30 ± 0.14*	0.92 ± 0.09**	0.57 ± 0.30
Nitrotyrosine			
Antrum	2.32 ± 0.11*	1.05 ± 0.10**	0.37 ± 0.26
Corpus	2.42 ± 0.12*	1.05 ± 0.86**	0.50 ± 0.33

Results are the mean ± SE
* $P < 0.01$, compared with group B or group C; ** $P < 0.05$, compared with group C

gastric carcinoma more than 2 years after the first endoscopic examination (cancer group). All of them tested positive for *H. pylori* infection. The expression of iNOS and nitrotyrosine in the gastric mucosa was examined by immunohistochemistry using gastric biopsy specimens obtained at the first endoscopic examination. For control subjects, we randomly chose 59 individuals (*H. pylori*-positive 51 cases, *H. pylori*-negative 8 cases) who were matched with cancer group in relation to age, gender, and follow-up time. The expression levels of iNOS and nitrotyrosine in the gastric mucosa is significantly higher in patients with *H. pylori* infection than in those without it. More interestingly, when we limited the analysis to *H. pylori*-positive patients, the expression of iNOS and nitrotyrosine in the cancer group was significantly higher than that in the *H. pylori*-positive control group (Table 2). The histological gastritis and *H. pylori* colonization were similar for these two groups. Therefore, increased production of iNOS and nitrotyrosine in the gastric mucosa infected with *H. pylori* may contribute to the carcinogenesis of gastric carcinoma.

H. pylori Infection and Inflammatory Cytokines

It is still unclear why the expression of iNOS and nitrotyrosine in the cancer group was higher than that in the *H. pylori*-positive control group. Blaser et al. reported that infection with *H. pylori* strains with the *cagA* gene is associated with an increased risk of developing adenocarcinoma of the stomach [5]. *H. pylori* strains with *cagA* gene induce inflammatory cytokines, including interleukin-1 (IL-1), IL-6, IL-8, and tumor necrosis factor (TNF), at high levels compared with *cagA*-negative strains. Because IL-1 and TNF are strong inducers of iNOS production by activating macrophages and neutrophils, *H. pylori* strains may be associated with differences in the grade of iNOS and nitrotyrosine.

Interleukin-8 is a chemotactic and activating factor for neutrophils. Crabtree et al. reported that *H. pylori* infection induces IL-8 production in the gastric epithelium [6]. Continued up-regulation of IL-8 and neutrophil activation by *H. pylori* infection may lead to increased free radical formation, which can induce DNA strand breaks and base modifications. IL-8 is a multifunctional cytokine known to induce angiogenesis, haptotactic migration, and proliferation of keratinocytes and melanoma cells. Angiogenesis is a prerequisite for tumor growth and metastasis. We have found that human gastric carcinomas overexpress IL-8, whose levels directly correlate with the vascularity in gastric carcinoma [7]. In addition, IL-8 influences the expression of metastasis-related genes, such as collagenase type IV, E-cadherin, and vascular endothelial cell growth factor (VEGF) by gastric carcinoma cells [8]. These findings indicate that IL-8 may act as an angiogenic factor and hence stimulate tumor progression.

Uemura et al. reported that *H. pylori* eradication inhibits the growth of the intestinal type of gastric carcinoma [9]. Because *H. pylori* eradication results in a decrease in the expression level of IL-8 and iNOS [3], inhibitors for IL-8 and iNOS might be used as chemopreventive drugs for human gastric carcinoma.

References

1. Tahara E (1993) Molecular mechanism of stomach carcinogenesis. J Cancer Res Clin Oncol 119:265–272
2. Komoto K, Haruma K, Kamada T, et al (1998) *Helicobacter pylori* infection and gastric neoplasia: correlations with histological gastritis and tumor histology. Am J Gastroenterol 93:1271–1276
3. Mannick EE, Bravo LE, Zarama G, et al (1996) Inducible nitric oxide synthase, nitrotyrosine, and apoptosis in *Helicobacter pylori* gastritis: effect of antibiotics and antioxidants. Cancer Res 56:3238–3243
4. Goto T, Haruma K, Kitadai Y, et al (1999) Enhanced expression of inducible nitric oxide synthase and nitrotyrosine in gastric mucosa of gastric cancer patients. Clin Cancer Res 5:1411–1415
5. Blaser MJ, Perez-Perez GI, Kleanthous H, et al (1995) Infection with *Helicobacter pylori* strains possessing cagA is associated with an increased risk of developing adenocarcinoma of the stomach. Cancer Res 55:2111–2115
6. Crabtree JE, Wyatt JI, Trejdosiewicz LK, et al (1994) Interleukin-8 expression in *Helicobacter pylori* infected, normal, and neoplastic gastroduodenal mucosa. J Clin Pathol 47:61–66
7. Kitadai Y, Haruma K, Sumii K, et al (1998) Expression of interleukin-8 correlates with vascularity in human gastric carcinomas. Am J Pathol 152:93–100
8. Kitadai Y, Haruma K, Mukaida N, et al (2000) Regulation of disease-progression genes in human gastric carcinoma cells by interleukin-8. Clin Cancer Res 6:2735–2740
9. Uemura N, Mukai T, Sumii K, et al (1997) Effect of *Helicobacter pylori* eradication on subsequent development of cancer after endoscopic resection of early gastric cancer. Cancer Epidemiol Biomarkers Prev 6:639–642

Does Cyclooxygenase-2 Down-Regulate Gastric Inflammation?

Shingo Tsuji[1,*], Wei-Hao Sun[1], Masahiko Tsujii[1], Sunao Kawano[2], and Masatsugu Hori[1]

Summary. This paper updates concepts on the role of cyclooxygenase (COX) in tissue inflammation. An inducible isoform of cyclooxygenase is expressed in various cell types by inflammatory promoters, mitogens, cytokines, their receptors, and pathogenic factors such as *Helicobacter.* Overexpressed COX-2 has been believed to serve as a proinflammatory enzyme that increases prostaglandin production and causes swelling, pain, and hyperemia. Recent data indicate that certain prostaglandins suppress immune responses and inflammatory cell infiltration. To test the hypothesis that COX-2 acts as antiinflammatory enzyme in a certain aspect, we examined the effects of specific and nonspecific COX-2 inhibitors on gastric mucosa. The results demonstrate that COX-2 inhibition activates inflammatory cell infiltration. Thus, the inducible isoform of cyclooxygenase may have antiinflammatory properties in the stomach.

Key words. Cyclooxygenase, Immunology, Inflammation, Mononuclear cells, Neutrophils, Prostaglandin

Introduction

Nonsteroidal antiinflammatory drugs (NSAIDs) have attracted the attention of physicians since ancient times, when leaves and barks of the family *Salicaseae* (e.g., willows) were used to alleviate pain and fever. Cyclooxygenase (COX), which catalyzes the conversion of arachidonic acid to prostaglandin (PG) G_2/H_2 (PGG_2/H_2), is the target of NSAIDs. COX-2, the inducible isoform of COX, is up-regulated in inflammatory tissue possibly by inflammatory cytokines and pathogenic factors such as lipopolysaccharides. Indeed, COX-2 products, PGs, are elevated in inflammatory tissues and are recognized as proinflammatory mediators. However, certain NSAIDs are known to

[1]Department of Internal Medicine and Therapeutics, Osaka University Graduate School of Medicine (A8), [2]Department of Clinical Laboratory Sciences, School of Allied Health Sciences, Osaka University Medical School, 2-2 Yamadaoka, Suita, Osaka 565-0871, Japan
* e-mail: tsuji@medone.med.osaka-u.ac.jp

cause damage and induce inflammatory cell infiltration in gastrointestinal tissues. In this paper, we discuss the role of COX-2 in gastric inflammation.

COX-2 Expression and Its Consequences in the Gastrointestinal Tract

Previous data indicated that COX-2 was not well expressed or less well expressed in unstimulated gastric mucosa. Recent studies have demonstrated that gastrointestinal epithelium is able to express COX-2 in response to various stimuli [1,2]. Acid-induced injury also up-regulates COX-2 in gastric epithelium and contributes to the healing process of the damaged tissue [3]. Stromal and inflammatory cells are also able to express COX-2 in response to growth factors or cytokines such as interleukin-1α (IL-1α).

COX-2 coordinates with phospholipase A_2 and prostaglandin synthases (e.g., PGE_2 synthase, etc.) to produce numerous PGs, such as PGE_2, PGI_2, and 15-deoxy-$\Delta^{12,14}$-PGJ_2 (15d-PGJ_2). These PGs bind cell surface receptors such as EP_2 and nuclear receptors including peroxisome proliferator-activated receptor gamma (PPARγ). Until recently, PGs have been recognized as proinflammatory mediators. Indeed most major PGs dilate arterioles to increase tissue blood flow, participate in increased vascular permeability, and lower the threshold for pain, consistent with the classic inflammation triad: reddishness, edema, and pain.

On the other hand, there are other criteria for inflammation: inflammatory cell infiltration and tissue injury due to these cells. Although they have not yet been characterized in detail, consequences of PGs on cellular inflammation and immunity have been distinct from those of the classic findings for inflammation. PGE_2 release and the subsequent increase in intracellular cyclic adenosine monophosphate (cAMP) level. For example, they are known to inhibit the production of IL-2 and interferon-γ (IFNγ) in T-helper-1 (Th1) cells but not to suppress IL-4 in Th2 cells [4]. Another study has demonstrated that PGE_2 blunts IFNγ and IL-12 and therefore shifts the immune balance toward Th2 and humoral immunity [5].

An immunomodulatory role for PPARγ was described in cells critical to the innate immune system, the monocytes/macrophages. For example, PPARγ is up-regulated in activated macrophages and 15d-PGJ_2, and synthetic PPARγ ligands inhibit expression of the inducible nitric oxide (NO) synthase and gelatinase B in these cells [6]. In addition, PPARγ ligands including 15d-PGJ_2 are reported to dramatically attenuate cytokine gene expression in colon cancer cell lines by inhibiting the activation of NF-κB via an IκB-α-dependent mechanism [7]. The expression of PPARγ1 has been demonstrated in murine helper T cells and isolated splenocytes [8]. PPARγ ligands, 15d-PGJ_2, and ciglitazone mediate significant inhibition of proliferative responses of both T cells and splenocytes [9]. Another study demonstrated that certain PGs directly inhibit IκB kinase by interacting with its α-subunit [8]. These results suggest that excessive expression of COX-2 results in suppression of tissue infiltration of immune cells and inflammatory cells. Therefore, we hypothesized that COX-2 up-regulation also suppressed inflammatory cell infiltration in the stomach.

To test the above hypothesis, we administered NS-398 and indomethacin to rats and examined the inflammatory cell infiltration in the stomach. As shown in Fig. 1, pretreatment with either NS-398 or indomethacin caused significant inflammatory

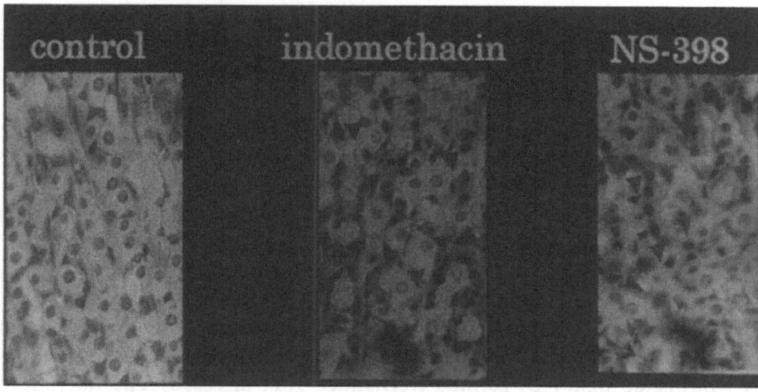

FIG. 1. Influence of NS-398 and indomethacin on rat gastric mucosa. *Arrowheads* indicate acute inflammatory cells infiltrated into the gastric mucosa

cell infiltration. Recently Gilroy et al. demonstrated that with carrageenin-induced inflammation COX-2 is up-regulated 2h and 48h after the inflammatory stimuli. The second up-regulation coincides with the inflammatory resolution. Interestingly, NS-398, a COX-2-specific inhibitor, augmented inflammatory cell infiltration in carrageenin-induced inflammation. These results consistently suggest that COX-2 inhibition aggravates the cellular inflammation (i.e., tissue infiltration of inflammatory cells and tissue injury due to these cells).

Conclusions

COX-2 inhibitors successfully relieve pain, swelling, and heat due to arthritis and other inflammation, suggesting that COX-2 up-regulation results in augmentation of classic inflammation. NSAIDs are not effective in suppressing injury to the joint due to inflammatory cells. Our own study and some others indicate that COX-2 up-regulation is a key event in the resolution of cellular inflammation. Thus, COX-2 is both proinflammatory and antiinflammatory in the humoral and cellular systems, respectively.

Acknowledgments. This work was partly supported by Grants-in-Aid from the Ministry of Health and Welfare, the Ministry of Culture and Education, and the Smoking Research Foundation.

References

1. Sawaoka H, Tsuji S, Tsujii M, et al (1997) Expression of the cyclooxygenase-2 gene in gastric epithelium. J Clin Gastroenterol 25(Suppl 1):S105–S110
2. Sawaoka H, Kawano S, Tsuji S, et al (1998) *Helicobacter pylori* infection induces cyclooxygenase-2 expression in human gastric mucosa. Prostaglandins Leukotrienes Essential Fatty Acids 59:313–316

3. Sun W-H, Tsuji S, Tsujii M, et al (2000) Cyclooxygenase-2 inhibitors suppress epithelial cell kinetics and delay gastric wound healing in rats. J Gastroenterol Hepatol 15:751–761
4. Betz M, Fox BS (1991) Prostaglandin E_2 inhibits production of Th1 lymphokines but not of Th2 lymphokines. J Immunol 146:108–113
5. Graf BA, Nazarenko DA, Borrello MA, et al (1999) Biphenotypic B/macrophage cells express COX-1 and up-regulate COX-2 expression and prostaglandin E_2 production in response to pro-inflammatory signals. Eur J Immunol 29:3793–3803
6. Ricote M, Li AC, Willson TM, et al (1998) The peroxisome proliferator-activated receptor-γ is a negative regulator of macrophage activation. Nature 391:79–82
7. Su CG, Wen X, Bailey ST, et al (1999) A novel therapy for colitis utilizing PPARγ ligands to inhibit the epithelial inflammatory response. J Clin Invest 104:383–389
8. Rossi A, Kapahi P, Natoli G, et al (2000) Anti-inflammatory cyclopentenone prostaglandins are direct inhibitors of IκB kinase. Nature 403:103–108
9. Clark RB, Bishop-Bailey D, Estrada-Hernandez T, et al (2000) The nuclear receptor PPARγ and immunoregulation: PPARγ mediates inhibition of helper T cell responses. J Immunol 164:1364–1371

Regulation of Mucin Synthesis by Neuronal Nitric Oxide Synthase in Gastric Pit Cells

KAZUHITO ROKUTAN*, SHIGETADA TESHIMA, TOMOKO KAWAI, TSUKASA KAWAHARA, KENJI KUSUMOTO, and KYOICHI KISHI

Summary. We investigated the stimulatory actions of epidermal growth factor (EGF) and a cytoprotective compound, geranylgeranylacetone (GGA), on mucin synthesis of guinea pig gastric pre-pit cells, maintained in a serum-free culture system. GGA increased [^{3}H]glucosamine uptake and accumulation of mucous granules positive for galactose oxidase-Schiff reaction in the cells. This stimulatory action of GGA was equivalent to that of EGF, whereas GGA did not stimulate cell growth. EGF and GGA increased the release of nitric oxide (NO) degeneration products, NO_2^- and NO_3^-. [^{3}H]Glucosamine uptake by the cells was completely inhibited by the non-selective NO synthase (NOS) inhibitors, N^G-nitro-L-arginine, and N^G-monomethyl-L-arginine; and it was only partially inhibited by a more selective inhibitor for inducible NOS isoform, aminoguanidine. Immunoblot analysis with antibodies against three isozymes of NOS showed that GGA and EGF induced neuronal NOS but not endothelial NOS or inducible NOS. Our results suggest that GGA and EGF stimulate mucin synthesis at least in part through the NO-dependent pathway, leading to increased integrity of the gastric mucosa.

Key words. Gastric pit cells, Mucin synthesis, Nitric oxide, Neuronal nitric oxide synthase, Geranylgeranylacetone

Introduction

Gastric surface mucous cells originate from the granule-free progenitor cells located at the isthmus of the gastric unit. During upward migration the granule-free pre-pit cell precursor acquires secretory granules at a pre-pit cell stage; secretory granules then increase in number and size along with maturation into pit cells. The matured cells were characterized by their large granules, consisting of two major components: mucin positive for the galactose oxidase-Schiff (GOS) reaction and surface-active phospholipids.

Department of Nutritional Physiology, School of Medicine, The University of Tokushima, 3-18-15 Kuramoto-cho, Tokushima 770-8503, Japan
* e-mail: rokutan@nutr.med.tokushima-u.ac.jp

We developed a serum-free culture of guinea pig gastric epithelial cells [1] that could completely eliminate fetal calf serum (FCS)-dependent proliferation and maturation of pit cell lineage. Using this culture system, we examined the effect of epidermal growth factor (EGF) and geranylgeranylacetone (GGA) on nitric oxide (NO)-mediated mucin synthesis in a pit cell lineage.

Materials and Methods

Reagents and Media

Geranylgeranylacetone (a gift from Eisai Co., Tokyo, Japan) was dissolved at a concentration of 3mM in absolute ethanol. This stock solution was supplemented with 2μg/ml α-tocopherol as an antioxidant. α-Tocopherol-free or GGA-free ethanol solution was provided by Eisai Co. Unless otherwise indicated, the GGA used was α-tocopherol-supplemented.

Preparation and Culture of Gastric Mucosal Cells

Gastric mucosal cells were aseptically isolated from male guinea pigs and were cultured in the serum-free medium, as described previously [1]. Briefly, the isolated cells were cultured in type 1 collagen-coated dishes in Dulbecco modified Eagle medium (DMEM)/Ham's F-12 (1:1) mixture, containing 15mM HEPES, 0.2% bovine serum albumin (BSA), 10μg/ml transferrin, and 2.5ng/ml sodium selenite. After cultivation for 2 days, floating cells were removed by washing with MEM, and attached cells were used for the experiments. Control cells were treated with GGA-free solution (vehicle) containing ethanol and α-tocopherol at final concentrations of 0.033% and 0.67ng/ml, respectively.

Cell growth was analyzed as described previously [1]. The attached cells did not replicate in serum-free conditions, and cytochemical and electron microscopic studies showed that most cells (80%–90%) displayed features characteristic of a pre-pit cell stage [1].

Measurement of [^{3}H]Glucosamine Uptake and NO_2^-/NO_3^- Release by Cells

The incorporation of [^{3}H]glucosamine into cells was measured as previously described [1]. For measurement of NO_2^- and NO_3^- concentrations, the attached cells were incubated in 1ml of Hank's balanced salt solution (HBSS) for 1h without any stimulus. The concentrations of NO_2^- and NO_3^- in the medium were determined by a fluorometric assay using a fluorometric assay kit (Dojindo, Tokyo, Japan).

Western Blot Analysis

The levels of neuronal nitric oxide synthase (nNOS), endothelial NOS (eNOS), and inducible NOS (iNOS) were measured by immunoblot analysis with polyclonal antibodies against the respective NOS isozymes (Wako, Tokyo, Japan). Bound antibodies were detected by an enhanced chemiluminescence system (Amersham Japan, Tokyo, Japan).

Results and Discussion

Effect of GGA on Cell Growth and Mucin Synthesis

The GGA at 10^{-10} to 10^{-5} M did not stimulate cell growth of pre-pit cells (data not shown). However, treatment with GGA at 10^{-8} M or higher significantly increased the [^{3}H]glucosamine uptake within 24h; and GGA at 1µM maximally increased the uptake about 2.7-fold on day 2. This action was equivalent to that of EGF (Table 1). In association with the increase in [^{3}H]glucosamine uptake, the percentages of mature pit cells on day 2 in EGF-, GGA-, and vehicle-treated cells were determined to be 89% ± 5% ($n = 5$), 85% ± 10% ($n = 5$), and 5% ± 2% ($n = 5$), respectively.

Effects of NOS Inhibitors on [^{3}H]Glucosamine Uptake

Pre-pit cells cultured in the serum-free medium were treated with 20nM EGF or 1µM GGA in the presence of nonselective inhibitors of NOS: N^G-nitro-L-arginine (L-NNA) and N^G-monomethyl-L-arginine (L-NMMA), or aminoguanidine (AG). L-NNA and L-NMMA completely blocked the uptake during 24–48h of culture, and AG partially

TABLE 1. Effects of NOS inhibitors on EGF- or GGA-stimulated [^{3}H]glucosamine uptake

Treatment	[^{3}H]Glucosamine (cpm/mg protein/24h)
None	3815 ± 876
EGF (20nM)	10270 ± 1322
+100µM L-NNA	3310 ± 385*
+100µM L-NMMA	2409 ± 364*
+100µM AG	6483 ± 336*
GGA (1µM)	10047 ± 1709
+100µM L-NNA	2662 ± 590*
+100µM L-NMMA	2586 ± 398*
+100µM AG	9436 ± 1135*

After isolated cells were cultured for 2 days in collagen-coated 35mm diameter dishes under serum-free conditions, the attached cells were treated with 20nM EGF or 1µM GGA. [^{3}H]glucosamine (1µCi/ml) and one of the NOS inhibitors were added 24h after addition of EGF or GGA. After incubation for 24h in the presence of 100µM L-NNA, L-NMMA, or AG, the radioactivity incorporated into cells was measured, as described in Materials and Methods

Values are means ± SD for six cultures in two experiments

NOS, nitric oxide synthase; EGF, epidermal growth factor; GGA, geranylgeranylacetone; L-NNA, N^G-nitro-L-arginine; L-NMMA, N^G-monomethyl-L-arginine; AG, aminoguanidine

* Significantly different versus NOS inhibitor-untreated cells ($P < 0.05$ by ANOVA and Shcheffé's test)

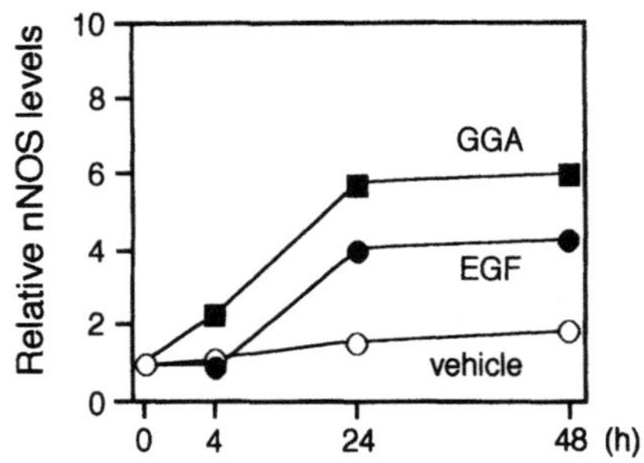

FIG. 1. Effects of epidermal growth factor (*EGF*) or geranylgeranylacetone (*GGA*) on nitric oxide synthase (NOS) inductions. Whole-cell proteins were prepared from the cells, treated with vehicle (*open circles*), 20 nM EGF (*squares*), or 1 μM GGA (*filled circles*) for the indicated times. The samples (30 μg protein per lane) were separated by 8% sodium dodecyl sulfate-polyacrylamide gel electrophoresis (SDS-PAGE) and transferred to a polyvinylidene difluoride filter. Immunoblotting with an antibody against neuronal nitric oxide synthase (*nNOS*) was performed. The amount of nNOS was quantified by densitometry, and the relative nNOS levels to that in untreated control cells are shown

inhibited it (Table 1). AG is not specific for iNOS at high concentrations [2]; therefore, it was likely that AG might partially inhibit the [^{3}H]glucosamine uptake by acting on constitutive forms of NOS. These three inhibitors exerted their actions on the EGF-stimulated [^{3}H]glucosamine uptake in a similar fashion (Table 1). Thus, the NO derived from a constitutive NOS isozyme appeared to be involved in the mucin synthesis stimulated by both EGF and GGA.

Effect of GGA on Induction of NOS Isoforms and NO Production

It was reported that surface mucous epithelial cells express nNOS but not eNOS [3]. We studied the effects of EGF and GGA on the expression of NOS isoforms. Gastric pit cells contained a 155-kDa protein that was immunoreactive to the anti-nNOS antibody. EGF and GGA increased the nNOS level about fourfold and sixfold on day 2, respectively (Fig. 1). iNOS and eNOS proteins were not detected by immunoblot analysis even after treatment with EGF or GGA (data not shown).

Pre-pit cell-rich cultures secreted NO_2^- and NO_3^- into the medium at 1.63 ± 0.05 nmol/mg protein/h (mean ± SD, $n = 6$). Treatment with GGA and EGF for 24 h significantly increased the value to 2.40 ± 0.36 ($n = 6$) and 2.10 ± 0.08 nmol NO_2^- and NO_3^-/mg protein/h ($n = 6$), respectively.

Nitric oxide is known to play an important role in the regulation of synthesis and secretion of gastric mucin [4]. The present study suggests that GGA and EGF may stimulate the nNOS-dependent metabolic pathways and increase the integrity of the gastric mucosa, at least in part, through stimulation of mucin synthesis in pit cells.

References

1. Rokutan K, Yamada M, Torigoe J, et al (1998) Tansforming growth factor-β inhibits proliferation and maturation of cultured guinea pig gastric pit cells. Am J Physiol 275:G526–G533

2. Griffith OW, Stuehr DJ (1995) Nitric oxide synthases: properties and catalytic mechanism. Annu Rev Physiol 57:707–736
3. Price KJ, Hanson PJ, Whittle BJR (1996) Localization of constitutive isoforms of nitric oxide synthase in the gastric glandular mucosa of the rat. Cell Tissue Res 285:157–163
4. Brown JF, Keates AC, Hanson PJ, et al (1993) Nitric oxide generators and cGMP stimulate mucus secretion by rat gastric mucosal cells. Am J Physiol 265:G418–G422

Role of Nitric Oxide and Capsaicin-Sensitive Sensory Nerves in Gastric Receptive Relaxation and Adaptive Relaxation in Isolated Stomachs of Guinea Pigs

HIRONORI UNO[1,2] and KAZUHIDE HIGUCHI[1]

Summary. We investigated the role of nitric oxide (NO) and capsaicin-sensitive sensory nerves (CPSNs) in gastric receptive relaxation and adaptive relaxation in isolated stomachs of guinea pigs. Changes in intragastric volume and pressure were recorded simultaneously in isolated stomachs in baths containing atropine and guanethidine. Receptive relaxation was induced by electrical vagal stimulation, and adaptive relaxation was induced by luminal distension. We found that receptive relaxation and adaptive relaxation were reduced by tetrodotoxin and N^G-nitro-L-arginine (LNNA). The effect of LNNA was partially reversed by co-incubation with L-arginine. Hexamethonium inhibited receptive relaxation but not adaptive relaxation. Desensitization to capsaicin inhibited adaptive relaxation but not receptive relaxation. Extraluminal capsaicin induced gastric relaxation. Capsaicin-induced relaxation also was reduced by tetrodotoxin and LNNA but not by hexamethonium. Neither $CGRP_{(8-37)}$, an antagonist of calcitonin gene-related peptide (CGRP) receptors, nor $VIP_{(10-28)}$, an antagonist of vasoactive intestinal peptide (VIP) receptors, inhibited all responses of receptive relaxation and adaptive relaxation or capsaicin-induced relaxation. These findings suggest that NO, but not CGRP or VIP, may be involved in the mechanisms of receptive relaxation and adaptive relaxation, and that activation of CPSNs may be involved in adaptive relaxation.

Key words. Nitric oxide, Receptive relaxation, Adaptive relaxation, Capsaicin-sensitive sensory nerve, Gastric reservoir function

Introduction

The stomach has reservoir functions, such as receptive relaxation and adaptive relaxation. These physiological responses are important to accommodate the intake of food or liquid. Disorders of gastric reservoir functions result in symptoms of early satiety

[1] Third Department of Internal Medicine, Osaka City University Medical School, 1-5-7 Asahi-machi, Abeno-ku, Osaka 545-8586, Japan
[2] Department of Internal Medicine, Ohno Memorial Hospital, 1-10-26 Minamihorie, Nishi-ku, Osaka 550-0015, Japan

and anorexia, which are the major symptoms of patients with functional dyspepsia [1]. To clarify the mechanisms of gastric reservoir functions, we investigated the role of nitric oxide (NO) and capsaicin-sensitive sensory nerves (CPSNs) in receptive relaxation and adaptive relaxation in isolated whole stomachs of guinea pigs.

Assessment of Gastric Receptive Relaxation and Adaptive Relaxation

We made a device to record gastric receptive relaxation and adaptive relaxation using stomachs isolated from guinea pigs in vitro according to Desai et al.'s reports [2,3]. Briefly, the canulated stomach is placed in a warmed (37°C) organ bath (500 ml) filled with oxygenated Krebs solution [4]. The cannula in the stomach was connected to both a wide reservoir bottle (2 l) containing oxygenated Krebs solution and a pressure transducer to monitor the intragastric pressure. The reservoir was mounted on a movable rack and sealed by a float recorder to record changes in gastric volume. The gastric volume was measured with a float recorder attached to an isotonic transducer. Serial changes in pressure and volume were recorded on a chart recorder. To inhibit cholinergic (muscarinic) and adrenergic effects, experiments were performed in Krebs solution containing atropine (3 μM) plus guanethidine (5 μM).

Receptive relaxation was induced by electrical vagal stimulation. The intragastric pressure was increased to 2 cm H_2O, a pressure at which adaptive relaxation did not occur. The vagus nerve was stimulated for 30 s with square wave pulses (supramaximal voltage) of 1 ms duration at 20 Hz. This electrical vagal stimulation induced gastric relaxation (Fig. 1).

Adaptive relaxation was induced by gastric luminal distension. The reservoir was elevated stepwise (in 1-cm increments), and Krebs solution entered the stomach as the pressure increased. Adaptive relaxation was found as a response wherein the fundus suddenly relaxed at a certain intragastric pressure and a large volume of Krebs solution entered the stomach (Fig. 1). This response occurred at intragastric pressures of 3.9 ± 0.1 cm H_2O.

Results

Preincubation with N^G-nitro-L-arginine (LNNA) (0.1 mM), an NO synthase inhibitor, for 30 min significantly inhibited receptive relaxation and adaptive relaxation. The effect of LNNA was partially reversed by co-incubation with L-arginine (1 mM), a precursor of NO synthesis, during adaptive relaxation and receptive relaxation. Preincubation with tetrodotoxin (1 μM) for 30 min significantly inhibited adaptive and receptive relaxation. Adaptive relaxation was not affected by the presence of hexamethonium (0.5 mM), an antagonist of ganglionic nicotinic receptors, although receptive relaxation was significantly inhibited by this agent. (Fig. 2)

Desensitization to capsaicin significantly reduced adaptive relaxation but had no effect on receptive relaxation (Fig. 2). After an equilibration period of 5 min under a tension of 2 cm H_2O, extraluminal capsaicin (0.1 μM) induced transient gastric relaxation. This effect was abolished by desensitization to capsaicin. Preincubation with

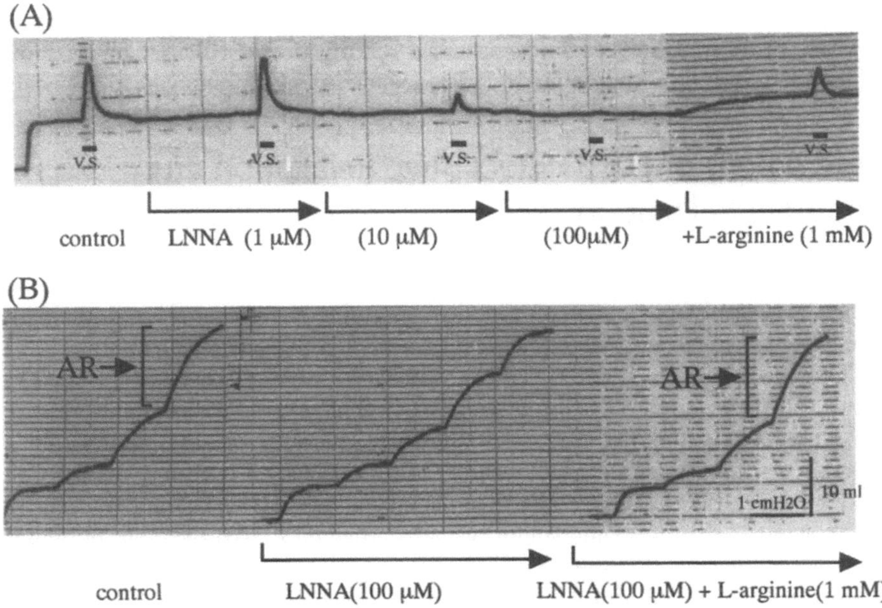

FIG. 1. Effects of N^G-nitro-L-arginine (LNNA) on receptive relaxation (**A**) and adaptive relaxation (**B**) in an isolated guinea pig stomach. *V.S.*, vagal stimulation; *AR*, adaptive relaxation

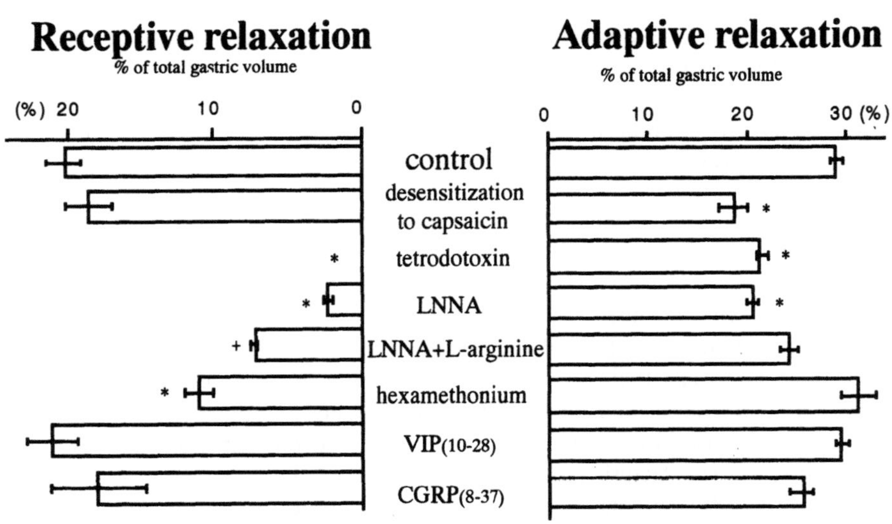

FIG. 2. Effects of desensitization to capsaicin, tetrodotoxin, LNNA, hexamethonium, $CGRP_{(8-37)}$, an antagonist of calcitonin gene-related peptide (CGRP) receptors, and $VIP_{(10-28)}$, an antagonist of vasoactive intestinal peptide (VIP) receptors, on receptive relaxation and adaptive relaxation in an isolated guinea pig stomach. Data are expressed as means ± SEM. $^*P < 0.01$ vs. control; $^{\dagger}P < 0.05$ vs. LNNA alone

tetrodotoxin (1 μM) or LNNA (0.1 mM) for 30 min significantly inhibited capsaicin-induced gastric relaxation. The effect of LNNA was partially reversed by co-incubation with L-arginine (1 mM). Capsaicin-induced gastric relaxation was not affected by the presence of hexamethonium (0.5 mM).

To investigate the effects of calcitonin gene-related peptide (CGRP) and vasoactive intestinal peptide (VIP) on the three types of gastric relaxation, the stomach was preincubated intra- and extraluminally for 10 min with $CGRP_{(8-37)}$, an antagonist of CGRP receptors (1 μM), and $VIP_{(10-28)}$, an antagonist of VIP receptors (1 μM). $CGRP_{(8-37)}$ and $VIP_{(10-28)}$ affected neither receptive relaxation nor adaptive gastric relaxation (Fig. 2).

Conclusions

We speculated on the possible mechanisms of receptive relaxation and adaptive relaxation of the stomach. Adaptive relaxation is an intragastric pressure-induced reflex. Stretching the gastric wall activates mechanoreceptors in the gastric mucosa, which generate impulses carried by the sensory neuron. The sensory neuron can synapse on the inhibitory efferent neuron directly or activate it via interneurons of the myenteric plexus. This leads to the release of NO from the nitroxergic efferent neuron, which causes relaxation of circular muscle and hence of the fundus. Alternatively, an axonal reflex causes NO release from the sensory neuron, resulting in hexamethonium-resistant gastric relaxation. The neurons involved in the extrinsic reflex responsible for receptive relaxation of the stomach enter the stomach wall as vagal motor fibers. The impulses carried by these fibers activate nitroxergic efferent neurons, resulting in generation of NO. In contrast with pressure-induced adaptive relaxation, ganglionic nicotinic transmission is essential for vagally induced relaxation. VIP and CGRP are important neurotransmitters of inhibitory sensory neurons, but these substances may not mediate both receptive relaxation and adaptive relaxation because these two types of gastric relaxation are resistant to antagonists of VIP and CGRP.

Our results showed that NO, but not CGRP or VIP, may be involved in the mechanisms of adaptive relaxation and receptive relaxation. Moreover, activation of CPSNs may be involved in adaptive relaxation but not receptive gastric relaxation.

References

1. Troncon LEA, Thompson DG, Ahluwalia NK, et al (1995) Relations between upper abdominal symptoms and gastric distension abnormalities in dysmotility like functional dyspepsia and after vagotomy. Gut 37:17–22
2. Desai KM, Sessa WC, Vane JR (1991) Involvement of nitric oxide in the reflex relaxation of the stomach to accommodate food or fluid. Nature 351:477–479
3. Desai KM, Zembowicz A, Sessa WC, et al (1991) Nitroxergic nerves mediate receptive relaxation in the isolated stomach of the guinea pig. Proc Natl Acad Sci USA 88: 11490–11494
4. Uno H, Arakawa T, Fukuda T, et al (1997) Involvement of capsaicin-sensitive sensory nerves in gastric adaptive relaxation in isolated guinea-pig stomachs. Digestion 58: 232–239

Role of Inducible Nitric Oxide Synthase in Murine Colitis

HIROYUKI OGAWA*, MITSUNARI YAMAMOTO, HIDEJI NAKAMURA, and HIROAKI ITO

Summary. To examine the role of inducible nitric oxide synthase (iNOS) in the development of colitis, we characterized the expression of iNOS in a murine colitis model and the effects of a selective inhibitor of iNOS production, aminoguanidine (AMG). Furthermore, we examined the correlation between the production of inflammatory cytokines and nitric oxide (NO) in human colonic epithelial cells. Colitis was induced in C.B-17-SCID mice transferred with $CD45RB^{high}$ $CD4^{+}$ T cells from BALB/c mice. Expression of iNOS in the intestine was determined by reverse transcriptase polymerase chain reaction and immunohitochemistry. Anti-interleukin-6 receptor (anti-IL-6R) monoclonal antibody (mAb) or AMG was administered after T cell transfer. Furthermore, NO activity and iNOS production in HT-29 cells were examined after stimulation with interferon-γ (IFNγ), tumor necrosis factor-α (TNFα), IL-1β, IL-6, and soluble (s) IL-6R. There was increased expression of iNOS in colonic epithelial cells in the murine colitis model, but expression of iNOS and development of colitis were suppressed by administration of anti-IL-6R mAb. Severe colitis was induced when iNOS was inhibited by administration of AMG. In HT-29 cells, production of iNOS was induced in the presence of IFNγ. Although no induction of iNOS production was observed in the presence of IL-6 alone, NO production mediated by INFγ was increased in the presence of INFγ plus IL-6 and soluble IL-6R. The production of NO induced by IFNγ was thus stimulated by the addition of IL-6 in human colonic epithelial cells. In the colitis model, NO induced by inflammatory cytokines at the onset of colitis may suppress the development of inflammation.

Key words. iNOS, HT-29, Murine colitis, Interleukin-6, Aminoguanidine

Introduction

Proinflammatory cytokines such as interferon-γ (IFNγ), tumor necrosis factor-α (TNFα), interleukin-1β (IL-1β), and IL-6 have been shown to be associated with the

---

Department of Molecular Medicine, Osaka University Medical School, 2-2 Yamadaoka, Suita, Osaka 565-0871, Japan
* e-mail: hogawa@ucsd.edu

pathogenesis of Crohn's disease (CD). The increase of these cytokines and the induction of inducible nitric oxide synthase (iNOS) were observed in CD. However, there are many undetermined factors concerning whether NO production aggravates or suppresses the development of inflammation, which is affected greatly by release concentrations, release profiles, or differences in metabolic processes. Recently, an effectiveness of anti-IL-6 receptor monoclonal antibody (anti-IL-6R mAb) has been shown to be useful in CD45RB^{high} CD4^{+} T cells transferred to a murine colitis model [1,2]. To investigate the effect of NO (an important mediator for various biological functions) on the development of colitis, the role of iNOS in the intestine was examined using this colitis model.

Material and Methods

Mice and Materials. BALB/c and C.B-17 SCID mice were purchased from Charles River Breeding Laboratories (Shiga, Japan). Anti-IL-6R mAb, which is rat immunoglobulin G1 (IgG1) mAb against murine IL-6R and recombinant human (rh) soluble (s) IL-6R was provided by Chugai Pharmaceutical Co. (Gotemba, Japan). The rh IFNγ, TNFα, IL-1β, and IL-6 were purchased from Peprotech (London, UK).

Colon Epithelial Cell Line and Cell Culture. HT-29 human colonic epithelial cells were grown in McCoy's 5A (Nacalai Tesque, Japan) supplemented with 10% fetal calf serum (FCS) and penicillin/streptomycin (10 U/ml/10 mg/ml). Confluent cell cultures were treated with the appropriate concentrations of stimuli in medium without FCS.

Purification of Murine Splenocyte Subsets and Cell Transfer. The method has been described previously in detail [1].

Administration of Anti-IL-6R mAb or AMG. Mice were given anti-IL-6R mAb by intraperitoneal injection (2 mg at the time of T cell transfer and 1 mg weekly up to 8 weeks) or treated orally with 100 mM AMG (hemisulfate salt; Sigma, St. Louis, MO, USA).

Histological and Immunohistological Analyses. Sections were stained as described previously [1], and phycoerythrin (PE)-conjugated anti-iNOS (Santa Cruz Biotechnology, Santa Cruz, CA, USA) was used.

Nitrite and Nitrate Assays. Nitric oxide production in HT-29 cells was determined by measuring the stable end-product nitrite in culture supernatants using a fluorometric assay kit (Cayman Chemical, Ann Arbor, MI, USA) and a spectrophotofluorometer Biolumin 960 (Molecular Dynamics, Sunnyvale, CA, USA), with excitation at 405 nm and emission at 450 nm.

RT-PCR for iNOS Expression. The expression of iNOS was determined by reverse transcriptase-polymerase chain reaction (RT-PCR) as described previously [1]. The following primers were used for murine (m) and human (h) iNOS and glyceraldchyde-3-phosphate dehydrogenase (GAPDH): m-iNOS sense, 5′-ACA-ACA-GGA-

ACC-TAC-CAG-CTC-A-3′; m-iNOS antisense, 5′-GAT-GTT-GTA-GCG-CTG-TGT-GTG-TCA-3′; m-GAPDH sense, 5′-CGG-AGT-CAA-CGG-ATT-TGG-TCG-TAT-3′; m-GAPDH antisense, 5′-AGC-CTT-CTC-CAT-GGT-GGT-GAA-GAC-3′; h-iNOS sense, 5′-ATG-GAA-CAT-CCC-AAA-TAC-GA-3′; h-iNOS antisense, 5′-CAG-CAT-CTC-CTG-GTG-AAA-CA-3′; h-GAPDH sense, 5′-GGT-GAA-GTT-CGG-AGT-CAA-CGG-A-3′; h-GAPDH antisense, 5′-GAG-GGA-TCT-CGC-TCC-TGG-AAG-A-3′. The amplification cycle was 94°C for 1 min, 55°C for 30 s, and 72°C for 1 min for murine cDNA; and it was 95°C for 45 s, 54°C for 90 s, and 72°C for 90 s for HT-29 cells' cDNA. The PCR cycle numbers were chosen to ensure that the amplification of PCR products was in the exponential range: 28 cycles for iNOS and 22 cycles for GAPDH.

Results

Suppression of iNOS and Colitis After Anti-IL-6R mAb Administration in Murine Colitis

Results from the RT-PCR demonstrated increased induction of iNOS in the intestine with colitis, whereas expression of iNOS was suppressed by anti-IL-6 mAb administration. The development of colitis was prevented by the mAb histologically. Furthermore, immunohistological studies demonstrated that iNOS production was detected mainly in colonic epithelial cells in colitis and suppressed after anti-IL-6 mAb.

NO Activity and iNOS Induction in HT-29 Cells

The induction of iNOS was investigated after stimulation of HT-29 cells with INFγ, TNFα, IL-1β, IL-6, and sIL-6R by RT-PCR. The presence of IFNγ was essential for induction of iNOS. No induction was observed in the presence of IL-6 alone. When the activity of NO was determined using the Griess reaction method, it also demonstrated that NO production was induced by IFNγ, whereas it was not induced by IL-6 alone. However, NO production was increased in the presence of IFNγ plus IL-6 or IFNγ plus IL-6 and soluble IL-6R.

Development of Colitis After AMG Administration

When AMG was administered to murine colitis transferred $CD45RB^{high}$ $CD4^+$ T cells, all mice were dead by 4 weeks after the administration, whereas none of the control mice was dead. Hematoxylin-eosin staining demonstrated that a severe inflammation accompanied by partial deciduation of colonic epithelial cells was detected in the intestine receiving AMG after T cell transfer. Immunohistological studies demonstrated that the production of iNOS protein was greatly suppressed by AMG administration.

Discussion

A substantial amount of NO produced by iNOS has been receiving attention as a factor that causes dysfunction of the intestinal epithelial barrier, resulting in aggravation of colitis [3]. A murine colitis model transferred $CD45RB^{high}$ $CD4^+$ T cells develop T-helper type 1 (Th1) cell-mediated chronic colitis, which resembles human CD. Our study demonstrated increased iNOS induction in the intestine. The expression and production of iNOS was significantly suppressed once the development of colitis was prevented by treatment with anti-IL-6 mAb. The main cells responsible for iNOS production were colonic epithelial cells. IL-6 may stimulate the production of NO in human epithelial cells.

Based on these results it was originally thought that AMG might be able to suppress intestinal inflammation; but AMG administration, resulting in inhibition of iNOS, induced a more severe colitis. The following are possible explanations: First, induction of iNOS seems to be a critical protective response to injury in the intestine during an acute phase of colitis [4]. Therefore, if AMG is administered prior to the onset of colitis, it is difficult to inhibit the development of colitis at the onset. Second, overproduction of NO due to iNOS may mediate Th1 cells [5], so suppression of NO with AMG may cause overproduction of proinflammatory cytokines.

We believe it is necessary to investigate the effects of AMG administration after induction of chronic inflammation. In this model, NO may play a part in suppression of inflammatory development at the onset of colitis.

References

1. Yamamoto M, Yoshizaki K, Kishimoto T, Ito H (2000) IL-6 is required for the development of Th1 cell-mediated murine colitis. J Immunol 164:4878–4882
2. Atreya R, Mudter J, Finotto S, et al (2000) Blockade of interleukin 6 trans signaling suppresses T-cell resistance against apoptosis in chronic intestinal inflammation: evidence in Crohn disease and experimental colotis in vivo. Nat Med 6:583–588
3. Unno N, Wang H, Menconi MJ, et al (1997) Inhibition of inducible nitric oxide synthase ameliorates endotoxin-induced gut mucosal barrier dysfunction in rats. Gastroenterology 113:1246–1257
4. McCafferty DM, Mudgett JS, Swain MG, Kubes P (1997) Inducible nitric oxide synthase plays a critical role in resolving intestinal inflammation. Gastroenterology 112: 1022–1027
5. Karupiah G, Chen JH, Mahalingam S, et al (1998) Rapid interferon γ-dependent clearance of influenza A virus and protection from consolidating pneumonitis in nitric oxide synthase 2-deficient mice. J Exp Med 188:1541–1546

Role of Nitric Oxide in the Progression of Severe Acute Pancreatitis

Akihiko Satoh*, Atsushi Masamune, and Tooru Shimosegawa

Summary. A growing amount of evidence has been presented that nitric oxide (NO) exerts various effects in the pathobiology of acute pancreatitis, but the role of NO during acute pancreatitis remains controversial. To investigate the role of NO during the progression of severe acute pancreatitis, we employed rat taurocholate (TCA)-induced pancreatitis. Serum nitrate and nitrite (NOx) concentrations increased during the course of TCA pancreatitis. The elevation of serum was significantly inhibited by the administration of specific NOS inhibitors (both nonselective NOS inhibitors and iNOS selective inhibitor). Despite the strong inhibition of NO production, these agents did not ameliorate the gross pathological appearance of the pancreas or reduce the elevation of serum amylase. In addition, nonselective NOS inhibitors worsened the hematocrit, myeloperoxidase activity in the lung, and mortality during pancreatitis. Although iNOS selective inhibitor did not affect the hematocrit and mortality during pancreatitis, it significantly aggravated myeloperoxidase activity in the lung. The supernatant of TCA pancreatitis ascites could induce iNOS in the peritoneal macrophages of normal rats in vitro, whereas, it decreased the endothelial NOS mRNA level in umbilical vein endothelial cells (HUVECs). The expression of adhesion molecules and interleukin-8 in HUVECs induced by ascitic fluid were attenuated by NO donor, whereas the NOS inhibitor augmented them. The results suggest that NO plays a protective role during the progression of acute pancreatitis through modulation of the leukocytes and endothelial cell systems.

Key words. Acute pancreatitis, Nitric oxide, Inducible nitric oxide synthase, Endothelial nitric oxide synthase, Ascitic fluids

The most serious complication during severe acute pancreatitis is the occurrence of multiple organ failure (MOF) during the early stages of this disease. The mortality associated with acute pancreatitis is closely related to the development of early systemic complications, and the mortality rate for patients with such pathological con-

---

Department of Gastroenterology, Division of Internal Medicine, Tohoku University Graduate School of Medicine, 1-1 Seiryo-machi, Aoba-ku, Sendai 980-8574, Japan
* e-mail: asato@int3.med.tohoku.ac.jp

ditions has been reported to reach 20%–50%. Several mediators such as activated pancreatic enzymes, cytokines, endotoxins, superoxides, and arachidonate metabolites have been suggested to play important roles in the pathogenesis; but as the mechanism of MOF in severe acute pancreatitis is still unclear, it remains difficult to develop an effective therapy.

Nitric oxide (NO) is recognized as an important mediator of several physiological and pathophysiological processes. In the pancreas a growing amount of evidence has been presented that NO exerts various effects in the pathobiology of acute pancreatitis [1,2], but the role of NO during acute pancreatitis remains to be controversial.

To investigate the role of NO in the progression of severe acute pancreatitis, we employed rat taurocholate (TCA)-induced pancreatitis and studied the expression of inducible nitric oxide synthase (iNOS). Intraductal administration of TCA produced hemorrhagic necrotizing pancreatitis, characterized by massive hemorrhage, severe infiltration of inflammatory cells, and large areas of necrosis in the pancreas. Serum nitrate and nitrite (NOx) concentrations increased during the course of TCA pancreatitis. In the TCA pancreatitis rats, the concentrations of serum NOx at 12 and 18h after the induction of pancreatitis were 92.4 ± 8.8 and $93.5 \pm 9.4\,\mu$mol/l, respectively. These values were significantly higher than those in control rats that had received saline alone [3]. These results indicate overproduction of NO during severe acute pancreatitis.

iNOS immunoreactivity, demonstrated by cytoplasmic immunofluorescence, was not detected in the peritoneal inflammatory cells of normal rats. However, in the TCA pancreatitis rats it became visible in 25%–35% of the peritoneal inflammatory cells 12h after the induction of pancreatitis. The amount of NO produced by constitutive NOS is too small to be reflected in the changes in the serum levels of NO metabolites. Accordingly, the results suggested that inflammatory cells may be an important source of the excess NO during TCA pancreatitis [3].

The elevation of serum NOx 12h after the induction of TCA pancreatitis was significantly inhibited by the administration of specific NOS inhibitors (both nonselective NOS inhibitors and an iNOS selective inhibitor). Despite the strong inhibition of NO production, these agents did not ameliorate the gross pathological appearance of the pancreas or reduce the elevation of serum amylase. In addition, nonselective NOS inhibitors worsened the hematocrit, myeloperoxidase activity in the lung, and mortality during pancreatitis. Although iNOS selective inhibitor did not affect the hematocrit and the mortality during pancreatitis, it significantly aggravated myeloperoxidase activity in the lung. These results suggest that NO plays a protective role during the course of severe acute pancreatitis.

It has been shown that ascitic fluid obtained from necrotizing pancreatitis had lethal effects. In addition, some studies demonstrated that removal of pancreatic ascitic fluid by peritoneal lavage resulted in improved survival not only in experimental models of severe acute pancreatitis but also in human clinical trials. Based on these studies, some factors in the pancreatitis-associated ascitic fluid appear to be responsible for the severity of the condition, but the mechanism remains poorly understood.

We next examined the effects of ascitic fluid on the leukocytes and human umbilical vein endothelial cells (HUVECs) in vitro. The supernatant of TCA pancreatitis ascites could induce iNOS in the peritoneal macrophages of normal rats in vitro [3], whereas it decreased the endothelial NOS (eNOS) mRNA level in HUVECs. The supernatant of TCA pancreatitis ascites could also induce intercellular adhesion molecule-1 (ICAM-1), vascular cell adhesion molecule-1 (VCAM-1), and interleukin-8 (IL-8) in HUVECs [4]. The expression of adhesion molecules and IL-8 by ascitic fluid were attenuated by NO donor sodium nitroprusside, whereas the NOS inhibitor augmented them. These results suggest that NO inhibits the endothelial activation by ascitic fluid. The effects on the endothelial activation were paralleled by the altered adhesion of leukocytes to endothelium. Treatment of HUVECs with sodium nitroprusside significantly inhibited ascitic fluid-induced adhesion. In contrast, the NOS inhibitor increased the adhesion [5]. The results suggest that NO plays a protective role during the progression of acute pancreatitis through modulation of the leukocytes and endothelial cell systems.

References

1. Satoh A, Shimosegawa T, Abe T, et al (1994) Role of nitric oxide in the pancreatic blood flow response to caerulein. Pancreas 9:574–579
2. Satoh A, Shimosegawa T, Masamune A, et al (1999) Ascitic fluid of experimental severe acute pancreatitis modulates the function of peritoneal macrophages. Pancreas 19: 268–275
3. Satoh A, Shimosegawa T, Kimura K, et al (1998) Nitric oxide is overproduced by peritoneal macrophages in rat taurocholate pancreatitis: the mechanism of inducible nitric oxide synthase expression. Pancreas 17:402–411
4. Masamune A, Shimosegawa T, Kimura K, et al (1999) Specific induction of adhesion molecules in human vascular endothelial cells by rat experimental pancreatitis-associated ascitic fluids. Pancreas 18:141–150
5. Masamune A, Shimosegawa T, Satoh A, et al (2000) Nitric oxide decreases endothelial activation by rat experimental severe pancreatitis-associated ascitic fluids. Pancreas 20:297–304

Role of Nitric Oxide in the Progression of Acute Pancreatitis

TAKAYOSHI NISHINO[1,*], SHIN-ICHIRO WATANABE[2], HIROYASU OYAMA[2], YUJI FUKUYA[1], NAOAKI HAYASHI[1], and MAKIO KOBAYASHI[3]

Summary. To clarify the role of nitric oxide (NO) in the development and progression of acute pancreatitis, we investigated the effect of various NO synthase (NOS) inhibitors and NO donors on experimental pancreatitis in rats. Closed duodenal loop (CDL)-induced pancreatitis was produced in male Wistar rats, and the animals were treated with normal saline, the NOS substrate L-arginine, the NO donor *S*-nitroso-*N*-acetylpenicillamine, aminoguanidine [which is a more powerful inhibitor of inducible NOS (iNOS) than endothelial NO synthase (eNOS)], and *N*-nitro-L-arginine methyl ester (L-NAME), a more powerful inhibitor of eNOS than of iNOS. All drugs were infused intravenously during a period of 12h in each group. Pancreatic tissue was removed 12h after creating the CDL. L-Arginine, *S*-nitroso-*N*-acetyl-penicillamine, and aminoguanidine treatment had no effect on the elevation of serum pancreatic enzymes, whereas L-NAME administration significantly exacerbated their elevation. Pathologically, L-NAME treatment resulted in a significantly worse histological score at 12h, especially in terms of the degree of hemorrhage, acinar cell necrosis, and microvascular thrombosis. Addition of L-arginine clearly reversed the effect of L-NAME. Neither the NO substrate nor NO donor could inhibit the progression of hemorrhagic pancreatitis in CDL-induced pancreatitis. Aminoguanidine had no effect on the severity of the pancreatitis. We therefore concluded that NO production by eNOS may play a significant role in preventing the development and progression of acute pancreatitis.

Key words. Nitric oxide, Nitric oxide synthase inhibitor, L-NAME, Aminoguanidine, CDL-induced pancreatitis

[1]Department of Gastroenterology, [2]Department of Clinical Chemistry, [3]Department of Pathology, School of Medicine, Tokyo Women's Medical University, 8-1 Kawada-cho, Shinjuku-ku, Tokyo 162-8666, Japan
* e-mail: nisino@clabo.zengaku.twmu.ac.jp

Introduction

The pathogenesis and the mechanism of the development and progression of severe acute pancreatitis are not clearly understood. Some investigators have indicated that endogenous and exogenous nitric oxide (NO) plays a protective role in preventing the development of cerulein-induced acute pancreatitis [1]. On the other hand, a nitric oxide synthase (NOS) inhibitor has been reported to ameliorate acinar cell necrosis in sodium taurocholate-induced acute necrotizing pancreatitis [2].

The present study was undertaken to evaluate the significance of NO and NOS in the development and progression of closed duodenal loop (CDL)-induced acute pancreatitis in rats by treating them with L-arginine, the spontaneous NO donor *S*-nitroso-*N*-acetyl penicillamine (SNAP), and two NOS inhibitors: aminoguanidine and N^G-nitro-L-arginine methyl ester (L-NAME). Aminoguanidine has been shown to have considerably more activity as an inhibitor of inducible NOS (iNOS) than as an inhibitor of endothelial NOS (eNOS); and L-NAME is considered to be a more powerful inhibitor of eNOS than of iNOS.

Materials and Methods

Induction of CDL-Induced Acute Pancreatitis

After an 18-h fast, male Wistar rats (weighing 230–280g) were anesthetized by intramuscular injection of pentobarbital (50mg/kg). Induction of pancreatitis was performed aseptically as follows [3]. A midline incision was made to expose the duodenum and biliopancreatic duct, and a 2-cm closed duodenal loop was created by carefully ligating the duodenum on either side of the biliopancreatic duct. The right jugular vein of every rat was cannulated with a polyethylene catheter that was tunneled subcutaneously to exit dorsally through the skin in the interscapular region. The animals were then placed in individual close-fitting restraint cages.

Experiment 1: Effect of L-Arginine, SNAP, and NOS Inhibitors on CDL-Induced Acute Pancreatitis

The animals were randomly divided into six groups: (1) a normal control group (n = 12); (2) a normal saline (NS) group (n = 24), treated with normal saline (0.2ml bolus injection at the start of CDL creation followed by 0.5ml/h thereafter); (3) an arginine (ARG) group (n = 24), treated with the NOS substrate L-arginine 25mg/kg followed by 5mg/kg/h; (4) a SNAP group (n = 24), treated with the exogenous NO donor *S*-nitroso-*N*-acetyl penicillamine (0.2mg/kg/h); (5) an aminoguanidine (AG) group (n = 24), treated with aminoguanidine 20mg/kg followed by 5mg/kg/h (AG is a stronger inhibitor of iNOS than of eNOS); and (6) a NAME group (n = 24), treated with *N*-nitro-L-arginine methyl ester 10mg/kg followed by 2.5mg/kg/h thereafter (L-NAME is a stronger inhibitor of eNOS than of iNOS). Each drug was dissolved in normal saline.

Blood samples were collected from the jugular vein at 0, 3, 6, and 12h to measure the serum lipase concentration. Ascitic fluid was collected with a disposable syringe for 12 h, and the volume was measured. The rats were anesthetized with pentobarbital. Twelve rats in each group were killed 12 h after creating the CDL. After exsanguination the pancreas was quickly removed, and the whole pancreas was then immediately fixed with 20% buffered formalin.

Experiment 2: Effect of L-Arginine Addition to L-NAME Treatment of Pancreatitis

To confirm the specificity of the effects of L-NAME in inhibiting NOS, we examined the effect on pancreatitis of additing L-arginine to L-NAME. The animals were randomly divided into two groups: (1) a NAME group ($n = 16$), treated with L-NAME 10 mg/kg bolus injection at the start of CDL creation, followed by 2.5 mg/kg/h thereafter via the right jugular vein and infused with normal saline (0.2 ml) followed by 0.5 ml/h via the left jugular vein; and (2) a NAME + ARG group ($n = 16$), treated with L-NAME 10 mg/kg followed by 2.5 mg/kg/h thereafter via the right jugular vein and L-arginine 100 mg/kg followed by 25 mg/kg/h thereafter via the left jugular vein. Blood samples, ascitic fluid volume, and histological findings were assessed as in experiment 1.

Histological Assessment

The grading of interstitial edema was based on the following scale: grade 0, absent; grade 1, diffuse expansion of interlobar septa; grade 2, 1+ diffuse expansion of interlobular septa; grade 3, 2+ diffuse expansion of interacinar septa; grade 4, 3+ diffuse expansion of intercellular septa. Histological grading of acinar cell necrosis and vacuolation was based on the approximate percentage of cells involved: grade 0, 0%; grade 1, <5%; grade 2, 5% to <25%; grade 3, 25% to <50%; grade 4, ≥50%. The grading of thrombosis was based on the approximate percentage of microvessels involved: grade 0, 0%; grade 1, <5%; grade 2, 5% to <10%; grade 3, 10% to <25%; grade 4, ≥25%. The grading of inflammatory cell infiltration and hemorrhage was based on the following scale: grade 0, absent; grade 1, minimal; grade 2, mild; grade 3, moderate; grade 4, severe.

Results

Effect of L-Arginine, SNAP, and NOS Inhibitors on CDL-Induced Acute Pancreatitis

The NAME-treated animals showed significant increases in serum lipase concentrations compared to the animals in the NS, ARG, SNAP, and AG groups from 3 h onward: peak values: NAME group, 2550 ± 270; NS group, 910 ± 110; ARG group, 1010 ± 120; SNAP group, 840 ± 80; AG group, 1050 ± 120) ($P < 0.01$). The ascitic fluid volume was increased 6 h after creating the CDL, and there were no significant differences among the five pancreatitis groups. The L-NAME-treated animals showed a significant increase in ascitic fluid volume at 12 h compared to the animals in the NS, ARG, SNAP, and AG groups (data not shown).

TABLE 1. Histological findings 12h after creating the closed duodenal loop

Histological finding	NS	ARG	SNAP	AG	NAME	Statistical significance
Interstitial edema	2.5 ± 0.2 (2–3)	2.4 ± 0.2 (2–3)	2.4 ± 0.2 (2–3)	2.5 ± 0.2 (2–3)	3.0 ± 0.2 (2–4)	
Cell infiltration	2.3 ± 0.2 (2–3)	1.9 ± 0.2 (1–3)	1.8 ± 0.2 (1–3)	2.1 ± 0.2 (1–3)	3.0 ± 0.2* (2–4)	vs. NS, ARG, SNAP, AG
Hemorrhage	2.3 ± 0.3 (2–3)	1.8 ± 0.2 (1–3)	1.6 ± 0.2 (1–3)	2.2 ± 0.2 (2–3)	3.1 ± 0.2* (2–4)	vs. NS, ARG, SNAP, AG
Vacuolation	2.4 ± 0.2 (2–3)	2.0 ± 0.2 (1–3)	1.8 ± 0.2 (1–3)	2.3 ± 0.2 (2–3)	2.6 ± 0.2 (2–3)	
Necrosis	1.7 ± 0.3 (1–2)	1.4 ± 0.2 (1–2)	1.3 ± 0.2 (1–2)	1.7 ± 0.2 (1–2)	2.8 ± 0.2* (2–4)	vs. NS, ARG, SNAP, AG
Microvascular thrombosis	2.0 ± 0.3 (1–3)	1.6 ± 0.3 (1–2)	1.4 ± 0.2 (1–2)	2.1 ± 0.3 (1–3)	3.3 ± 0.2* (2–4)	vs. NS, ARG, SNAP, AG

Results are expressed as means ± SEM of the values in 12 rats in each group. Numbers in parentheses are ranges

L-NAME treatment significantly increased hemorrhage, vacuolation, necrosis, and microvascular thrombosis versus the normal saline (NS), arginine (ARG), *S*-nitroso-*N*-acetyl penicillamine (SNAP), and aminoguanidine (AG) groups ($P < 0.05$) (From [3] with permission)

Histological Findings 12 Hours After Creating the Closed Duodenal Loop

In addition to interstitial edema and vacuolation, acinar cell necrosis extending to whole lobules, and hemorrhage and micirovascular thrombosis were frequently observed in the NS group 12h after creation of the CDL (Table 1). L-NAME treatment significantly increased the acinar cell necrosis, inflammatory cell infiltration, hemorrhage, and microvascular thrombosis compared to the NS, ARG, SNAP, and AG groups. Degeneration or defects in arteriole and capillary walls and perinuclear vacuolation of the arteriole wall, indicating powerful vasoconstriction, were frequently observed in the L-NAME-treated animals. Leukocyte adhesion to endothelial cells was also frequently seen. Administration of L-arginine or SNAP slightly decreased the necrosis, hemorrhage, and microvascular thrombosis, but their effect was not significant. Aminoguanidine did not change the severity of the histological scores.

Effect of L-Arginine Addition to L-NAME Treatment of Pancreatitis

The increases in serum lipase by L-NAME were reversed by L-arginine administration from 3h onward. The ascitic fluid volume increased by L-NAME was reversed by L-arginine administration 12h after creating the CDL. Macroscopically, the marked hemorrhage induced by L-NAME treatment was significantly decreased by L-arginine addition at 6h and 12h.

TABLE 2. Histological findings 12h after creating the closed duodenal loop in NAME and NAME + ARG groups

Histological finding	NAME	NAME + ARG	*P*
Interstitial edema	2.8 ± 0.2 (2–3)	2.4 ± 0.2 (2–3)	
Cell infiltration	2.8 ± 0.2 (2–4)	2.2 ± 0.2 (2–3)	<0.05
Hemorrhage	3.2 ± 0.2 (2–4)	2.4 ± 0.2 (2–3)	<0.01
Vacuolation	2.7 ± 0.2 (2–3)	2.4 ± 0.2 (2–3)	
Necrosis	3.0 ± 0.3 (2–4)	2.0 ± 0.2 (1–3)	<0.01
Microvascular thrombosis	3.2 ± 0.2 (2–4)	2.4 ± 0.2 (2–3)	<0.01

Results are expressed as means + SEM of the values in eight rats in each group. Numbers in parentheses are the ranges [3]

Histological Findings 12 Hours After Creating the CDL

L-Arginine infused in combination with L-NAME significantly decreased inflammatory cell infiltration, hemorrhage, acinar cell necrosis, and microvascular thrombosis compared to the L-NAME group (Table 2). L-Arginine addition also reduced the degeneration and defects in arteriole and capillary walls enhanced by L-NAME treatment.

Discussion

The results of the present study can be summarized as follows. First, the eNOS inhibitor L-NAME significantly aggravated the elevation of serum pancreatic enzymes and histological scores, but the iNOS inhibitor AG did not change the severity of the pancreatitis. Second, L-arginine administration combined with L-NAME clearly reversed the effect of L-NAME on pancreatitis. Third, the NO donors L-arginine and SNAP failed to prevent the progression of CDL-induced pancreatitis to hemorrhagic pancreatitis.

The major results of this study are that L-NAME significantly aggravated pancreatitis based on the increased serum pancreatic enzyme levels, ascitic fluid, and especially the histological lesions, such as hemorrhage, micovascular thrombosis, and necrosis. Furthermore, L-arginine administration combined with L-NAME clearly reversed the effect of L-NAME on pancreatitis. Lui et al. [1] reported that nitric-L-arginine, a more powerful inhibitor of eNOS than of iNOS, the same as L-NAME, caused vasoconstriction, reduced pancreatic blood flow, and caused progression of cerulein-induced pancreatitis from edematous pancreatitis to hemorrhagic pancreatitis. These findings are consistent with our finding that pancreatitis was aggravated by infusion of the more powerful inhibitor of eNOS. The fact that such histological changes as fibrinoid degeneration of the walls of venules and arterioles, vascular wall destruction, and microvascular thrombosis were observed more frequently in L-NAME-treated animals also suggests marked impairment of pancreatic microcirculation during progression of pancreatitis.

There is accumulating evidence to suggesting that many of the toxic effects of NO, such as inactivation of mitochondrial aconitase [4] and activation of polyadenosine diphosphate ribosyl polymerase [5], are mediated by ONNO-. Aminoguanidine, a stronger inhibitor of iNOS than of eNOS, is thought to inhibit NO-derived cytotoxicity, and aminoguanidine administration is known to suppress colitis and myocarditis. In the present study we examined the effect of aminoguanidine on experimental pancreatitis for the first time. The results showed that aminoguanidine did not ameliorate CDL-induced pancreatitis at the level of serum pancreatic enzymes and histologic damage, nor did it exacerbate pancreatitis as observed in response to L-NAME treatment. Possible explanations why aminoguanidine does not ameliorate CDL-induced pancreatitis are as follows. First, because aminoguanidine is not a completely selective inhibitor of iNOS, it may act as a partial aggravating agent through inhibition of eNOS; and second, iNOS may not play a significant role in the progression of CDL-induced pancreatitis.

Conclusions

The eNOS inhibitor L-NAME significantly aggravated CDL-induced pancreatitis by increasing vascular injury. Addition of L-arginine to L-NAME clearly reversed the effect of L-NAME on pancreatitis. Administration of an iNOS inhibitor did not change the severity of the pancreatitis. We conclude that NO production by eNOS may play a significant role in preventing the progression of acute pancreatitis probably through maintenance of pancreatic perfusion and prevention of vascular injuries.

References

1. Liu X, Nakano I, Yamaguchi H, et al (1995) Protective effect of nitric oxide on development of acute pancreatitis in rats. Dig Dis Sci 40:2162–2169
2. Closa D, Hotter G, Prats N, et al (1994) Prostanoid generation in early stages of acute pancreatitis: a role for nitric oxide. Inflammation 18:469–480
3. Nishino T, Watanabe S, Oyama Y, et al (1999) An endothelial nitric oxide synthase inhibitor aggravates CDL-induced acute pancreatitis in rats. Pancreas 19:390–400
4. Castro L, Rodriguez M, Radi R (1994) Aconitase is readily inactivated by peroxynitrite, but not its precursor, nitric oxide. J Biol Chem 269:29409–29415
5. Szabo C, Zingarelli B, Salzman AL (1996) Role of poly-ADP ribosyltransferase activation in vascular and energetic failure elicited by exogenous and endogenous nitric oxide and peroxynitrite, Circ Res 78:1051–1063

Protective Effect of Nitric Oxide on Acute Liver Failure in Rats

Toru Kono[1,*], Hiromi Kotani[1], Toshiyuki Asama[1], Noriaki Mamiya[1], Nobutoshi Ando[1], Naoyuki Chisato[1], Kazunori Kamiya[1], Masashi Yoneda[2], Jun Iwamoto[3], and Shinichi Kasai[1]

Summary. The effect of low-dose lipopolysaccharide (LPS)-induced nitric oxide (NO) on liver damage and survival in rats with acute liver failure caused by a lethal dose of D-galactosamine (D-gal) was studied. There was marked elevation of serum aspartate aminotransferase and alanine aminotransferase levels 24 h after D-gal. These aminotransferases were significantly improved in low-dose LPS-pretreated rats at 24 h after the administration of D-gal. Ninety percent of control animals died within 4 days after D-gal injection but pretreatment of low-dose LPS significantly decreased mortality to 10%. N^G-Nitro-L-arginine-methyl ester, but not N^G-nitro-D-arginine-methyl ester, reversed this cytoprotection. In conclusion, pretreatment of low-dose LPS prevents experimental liver failure through activation of endogenous NO synthesis.

Key words. Nitric oxide, Liver failure, D-Galactosamine, Cytoprotection, Lipopolysaccharide

Introduction

Fulminant acute liver failure is a condition with a poor prognosis and a high mortality rate, and the development of an effective treatment is still a major current objective of clinical hepatology. The most appropriate treatment, apart from liver transplantation, is to prevent progressive hepatocyte necrosis. Although supplementation of glucagon and insulin has been well known therapy for fulminant hepatitis [1], at present the clinical effect of insulin and glucagon therapy is not satisfactory, perhaps because the glucagon receptors on hepatocytes are destroyed with severe hepatic damage. Moreover, insulin and glucagon therapy had no effect on the survival

[1] Second Department of Surgery, [3] Division of Applied Physiology, Asahikawa Medical College, 2-1 Midorigaoka-Higashi, Asahikawa, Hokkaido 078-8510, Japan
[2] Department of Gastroenterology, Dokkyo University, School of Medicine, Mibu, Tochigi 321-0293, Japan
* e-mail: kono@asahikawa-med.ac.jp

of rats with D-galactosamine (D-gal)-induced acute liver failure [2]. Therefore, other therapeutic agents or methods that have the potential to improve liver function and survival are required.

Nitric Oxide Production in the Liver During Low-Grade Endotoxemia

In previous studies we demonstrated that a sublethal dose (0.1 mg/kg) of LPS-induced intraabdominal nitric oxide (NO) reflected endogenous NO production by inducible NO synthase (iNOS) in the liver, and that induced NO was released from the liver surface during endotoxemia [3]. Our recent study showed that low doses (0.001 mg/kg) of LPS-induced intraabdominal NO production at 2h, and the intraabdominal NO concentration reached a maximal 10h after LPS injection without significant increases of serum transaminase levels. We are aware of no published in vivo studies that described NO production caused by low-dose LPS without liver damage. It is not clear whether LPS-induced endogenous NO is cytotoxic or cytoprotective. There are many controversial reports about the role of NO during endotoxemia.

Cytoprotective Effect of Nitric Oxide on Acute Liver Failure

We demonstrated that LPS-induced endogenous NO has a cytoprotective role until 10h after LPS injection, and this NO was mainly produced in the liver [4,5]. We also demonstrated that beneficial hepatic NO production started to increase at 2h and peaked at 8–10h after low-dose LPS injection (0.001 mg/kg) and after that NO production declined [4,5]. Moreover, the inhibition of low-dose LPS-induced NO during the first 10h after LPS injection caused significant liver damage. Therefore, we hypothesized that if the liver would start to produce beneficial NO before D-gal toxicity appeared liver injury might be prevented.

In the present study, we found that low-dose LPS administration 2, 6, or 12h before D-gal injection significantly avoided liver damage caused by a lethal dose of D-gal. Maximum improvement was observed during the 6-h interval between LPS and D-gal. This improvement was blocked by the NO blocker. Thus, we speculated that the cytoprotective effect of pretreatment of low-dose LPS might be mainly mediated by NO.

Although the mechanism of the beneficial role of the NO is unclear, it can be speculated based on previous reports of NO during endotoxemia that there is a cytoprotective effect. There have been reports of inhibitory effects of NO regarding adhesion of platelets to the endothelium and platelet aggregation. In previous reports, inhibition of NO formation increased neutrophil accumulation in mesenteric venules and in liver sinusoids. Furthermore, NOS inhibitors reduced liver blood flow during endotoxemia and aggravated liver damage in the *Corynebacterium parvum*/endotoxin model. It also has been reported that the mortality rate during endotoxemia is increased by N^G-nitro-L-arginine methyl ester (L-NAME) via organ ischemia and microvascular thrombosis. These observations are consistent with our present findings showing that inhibition of NO by L-NAME reversed the beneficial effect of pretreatment with low-dose LPS. Thus, we speculated that the beneficial NO might contribute to maintaining the microcirculation in the liver, providing protection against liver damage. Moreover, the efficacy of pretreatment with low-dose LPS might be correlated with the NO concentration induced by the low-dose LPS.

Cytotoxicity of Nitric Oxide During Endotoxemia

In contrast, in vitro studies have suggested that NO production by liver cells during endotoxemia are associated with inhibition of cell growth and DNA and protein synthesis, which were reversed by the NOS inhibitor. Other studies showed that endotoxin-induced vascular leakage and bacterial translocation are blocked by selective inhibition of inducible NO. Increased levels of NO also have been observed in patients whose recovery is complicated by sepsis after surgery, and that the NO level is well correlated with the severity of sepsis. These observations do not conflict with our results, as the previous studies were not focused on the early phase of endotoxemia.

Conclusions

Low-dose LPS-induced NO may have a beneficial role, which may be one of the self-defense systems for the liver. Further studies are necessary to confirm the mechanism of the beneficial roles of low-dose LPS-induced NO during the first 10h after LPS administration.

References

1. Okita K, Matsuda S, Hanta T, et al (1987) Clinical evaluation of glucagon and insulin in therapy of fulminant hepatitis. Gastroenterol Jpn 22:607–613
2. Nishiguchi S, Kuroki T, Takeda T, et al (1990) Effects of putrescine on D-galactosamine-induced acute liver failure in rats. Hepatology 12:348–353
3. Ando N, Kono T, Iwamoto J, et al (1998) Nitric oxide release from the liver surface to the intra-abdominal cavity during acute endotoxemia in rats. Nitric Oxide 2:481–488
4. Kamiya K, Kono T, Iwamoto J, et al (2000) The cytoprotective role of lipopolysaccharide-induced nitric oxide against liver damage during early phase of endotoxemia in rats. Shock 14:229–233
5. Kono T, Yoneda M, Ando N, et al (1998) Hepatic adaptive cytoprotection through the nitric oxide pathway. Gastroenterology 114:A1278–A1279

Regulatory Mechanism of Cationic Amino Acid Transporters in Hepatic Sinusoidal Ito Cells

TOSHIJI SAIBARA*, KOUJI OOKAWAUCHI, NAOAKI AKISAWA, SHINJI IWASAKI, TAKASHI MAEDA, and SABURO ONISHI

Summary. Nitric oxide (NO) is a potent mediator of hepatic sinusoidal hemodynamics. It is synthesized in and affects hepatic Ito cells. Although NO production may depend on the induction of inducible nitric oxide synthase (iNOS) and on transport of extracellular L-arginine, the precise mechanism controlling NO production in stellate cells has not been well characterized. Recently, however, the L-arginine transport system functioning in transformed hepatic stellate cells was identified. In this review, we show the regulatory mechanisms involved in system y+, which may be mediated by cationic amino acid transporter-1 (CAT-1) and CAT-2B during uptake of extracellular L-arginine as the substrate for NO synthesis.

Key words. Nitric oxide, Ito cells, Cationic amino acid transporter, Arginine, Hepatic sinusoid

Introduction

Hepatic Ito cells (stellate cells, fat-storing cells) are potent regulators of hepatic sinusoidal blood flow, because they become contractile when "activated." Endothelin-1 (ET-1) elicits hepatic sinusoid constriction in normal rats at sites in hepatic stellate cells. The effect of ET-1 is much more prominent in hepatic stellate cells isolated from the cirrhotic liver than in those from normal liver.

Nitric oxide (NO), a well-known smooth muscle relaxant, plays a significant role in liver sinusoidal hemodynamics, and its level is increased in hepatic tissue of patients with cirrhosis. NO attenuates ET-1-induced contraction of hepatic stellate cells in vitro and in vivo, as parenchymal cells and nonparenchymal cells produce NO and the distance between these NO-producing cells and transformed hepatic stellate cells are within a calculated distance of NO diffusion. Recently, however, transformed hepatic stellate cells were shown to produce NO in response to tumor necrosis factor-α (TNFα) plus interferon-γ (IFNγ).

First Department of Medicine, Kochi Medical School, Kohasu, Oko-cho, Nankoku, Kochi 783-8505, Japan
* e-mail: saibarat@kochi-ms.ac.jp

Production of NO depends mostly on inducible nitric oxide synthase (iNOS) and on the availability of extracellular L-arginine via system y+ transport. As is also true in transformed hepatic stellate cells, L-arginine availability from the extracellular pool such as the portal vein is critical. Corresponding transporter proteins for system y+, called cationic amino acid transporters (CATs), were identified recently. CAT-1, encoded by the *cat-1* gene, is a high-affinity basic amino acid transporter constitutively expressed in most cell types except hepatocytes. The mutually exclusive alternative splicing of the *cat-2* transcript is regulated in a cell-specific manner: Hepatocytes exclusively express a low-affinity basic amino acid transporter (CAT-2A), whereas lymphocytes express a high-affinity basic amino acid transporter (CAT-2B). Here we review the molecular mechanism of L-arginine transport regulation in relation to NO production in transformed hepatic stellate cells in the rat [1].

Characterization of Basic Amino Acid Transport

Saturable and stereospecific transport of L-[^{3}H]arginine was measured, and the transport velocity was plotted as a function of the velocity/L-arginine concentration ratio [2]. Substitution of Na^+ in the uptake buffer with choline at equimolar concentrations did not significantly affect the uptake of L-arginine. The Eadie-Hofstee plots proved that L-arginine uptake by hepatic stellate cells was biphasic, with two affinity states. A high-affinity component had a Michaelis constant (Km) of 42.4 ± 5.1 μM with a maximum transport velocity (Vmax) of 0.82 ± 0.17 nmol/mg protein/45 s. A low-affinity component was detected as well, with a Km of 1.57 ± 0.19 mM and a Vmax of 4.40 ± 0.37 nmol/mg protein/45 s.

When the transformed hepatic stellate cells were preincubated with TNFα (1000 U/ml) for 24 h, the Vmax of the high-affinity component increased significantly compared to that of the cells without addition of cytokines; the Vmax of the low-affinity component also increased. When the cells were cultured with IFNγ (500 U/ml) for 24 h, neither the Km nor the Vmax of the two components changed significantly. When both TNFα (1000 U/ml) and IFNγ (500 U/ml) were supplemented in the medium, not only the Vmax but also the Km of the high-affinity component increased significantly. Under these conditions the Vmax of the low-affinity component was significantly increased, but the Km was not.

cis-*Inhibition and* trans-*Stimulation of* L-*Arginine Uptake*

L-[^{3}H]Arginine uptake was inhibited by co-incubation with L-arginine, L-lysine, L-ornithine, or N^G-monomethyl-L-arginine (L-NMMA) during the test period. In contrast, the same group of amino acids augmented L-[^{3}H]arginine uptake significantly when supplemented in the medium during the preincubation period.

Detection of CAT mRNA and Its Enhancement in Cytokine Stimulation

The expression of CAT-1, CAT-2B, and iNOS mRNA was semiquantified when cells were stimulated for 24 h with TNFα or IFNγ alone or in combination. CAT-1 mRNA expression remained unchanged, whereas CAT-2B mRNA expression was enhanced by TNFα, especially in combination with IFNγ.

NO Production, iNOS mRNA Expression, and L-Arginine Transport in Transformed Hepatic Stellate Cells

Nonstimulated or TNFα-stimulated hepatic stellate cells induce neither iNOS mRNA expression nor NO production, whereas IFNγ treatment induced both, especially when stimulated in combination with TNFα. IFNγ with TNFα markedly stimulated L-arginine transport, iNOS mRNA expression, and NO production in transformed hepatic stellate cells; and the competitive inhibition assay, with an excessive dose of extracellular L-lysine, revealed that the NO production depended on extracellular L-arginine uptake. IFNγ enhanced NO production without obvious activation of L-arginine transport. In contrast, TNFα enhanced L-arginine transport possibly through an increase in the number of transporters without obvious enhancement of NO production.

Discussion

Basic amino acids are physiologically transported across the mammalian cell membrane by a limited well-defined physiological transport system, such as y+, b0,+, B0,+, and y + L. Kinetic studies of L-arginine uptake indicated the presence of a predominantly stereospecific and saturable high-affinity transporter compatible with the y+ system. The contribution of system b0,+(NBAT), B0,+, or y + L to the total L-arginine transport is probably insignificant, if it has any effect at all, because of the lack of Na^+-stimulated L-arginine or L-leucine uptake and the lack of inhibitory effect of L-leucine on Na^+-independent L-arginine uptake.

Two kinds of high-affinity system y+ transporter mRNA were expressed (i.e., CAT-1 and CAT-2B) in activated Ito cells. In addition, a low-affinity transporter activity (Km ~2 mM) was detected; whereas mRNA for CAT-2A, a low-affinity transporter expressed only in liver and muscle, was not detectable. L-Arginine concentration in plasma and tissues is 50–100 μM under physiological circumstances. The high-affinity transporter would mediate most of the L-arginine uptake in transformed hepatic stellate cells; even a small increase in the L-arginine level in hepatic sinusoids may considerably affect the rate of L-arginine influx in these cells.

It is difficult to ascertain exactly how CAT-1 and CAT-2B contribute to the overall L-arginine transport activity in these cells, as the two transporters show similar high-affinity uptake kinetics, and their mRNAs are readily detectable in the nonstimulated transformed hepatic stellate cells. The effect of TNFα was apparent in enhancing CAT-2B mRNA expression, increasing the Vmax of the high-affinity transporter and facilitating L-arginine transport without affecting the Km of the transporter and CAT-1 mRNA expression. In addition, combined treatment with TNFα and IFNγ resulted in increased Vmax and Km of the high-affinity transporter, and the increase was coincidental with increased CAT-2B mRNA expression. The effect of TNFα on transformed hepatic stellate cells was to increase the rate of L-arginine transport via an increase in the amount of CAT-2B transporter protein, suggesting a major contribution of CAT-2B in the increased activity of system y+. Indeed, in brain astrocytes CAT-2B expression was strongly associated with the increase in L-arginine uptake and NO production.

TNFα enhanced CAT-2B mRNA expression and L-arginine uptake but failed to induce iNOS mRNA expression and NO production. In contrarst, the effect of IFNγ was directed exclusively to the induction of iNOS mRNA expression and enhancement of overall NO production with neither enhancement of CAT-2B mRNA expression nor increased L-arginine uptake. It is noteworthy that L-arginine can be supplied from the intracellular pool by endogenous synthesis, in part because arginosuccinate synthetase, the rate-limiting enzyme in intracellular L-arginine biosynthesis, is known to be co-induced with iNOS. However, L-arginine supplied from extracellular sources through system y+ plasma membrane transporter plays a major role as the substrate in NO production, as enhanced NO production is considerably inhibited by an excessive amount of extracellular L-lysine, a potent competitor for system y+. For this reason, IFNγ treatment in combination with TNFα resulted in maximal NO production through iNOS expression and enhanced L-arginine uptake.

The NO secreted from hepatocytes and Kupffer cells was suggested to counteract the effect of ET-1 in the hepatic sinusoids. However, transformed hepatic stellate cells express iNOS mRNA and produce NO in response to IFNγ. Therefore, the autocrine regulatory mechanism of NO may function predominantly on transformed hepatic stellate cells in the hepatic sinusoids because infiltrating lymphocytes in the portal area in patients with chronic liver disease may produce inflammatory cytokines, including IFNγ, and may stimulate adjacent transformed hepatic stellate cells to produce NO. Indeed, disturbed distribution of blood flow in the hepatic lobules and increased production of ET-1 and NO are characteristic hemodynamic features in patients with liver cirrhosis. An empirical observation in human indicates that administration of L-arginine per os modulates the metabolism of NH_3 in hepatocytes. This L-arginine uptake into hepatocytes may be mediated through a low-affinity transporter, CAT-2A, because hepatocytes lack high-affinity transporters. L-Arginine concentration in the portal vein may be significantly increased above physiological concentrations. L-Arginine transport into transformed hepatic stellate cells through high-affinity transporter(s) drastically increases and results in increased NO production. This seems to be true in vivo, as sinusoidal diameter and blood flow are known to be modulated by the administration of L-arginine. Therefore, modulation of NO production via access to portal blood L-arginine concentration is an alternative, simple step in controlling disturbed hepatic sinusoidal blood flow in patients with chronic inflammation of the liver.

Conclusions

Induction of iNOS and enhancement of L-arginine transport in transformed hepatic stellate cells are regulated through two distinct signal transduction pathways, with co-activation of the two pathways by inflammatory cytokines. The y+ system, a high-affinity transporter, was expressed in transformed hepatic stellate cells, and the activity was enhanced by TNFα possibly through an increase in the number of CAT-2B molecules. The effect of IFNγ was exclusively directed to induction of iNOS mRNA expression and enhancement of overall NO production.

References

1. Ookawauchi K, Saibara T, Yoshikawa T, et al (1998) Characterization of cationic amino acid transporter and its gene expression in rat hepatic stellate cells in relation to nitric oxide production. J Hepatol 29:923–932
2. Durante W, Liao L, Schafer AI (1995) Differential regulation of L-arginine transport and inducible NOS in cultured vascular smooth muscle cells. Am J Physiol 268:H1158–H1164

Part 6
Transcription Factors in Digestive Organs

Novel NADPH Oxidase, Mox1, Expressed in Cultured Gastric Pit Cells: Modulation of NF-κB Activation

Shigetada Teshima*, Tsukasa Kawahara, Kyoichi Kishi, and Kazuhito Rokutan

Summary. Recently we showed that primary cultured guinea pig gastric pit cells have a phagocyte NADPH oxidase-like activity that is up-regulated by *Helicobacter pylori* lipopolysaccharide (LPS). We demonstrate here that pit cells expressed all of the phagocyte NADPH oxidase components (p22-, p67-, and p47-*phoxes*) and a non-phagocyte-specific isoenzyme of gp91-*phox* (Mox1). Overproduced superoxide anion (O_2^-) and related oxidants from *H. pylori* LPS-primed cells induced continuous activation of nuclear factor κB (NF-κB). We provide evidence here that gastric pit cells express a potent Mox1 oxidase and suggest that O_2^- and related oxidants derived from the oxidase might act as important signal molecules for NF-κB activation during *H. pylori* infection.

Key words. Mox1 oxidase, Superoxide anion, NF-κB, Gastric mucosal defense, *Helicobacter pylori*

Introduction

Phagocyte reduced nicotinamide adenine dinucleotide phosphate (NADPH) oxidase-derived superoxide anion (O_2^-) and related oxygen metabolites play a crucial role in microbial and tumoricidal activities. These oxygen metabolites are now considered to be an important signal for initiation of inflammatory and immune responses. The phagocyte NADPH oxidase consists of a membrane-bound cytochrome b_{558} heterodimer (gp91-*phox* and p22-*phox*) and three cytosolic components (p67-*phox*, p47-*phox*, p40-*phox*); it is modulated by Rac1/2 [1].

There is increasing evidence that distinct types of nonphagocytic cells, such as vascular smooth muscle cells, glomerular mesangial cells, endothelial cells, and fibroblasts, express p22-, p67-, and p47-*phox* and can produce small amounts of O_2^- [2]. These cells were suggested to have an unknown low potential cytochrome *b* in their

Department of Nutrition, School of Medicine, The University of Tokushima, 3-18-15 Kuramoto-cho, Tokushima 770-8503, Japan
* e-mail: teshima@nutr.med.tokushima-u.ac.jp

plasma membranes [2]. Recently, Suh et al. molecularly identified a novel, non-phagocyte-specific gp91-*phox* isoenzyme, termed Mox1 [3].

We previously reported that primary cultures of guinea pig gastric pit cells can release abundant O_2^- through a phagocyte NADPH oxidase-like system [4,5]. In the present study, we identified the O_2^--producing system in gastric pit cells as a Mox1 oxidase. Furthermore, we suggest that O_2^- derived from the oxidase may regulate the gastric mucosal response against *Helicobacter pylori* through modulating the nuclear factor κB (NF-κB)-dependent route.

Materials and Methods

Preparation and Culture of Gastric Mucosal Cells. Gastric mucosal cells were isolated aseptically from guinea pig fundic glands, as previously described [4].

Gel Mobility Shift Assay. Nuclear proteins were prepared from cultured gastric mucosal cells, and the activation of NF-κB was examined by gel mobility shift assay, as described previously [6].

Immunoblotting. Extracted whole-cell proteins (40 μg per lane) were separated by sodium dodecyl sulfate-polyacrylamide gel electrophoresis (SDS-PAGE) and transferred to a polyvinylidene difluoride filter. After blocking with 4% milk casein, the blot was incubated with antibody against each phox protein. The bound antibody was detected by an enhanced chemiluminescence (ECL) system (Amersham-Pharmacia Biotech, Tokyo).

Reverse Transcription and Polymerase Chain Reaction. The reverse transcription-polymerase chain reaction (RT-PCR) was performed using a TaKaRa RT-PCR kit (TaKaRa, Tokyo, Japan). The sequences of the primers used were as follows: human gp91-*phox*, 5′-CATCATCTCTTTGTGATCTTCT-3′ (sense) and 5′-CTTAGGTAGTTTC-CACGCATC-3′ (antisense); human *mox1*, 5′-GCTCATTTTGCAGCCGCA-3′ (sense) and 5′-AGAATGACCGGTGCAAGG-3′ (antisense). Amplified products were separated in a 6% polyacrylamide gel.

Results and Discussion

Expression of Mox1 Oxidase Components in Gastric Mucosal Cells

Our previous studies [4] showed that the O_2^--generating system in gastric pit cells shared functional and structural similarities with the phagocyte NADPH oxidase, as seen in cell-free reconstitution experiments and immunoblot analysis with antibodies against the human neutrophil p67-*phox* and p47-*phox* components. In this study, we identified the O_2^--generating system in gastric pit cells. As shown in Fig. 1A, gastric mucosal cells contained immunoreactive proteins corresponding to all of the NADPH oxidase component proteins.

We focused on the gp91-*phox* subunit expressed in gastric mucosal cells, as a non-phagocyte-specific isoenzyme of gp91-*phox* (Mox1) was molecularly identified [3].

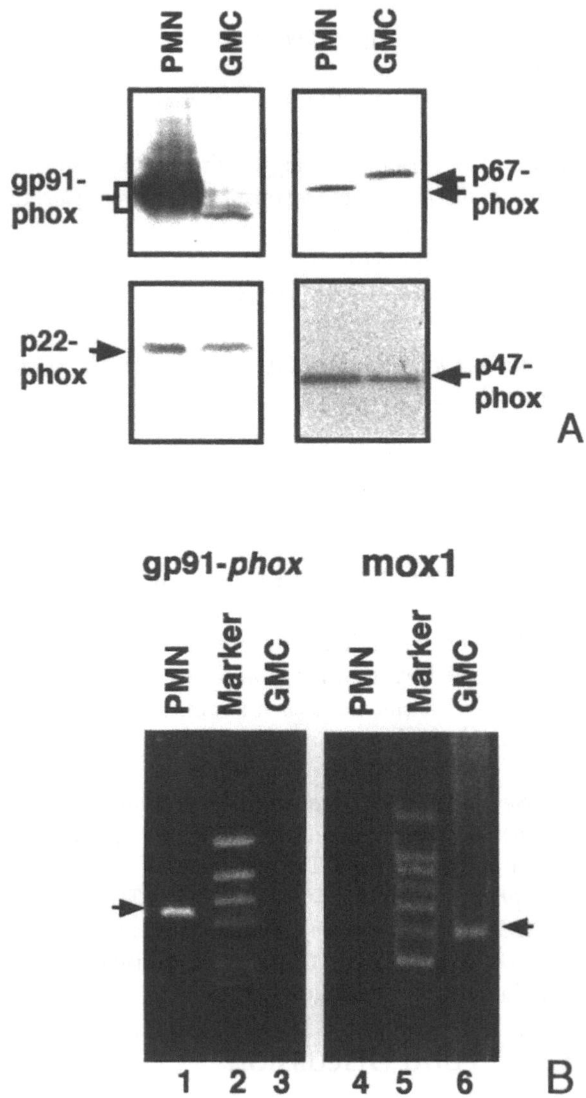

Fig. 1. Expression of the Mox1 oxidase system in gastric mucosal cells. **A** Expression of the phagocyte NADPH oxidase components in gastric mucosal cells. Whole-cell proteins were prepared from guinea pig neutrophils (*PMN*) and guinea pig gastric mucosal cells (*GMC*). Immunoblot analysis with antibody against each *phox* protein was performed. **B** Expression of *mox1* transcripts in gastric mucosal cells. Total RNA was prepared from PMN and GMC. Extracted total RNA (1 µg) was reverse transcribed into cDNA with oligonucleotide antisense primer specific for gp91-*phox* or *mox1*. Generated cDNA was used as a template in PCR for gp91-*phox* (lanes *1* and *3*) and *mox1* (lanes *4* and *6*)

The amino acid sequence of the epitope of anti-human gp91-*phox* antibody is 48% identical to that of human Mox1; therefore, it was possible that the antibody recognized Mox1 but not gp91-*phox*. To address this issue, we designed primer sets that specifically hybridize the gp91-*phox* or *mox1* mRNA, respectively. RT-PCR with the primer set for gp91-*phox* did not amplify any products in gastric mucosal cells (Fig. 1B, lane 3), whereas RT-PCR for *mox1* resulted in generation of a single product corresponding to the predicted basepair (bp) size for the *mox1* transcript in gastric mucosal cells (lane 6). The *mox1* transcript could not be detected in guinea pig neutrophils (lane 4). The amplified PCR product from gastric mucosal cells was confirmed to be a guinea pig *mox1* by DNA sequencing; the sequence of the product showed 84% identity with the human *mox1* cDNA (454–1042 bp, data not shown), and the expression of *mox1* mRNA in gastric mucosal cells was confirmed by Northern blot analysis [6].

NF-κB Activation

Gastric pit cells have oxidant-sensitive transcription factor NF-κB [7]. Thus, we examined whether Mox1-derived reactive oxygen intermediates could activate NF-κB. The gel mobility shift assay showed that untreated cells constitutively contained low levels of NF-κB binding activity (Fig. 2, lane 1). When cells were treated with *H. pylori* LPS to enhance the Mox1 oxidase activity [4,5], this binding activity was markedly increased in a time-dependent manner (Fig. 2, lanes 2–6). The NF-κB activity was completely suppressed by inclusion of superoxide dismutase (SOD) plus catalase (lane 8), which could not penetrate plasma membrane, suggesting that overproduction of O_2^- and related oxidants from the LPS-treated cells strongly activate NF-κB. We also demonstrated that Mox1-induced NF-κB induced cyclooxygenase-2 mRNA, which is known to be regulated mainly by NF-κB (data not shown).

The activation of NF-κB plays an important role in initiation of inflammation through expression of inflammatory response genes, such as chemokines, cytokines, and adhesion molecules. All of these products initiate recruitment and activation of inflammatory cells and the evolution of inflammation. The evidence that gastric pit cells have a Mox1 oxidase system may provide a previously unrealized pathway for initiating the inflammatory responses in gastric mucosa. The findings reported here are compatible with (but do not prove) the concept that gastric pit cells them-

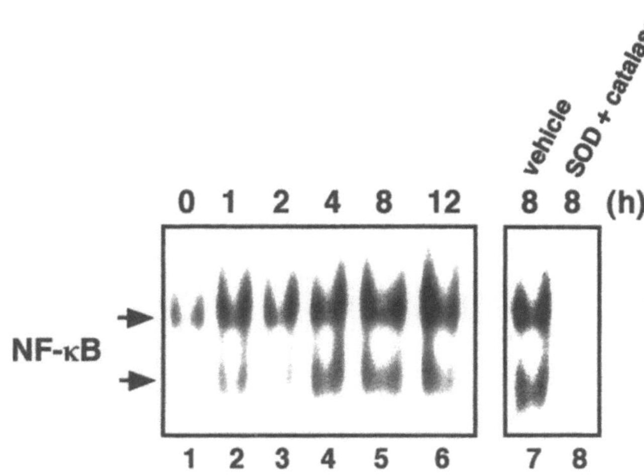

FIG. 2. Activation of nuclear factor κB (NF-κB). After cells were primed with *Helicobacter pylori* lipopolysaccharide (LPS) at 10 ng/ml for 12 h, cells were washed to remove the LPS and further incubated for the indicated times in serum-free medium alone (lanes *1–6*) or with vehicle (lane *7*) or superoxide dismutase (*SOD*) 200 U/ml plus catalase 350 U/ml (lane *8*). Nuclear extracts were prepared from the cells and analyzed by the gel mobility shift assay as described in Materials and Methods

selves may actively regulate the inflammatory and immune responses against *H. pylori* infection.

References

1. Babior BM (1999) NADPH oxidase: an update. Blood 93:1464–1476
2. Cross AR, Jones OTG (1991) Enzymic mechanisms of superoxide production. Biochim Biophys Acta 1057:281–298
3. Suh Y-A, Arnold RS, Lassegue B, et al (1999) Cell transformation by the superoxide-generating oxidase Mox1. Nature 401:79–82
4. Teshima S, Rokutan K, Nikawa T, et al (1998) Guinea pig gastric mucosal cells produce abundant superoxide anion through an NADPH oxidase-like system. Gastroenterology 115:1186–1196
5. Teshima S, Tsunawaki S, Rokutan K (1999) *Helicobacter pylori* lipopolysaccharide enhances the expression of NADPH oxidase components in cultured guinea pig gastric mucosal cells. FEBS Lett 452:243–246
6. Teshima S, Kutsumi H, Kawahara T, et al (2000) Regulation of cell growth and apoptosis of gastric pit cells by Mox1 oxidase. Am J Physiol 279:G1169–G1176
7. Rokutan K, Teshima S, Miyoshi M, et al (1997) Oxidant-induced activation of nuclear factor-kappa B in cultured guinea pig gastric mucosal cells. Dig Dis Sci 42:1880–1889

Role of PPARγ in the Growth and Differentiation of Gastric and Colorectal Cancers

YOSHIJI MIYAZAKI*, SHINJI KITAMURA, YASUHISA SHINOMURA, and YUJI MATSUZAWA

Summary. Several colonic and gastric cancer cell lines express peroxisome proliferator activated receptor γ (PPARγ), a member of the nuclear receptor superfamily. The thiazolidinedione class of antidiabetic drugs including troglitazone and rosiglitazone are known to be ligands for PPARγ. Treatment with troglitazone inhibits the growth of colonic cancer cells and promotes their differentiation. Troglitazone also inhibits the growth of MKN-45 gastric cancer cells, which overexpress c-Met tyrosine kinase. Thus PPARγ ligands may be candidates for a novel approach to the treatment of gastric and colorectal cancers. Ligand activation of PPARγ reduces the expression of c-Met tyrosine kinase, which is suggested to be one mechanism by which troglitazone inhibits the growth of MKN-45 cells. The mechanisms whereby PPARγ inhibits the growth of gastric and colorectal carcinoma cells in general remain unknown. Further investigations are needed to clarify the role of PPARγ in the proliferation and differentiation of gastrointestinal epithelial cells.

Key words. PPARγ, Stomach, Colon, Cancer, Transcription factor

Introduction

Peroxisome proliferator activated receptor γ (PPARγ) is a member of the nuclear receptor superfamily, which forms a heterodimeric DNA-binding complex with the 9-*cis*-retinoic acid receptor. Adipose tissue has been recognized as a principal site of PPARγ expression. PPARγ not only functions as a transcriptional regulator of genes linked to lipid metabolism, it plays a key role in adipocyte differentiation [1]. In addition to adipose tissue, PPARγ is expressed in some other tissues including gastrointestinal epithelial cells.

Department of Internal Medicine and Molecular Science, Graduate School of Medicine, Osaka University, 2-2 Yamadaoka, Suita, Osaka 565-0871, Japan
* e-mail: miyazaki@imed2.med.osaka-u.ac.jp.

Ligands for PPARγ and Adipocyte Differentiation

PPARγ recognizes the peroxisomal proliferator response element (PPRE) in the promoter of its target genes. Several polyunsaturated fatty acids, the nuclear prostanoid 15-deoxy-delta^{12,14}-prostaglandin J_2, nonsteroidal antiinflammatory drugs (NSAIDs), and the thiazolidinedione class of antidiabetic drugs (e.g., troglitazone and rosiglitazone) have been identified as ligands for PPARγ. Ligand activation of PPARγ induces cell cycle withdrawal of preadipocytes, promotes adipogenesis [1], and even causes growth inhibition of liposarcoma. In a clinical trial of patients with advanced liposarcoma, administration of troglitazone induced the differentiation of such tumors in vivo.

PPARγ in Colon Cancer

One early immunohistochemical study demonstrated that high expression of PPARγ is observed in the more differentiated murine colonic epithelial cells facing the intestinal lumen compared with cells in the lower parts of the crypts. Subsequent studies have shown that PPARγ is expressed in azoxymethane-treated rat colonic carcinoma cells and several colon cancer cell lines. PPARγ expressed in colon cancer cell lines is functional because treatment with troglitazone activates the transcription of PPRE-containing luciferase reporter genes transfected into the cells.

Investigations, including ours, have shown that activation of PPARγ causes growth inhibition and induces differentiation of colon cancer cells [2]. In addition, in vivo animal studies have shown that xenograft tumor growth can be markedly suppressed by treatment with PPARγ ligands. In contrast, it has been reported that activation of PPARγ can promote the development of colon tumors in C57BL/6J-APC^{Min}/+ mice, an animal model of familial adenomatous polyposis coli [3,4]. The reason for this discrepancy is unknown, and further investigations are needed.

PPARγ in Gastric Cancer

Two reports indicated that MKN-45 gastric cancer cell lines express PPARγ, and that troglitazone can activate transcription of PPRE-containing luciferase reporter genes. In addition, ligand activation of PPARγ inhibits the growth and induces apoptosis of MKN-45 cells. Because of its gene amplification, c-Met tyrosine kinase is constitutively phosphorylated and supposed to be involved in the proliferation and apoptosis resistance of MKN-45 cells. Our study demonstrated that treatment with troglitazone reduces the levels of c-Met mRNA and protein and inhibits its autophosphorylation in MKN-45 cells [5]. Reduction of c-Met tyrosine kinase may be one mechanism by which troglitazone inhibits the growth of MKN-45 cells.

Interaction with Other Transcription Factors

PPARγ directly regulates the expression of numerous genes of lipid metabolism by binding to its response element in the promoter. In addition, evidence suggests that

PPARγ may regulate the expression of several genes by interacting with other transcription factors. Our study indicated that PPARγ activation suppresses Ets-induced c-MET gene transcription in a gastric cancer cell line [5]. In adipogenic HIB1B cells, the DNA binding and transcriptional activity of the cell growth-promoting E2F/DP transcription factors is inhibited following PPARγ activation [6]. Activation of PPARγ in peripheral macrophages leads to inhibition of phorbol ester-induced nitric oxide and cytokine production [7]. This antiinflammatory action is elicited by antagonizing activities of transcription factors, activated protein-1 (AP-1), and nuclear factor (NF)-κB. In differentiated human monocyte-derived macrophages, ligand activation of PPARγ induces apoptosis and inhibits the transcriptional activity of the NF-κB p65/ RelA subunit [8]. These results suggest that PPARγ activators induce macrophage apoptosis by negatively interfering with the antiapoptotic NF-κB signaling pathway.

The molecular mechanisms by which activation of PPARγ reduces the transcriptional activity of several transcription factors are not well understood. One possibility is that PPARγ directly interacts with other transcription factors. A recent report indicated that activated PPARγ physically associates with the T cell-specific transcription factor, NF-AT, and blocks NF-AT DNA binding and transcriptional activity [9]. It is unknown whether PPARγ directly associates with the other transcription factors. Another possibility is that PPARγ competes with the other transcription factors for interacting with common co-activators such as CBP/p300. Previous studies suggested that inhibition of AP-1 activity by several nuclear receptors is the apparent result of competition for limited amounts of CBP/p300. Although PPARγ is known to interact with several co-activators [10], it is unknown whether this mechanism is true for PPARγ inhibition of several transcription factors.

References

1. Chawla A, Schwarz EJ, Dimaculangan DD, et al (1994) Peroxisome proliferator-activated receptor (PPAR) γ: adipose-predominant expression and induction early in adipocyte differentiation. Endocrinology 135:798–800
2. Kitamura S, Miyazaki Y, Shinomura Y, et al (1999) Peroxisome proliferator-activated receptor γ induces growth arrest and differentiation markers of human colon cancer cells. Jpn J Cancer Res 90:75–80
3. Lefebvre AM, Chen I, Desreumaux P, et al (1998) Activation of the peroxisome proliferator-activated receptor γ promotes the development of colon tumors in C57BL/6J-APCMin/+mice. Nat Med 4:1053–1057
4. Saez E, Tontonoz P, Nelson MC, et al (1998) Activators of the nuclear receptor PPARγ enhance colon polyp formation. Nat Med 4:1058–1061
5. Kitamura S, Miyazaki Y, Hiraoka S, et al (1999) PPARγ inhibits the expression of c-MET in human gastric cancer cells through the suppression of Ets. Biochem Biophys Res Commun 265:453–456
6. Altiok S, Xu M, Spiegelman BM (1997) PPARγ induces cell cycle withdrawal: inhibition of E2F/DP DNA-binding activity via down-regulation of PP2A. Genes Dev 11: 1987–1998
7. Ricote M, Li AC, Willson TM, et al (1998) The peroxisome proliferator-activated receptor-γ is a negative regulator of macrophage activation. Nature 391:79–82
8. Jiang C, Ting AT, Seed B (1998) PPAR-γ agonists inhibit production of monocyte inflammatory cytokines. Nature 391:82–86

9. Yang XY, Wang LH, Chen T, et al (2000) Activation of human T lymphocytes is inhibited by peroxisome proliferator-activated receptor γ (PPARγ) agonists: PPARγ co-association with transcription factor NFAT. J Biol Chem 275:4541–4544
10. Gelman L, Fruchart JC, Auwerx J (1999) An update on the mechanisms of action of the peroxisome proliferator-activated receptors (PPARs) and their roles in inflammation and cancer. Cell Mol Life Sci 55:932–943

PPARγ Ligand and Induction of Growth Arrest in Pancreatic Cancer Cells

AYMAN ELNEMR[1,*], TETSUO OHTA[1], SACHIO FUSHIDA[1], ITASU NINOMIYA[1], GENICHI NISHIMURA[1], HIROHISA KITAGAWA[1], MASATO KAYAHARA[1], TADASHI TERADA[2], and KOICHI MIWA[1]

Summary. Peroxisome proliferator-activated receptor γ (PPARγ), one of the nuclear receptors expressed in adipose tissue, plays an important role in adipocyte differentiation. In this study, we investigated the expression of PPARγ and its role in cellular growth in five pancreatic cancer cell lines: Capan-1, AsPC-1, BxPC-3, PANC-1, and MIA PaCa-2. All five expressed PPARγ mRNA and protein, shown respectively on reverse transcriptase-polymerase chain reaction (RT-PCR) and Western blot analysis. Clonogenic assays showed that thiazolidinedione (TZD), the parent compound of PPARγ ligands, completely inhibits colony formation of these cells at a concentration of 10 μM. Moreover, treatment of these cells with 10 μM TZD resulted in G_0/G_1 cell cycle arrest. In conclusion, pancreatic cancer cell lines express PPARγ, and PPARγ ligand cytostatically inhibits cell growth.

Key words. Peroxisome proliferator-activated receptor γ, Nuclear receptor, Thiazolidinedione, Pancreatic cancer, Growth arrest

Introduction

Adenocarcinoma of the pancreas is one of the most lethal malignancies. Unfortunately, more than 90% of pancreatic cancer patients present with metastatic disease or advanced local disease, precluding curative surgical resection. Chemotherapy has not resulted in a significant survival benefit [1]. On the basis of these observations, it is clear that new molecular targets are needed for the prevention and treatment of pancreatic cancer.

Peroxisome proliferator-activated receptor γ (PPARγ), a transcription factor belonging to the nuclear receptor superfamily, forms functional heterodimers with the retinoid X receptor [2]. PPARγ is of great current interest because it mediates the antidiabetic effects of several thiazolidinediones (TZDs) that are now in widespread

[1]Department of Surgery II, School of Medicine, Kanazawa University, 13-1 Takara-machi, Kanazawa 920-0934, Japan
[2]Department of Pathology II, School of Medicine, Tottori University, 86 Nishi-machi, Yanago, Tottori 683-8503, Japan
* e-mail: aymann1@yahoo.com

clinical use for treating type 2 diabetes [3]. Interestingly, PPARγ has a preference for polyunsaturated fatty acids and dietary components that have shown to lower the incidence of cancer in experimental animals [4], although the clinical relevance of these observations remains unclear.

Synthetic PPARγ ligands have been shown to inhibit the growth of several human tumor cell lines and, most notably, to induce growth arrest and differentiation in primary cultures of human liposarcoma and breast cancer cells in vitro and in vivo [5,6]. In contrast, there have been conflicting reports on the effects of the TZD class of PPARγ ligands in experimental colon carcinogenesis [7,8]. To our knowledge, this is the first report focusing on PPARγ expression in pancreatic cancer and induction of growth arrest by its ligand treatment.

Expression of PPARγ in Pancreatic Cancer

We initially examined the expression of PPARγ in pancreatic cancer cell lines using reverse transcriptase polymerase chain reaction (RT-PCR). Five pancreatic cancer cell lines—Capan-1, AsPC-1, BxPC-3, PANC-1, MIA PaCa-2—expressed PPARγ mRNA at significant levels (Fig. 1A). Moreover, in the surgically resected specimens PPARγ mRNA was strongly expressed in cancerous tissues compared to their normal coun-

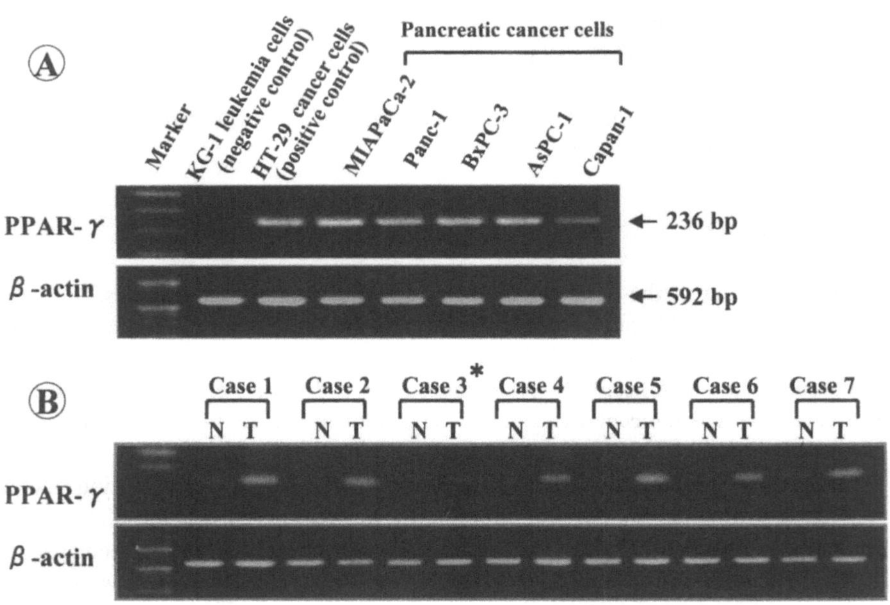

FIG. 1. Expression of peroxisome proliferator-activated receptor γ (PPARγ) mRNA in pancreatic cancer. **A** Expression of PPARγ mRNA in pancreatic cancer lines. A 236-bp band corresponds to nucleotides 545–778 of the PPARγ cDNA. **B** Expression of PPARγ mRNA in representative pancreatic cancer tissues of seven patients. PPARγ mRNA was strongly expressed in cancerous tissue (*T*) when compared to their noncancerous counterparts (*N*)

terparts (Fig. 1B). Western blotting showed that PPARγ protein was expressed as a doublet (PPARγ1 and PPARγ2) with an approximate molecular mass of 60kDa in all cell lines. Interestingly, PPARγ expression was high in cell lines that are known to be poorly differentiated, such as PANC-1 and MIA PaCa-2. Meanwhile, it was low in Capan-1 cells, a well-differentiated cell line. However, expression of this receptor in a differentiation-related fashion has not been established (Fig. 2A). PPARγ-positive immunocytochemical staining was detected in the nuclei of all cell lines. As shown in Fig. 2B, representative PANC-1 cells show intense nuclear staining.

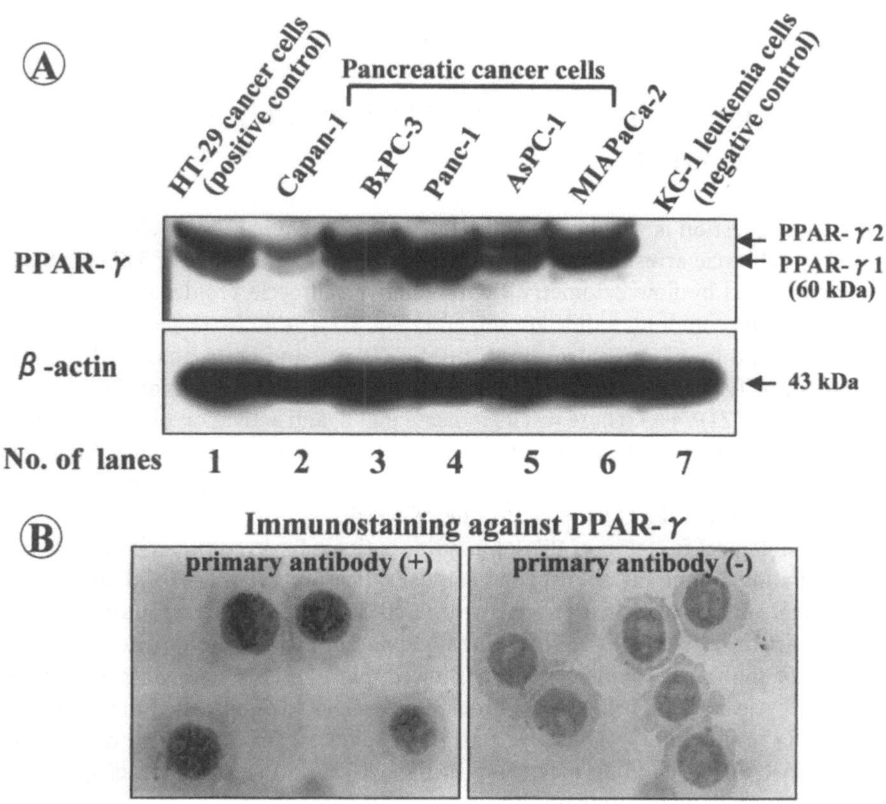

FIG. 2. PPARγ protein expression in pancreatic cancer. **A** PPARγ expression in pancreatic cancer cell lines. KG-1 leukemia cell line was used as negative control (lane *7*); HT-29 colon cancer cell line was used as a positive control (lane *1*). PPARγ protein was expressed as a doublet with an approximate molecular mass of 60kDa in all cell lines, consistent with the predicted mass of PPARγ1 and PPARγ2. **B** Immunocytochemical staining using anti-PPARγ rabbit polyclonal antibody on cytospin preparations. Slides were counter-stained with hematoxylin and eosin. *Right*: PPARγ-positive immunocytochemical nuclear staining is shown in representative PANC-1 cells. *Left*: Negative control cells were treated with nonimmune serum instead of the primary antibody. (×1200)

PPARγ Ligand Treatment and Inhibition of Clonogenic Growth

We confirmed that the high PPARγ expression in pancreatic cancer cell lines is relevant, so we examined the effect of activating PPARγ on the ability of the pancreatic cell lines to form colonies when plated at low seeding densities in soft agar. The clonogenic capacity of all five cell lines was potently inhibited by a TZD (the parent compound of thiazolidinediones), a specific and high-affinity agonist for PPARγ, in a dose-related fashion, with an inhibitory concentration of 50% (IC_{50}) at a concentration of 5μM and complete inhibition at a concentration of 10μM. The dose of TZD that effectively inhibits cell growth of pancreatic cancer cells in this study is the same as that needed to induce growth inhibition of human colon cancer cells, as shown by Saraf et al. [7]. The mechanism by which TZD induces growth inhibition in pancreatic cancer cells remains to be clarified.

PPARγ Ligand Treatment and Induction of Cell Cycle Arrest

A critical question is whether TZD treatment of pancreatic cancer cells is accompanied by cell cycle arrest. Cells cultured in the presence or absence of TZD for 8 days were analyzed by flow cytometry. Representative cell cycle profiles of BxPC-3 cells stained with propidium iodide are shown in Fig. 3D. The TZD-treated cells exhibited a decreased S fraction (control 14%; 10μM TZD 8%) and G_2/M-phase cells (control 22%; 10μM TZD 14%) resulting from increased accumulation of cells at G_0/G_1 (control 60%; 10μM TZD 74%). These results indicate that ligand activation of PPARγ inhibits cellular growth and induces cell cycle arrest at G_0/G_1 in pancreatic cancer. Treatment of cancer cells with 10μM TZD for 8 days resulted in a significant increase in the number of cells in the G_0/G_1 phase of the cell cycle.

The biological function of PPARγ in adipose tissue has traditionally been defined as regulation of lipid metabolism and adipose differentiation [3]. We did not find that treatment of pancreatic cancer cells with TZD stimulated differentiation along the adipose pathway (based on our finding no apparent increase in lipid accumulation) (data not shown). A couple of reports showed that PPARγ is closely associated with the cell cycle, altering cell growth. Brockman et al. [9] demonstrated that activation of PPARγ resulted in G_0/G_1 cell cycle arrest in colon cancer cells. These data suggest that PPARγ ligand binding may result in the activation or expression of genes that modulate cell cycle progression.

Conclusions

The results described here demonstrate that PPARγ expression is elevated in pancreatic cancer cell lines and tissues, at both the RNA and protein levels. Most importantly, these receptors are functioning, as PPARγ ligand treatment caused a pronounced inhibitory effect on the clonogenic growth of these cells. This tumor-suppressive effect of PPARγ may provide a nontoxic therapeutic approach to the treatment of pancre-

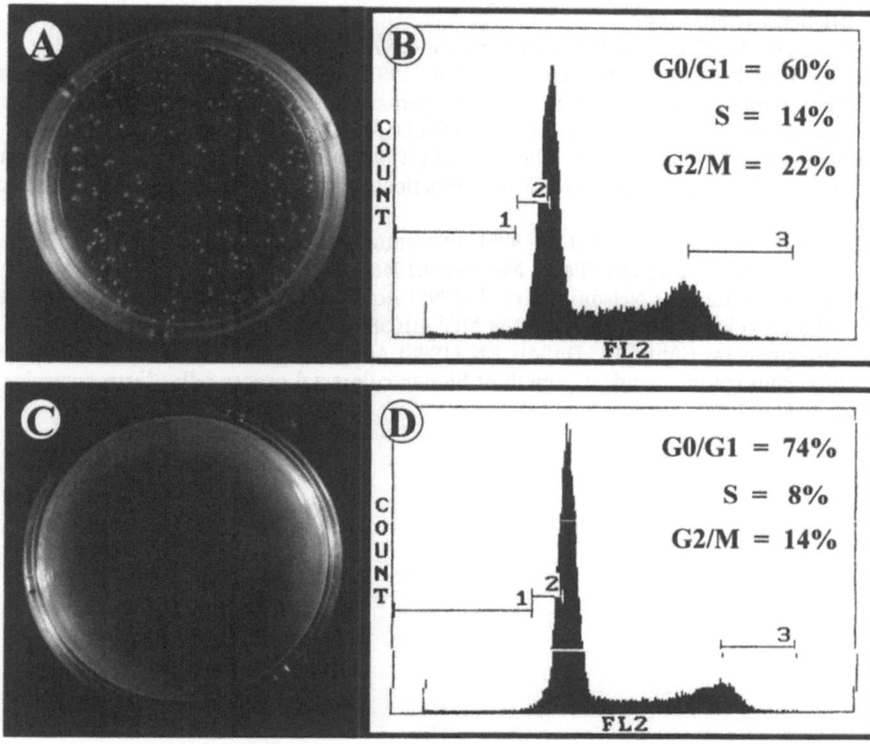

FIG. 3. **A,C** Clonogenic growth of B×PC-3 cells in two-layer soft agar after 16 days. **A** Cells were cultured in the presence of vehicle [0.1% dimethylsulfoxide (DMSO)]. **C** Cells were cultured in the presence of 10 μM thiazolidinedione (TZD) show complete inhibition of colony formation. **B,D** PPARγ activation induces G_0/G_1 cell cycle arrest. Cells were harvested, stained with propidium iodide, and analyzed for DNA content by fluorescence-activated cell sorter analysis. The values represent the number of cells in each phase of the cell cycle as a percentage of total cells. **B** B×PC-3 cells were treated with 0.1% DMSO. **D** B×PC-3 cells were treated with 10 μM TZD for 8 days. These experiments were repeated three times with similar results

atic cancer. Moreover, it could provide a key link between dietary fatty acid precursors and the transcriptional regulation that may be involved in pancreatic carcinogenesis. Work is under way to determine the mechanisms of action and biological relevance of this aberrant expression of PPARγ in pancreatic cancer.

References

1. Ahlgren JD (1996) Epidemiology and risk factor in pancreatic cancer. Semin Oncol 23:241–250
2. Kliewer SA, Umesono K, Noonan DJ, et al (1992) Convergence of *9-cis* retinoic acid and peroxisome proliferator signaling pathways through heterodimer formation of their receptors. Nature 358:771–774

3. Spiegelman BM (1998) PPARγ: adipogenic regulator and thiazolidinedione receptor. Diabetes 47:507–514
4. Rose DP (1997) Dietary fatty acids and cancer. Am J Clin Nutr 66:998S–1003S
5. Tontonoz P, Singer S, Forman BM, et al (1997) Terminal differentiation of human liposarcoma cells induced by ligands for peroxisome proliferator-activated receptor γ and retinoid X receptor. Proc Natl Acad Sci USA 94:237–241
6. Demetri GD, Fletcher CD, Mueller E, et al (1999) Induction of solid tumor differentiation by the PPARγ ligand trogliazone in patients with liposarcoma. Proc Natl Acad Sci USA 95:3951–3956
7. Saraf P, Mueller E, Jones D, et al (1998) Differentiation and reversal of malignant changes in colon cancer through PPARγ. Nat Med 4:1046–1052
8. Saez E, Tontonoz P, Nelson MC, et al (1998) Activators of the nuclear receptor PPARγ enhance colon polyp formation. Nat Med 4:1058–1061
9. Brockman JA, Gupta RA, DuBois RN (1998) Activation of PPARγ leads to inhibition of anchorage-independent growth of human colorectal cancer cells. Gastroenterology 115:1049–1055

Role of β-Catenin During Early Colorectal and Hepatic Carcinogenesis

MASARU MURATA[1,*] and YASUO MIYOSHI[2]

Summary. β-Catenin has been identified as an oncogene in several tumors including colorectal and hepatocellular carcinomas. The β-catenin gene is activated by interstitial deletions involving exon 3 in 3% of colorectal cancers in the Japanese population, by missense mutations in critical serine/threonine residues including exon 3 in 16% of colorectal cancers in Caucasians, and by missense mutations or interstitial deletions in 19%–26% of hepatocellular carcinomas. The type and frequency of the mutation of this gene in colorectal adenomas in Japanese and Caucasians are similar to those in colorectal cancers in each population. As for hepatic tumors, expression of β-catenin correlates with its accumulation in the cytoplasm and nuclei, which implies activation of the Wnt/Wingless signal transduction pathway in adenomatous hyperplasias and for each differentiation grade of hepatocellular carcinomas with similar frequency. In conclusion, activation of the β-catenin gene by interstitial deletions or missense mutations in the Japanese and Caucasian populations, respectively, may be less frequent than alterations of the adenomatous polyposis coli (*APC*) gene, but it may be an early event in colorectal tumorigenesis that is equivalent to *APC* gene alterations. The Wnt/Wingless signal transduction pathway may be activated during early hepatic carcinogenesis.

Key words. β-Catenin, Colorectal carcinogenesis, Hepatic carcinogenesis, Colorectal adenoma, Adenomatous hyperplasia

Introduction

β-Catenin is known to have two principal functions; first, it acts as a cell–cell adhesion regulatory protein that binds cadherin. In various cancers including colorectal and hepatocellular carcinomas, reduction of β-catenin expression correlates with dif-

[1] Department of Surgery, Ikeda Municipal Hospital, 3-1-18 Jonan, Ikeda, Osaka 563-8510, Japan
[2] Division of Clinical Genetics, Department of Medical Genetics, Biomedical Research Center (B9), Osaka University Medical School, 2-2 Yamadaoka, Suita, Osaka 565-0871, Japan
* e-mail: muratamasaru@mth.biglobe.ne.jp

ferentiation and invasiveness of the tumor. Second, β-catenin is involved in the Wnt/Wingless signal transduction pathway. Abnormally accumulated β-catenin in the cytoplasm, caused by dysfunction of the *APC* gene or activation of β-catenin by mutation of its gene, translocates into the nucleus by binding with high mobility group box factors of the Lef/Tcf (lymphoid enhancer binding factor/T cell specific transcriptional factor) family, a DNA binding protein, where it serves as a transcriptional factor for target genes such as c-*myc* or *cyclin D1*. Activation of the β-catenin gene by somatic alterations such as amino acid substitutions and interstitial deletions involving critical serine or threonine residues in exon 3 have been recognized in colorectal carcinomas, melanomas, hepatocellular carcinomas, endometrial cancers, medulloblastomas, endometrioid ovarian cancers, prostate cancers, and desmoid tumors. In this chapter we review these data and discuss the role of β-catenin during early colorectal and hepatic carcinogenesis.

Role of β-Catenin in Colorectal Carcinogenesis

The genetic changes underlying the multistep process of development and progression of colorectal carcinogenesis are relatively well defined. For example, mutations of the adenomatous polyposis coli (*APC*) tumor-suppressor gene result in a series of sequential genetic alterations such as activation or dysfunction of K-*ras*, *p53*, and deleted colorectal cancer (*DCC*) genes (adenoma–carcinoma sequence). Among these events, mutations of the *APC* gene is believed to play a crucial role during the early process in association with β-catenin and glycogen synthase kinase 3-β.

Most truncated APC protein generated by somatic or germ-line mutation lacks a β-catenin binding domain, resulting in disturbance of degradation of β-catenin. β-Catenin then accumulates in the cytoplasm. In colorectal cancers, *APC* gene mutations are recognized in about 70% cases [1,2].

β-Catenin can also accumulate in the cytoplasm via oncogenic activation of the β-catenin gene itself. It has been reported that the β-catenin gene is activated by interstitial deletions in the Japanese population or missense mutations in Caucasians involving exon 3 in about 3% [1] and 16% [2], respectively, of primary colorectal carcinomas without *APC* abnormalities. The type and frequency of mutations of this gene in colorectal adenomas are similar to those in colorectal cancers among each population, respectively (Table 1). Activation of the β-catenin gene by interstitial deletions in the Japanese population and missense mutations in Caucasians may be less frequent compared with the frequent alterations of the *APC* gene, but it can be an early event in colorectal tumorigenesis equivalent to *APC* gene alterations.

Role of β-Catenin in Hepatocellular Carcinogenesis

It was recently demonstrated that 16%–26% of hepatocellular carcinomas (HCCs) are targeted for oncogenic activation of the β-catenin gene via somatic alterations involving exon 3 [3,4]. These alterations include amino acid substitutions in serine or threonine residues in exon 3 at codons 33, 37, 41, and 45 or residues flanking the serine residues at codon 33 as well as interstitial deletions involving some of these residues in exon 3, which result in the cytoplasmic accumulation of β-catenin. Meanwhile,

TABLE 1. β-Catenin gene mutations in primary colorectal tumors

Colorectal tumors in Japanese or Caucasians	Frequency of β-catenin gene mutations
Colorectal adenomas	
Japanese	3/100 (3%)[a]
Caucasians	2/16 (13%)[b]
Colorectal cancers	
Japanese	7/222 (3.2%)[c]
Caucasians	4/25 (16%)[d]

[a] Type of β-catenin gene mutation of all three cases were interstitial deletions
[b] One case contained missense mutation, and another case contained interstitial deletion
[c] Type of β-catenin gene mutation of all seven cases were interstitial deletions
[d] Type of β-catenin gene mutation of all four cases were missense mutations

accumulation of β-catenin in the cytoplasm and nuclei is more frequent than the gene mutation among HCCs. *AXIN1* mutations recognized in 5% of HCCs can explain the discrepancy of the frequency of *CTNNB1* mutation and β-catenin accumulation [4]. Accumulation of β-catenin in the cytoplasm and nuclei is observed in more than 30% of HCCs, and the frequency is similar among each differentiation grade as well as in adenomatous hyperplasias, which are precancerous lesions of the liver. Considering these data, the Wnt/Wingless signal transduction pathway may be activated during early hepatic carcinogenesis.

β-Catenin Gene Mutation in Other Cancers from Various Anatomic Sites

Activation of the β-catenin gene by somatic alteration has previously been recognized in various tumors. Among them, most cases with β-catenin gene abnormalities is concentrated in missense mutations at serine/threonine phosphorylation sites and the flanking residues. Another important mechanism of oncogenic activation of the β-catenin gene is interstitial deletion involving exon 3. Such a mutation has been recognized in colorectal cancers [1], adenomas, and a case of small intestinal cancer [5] in the Japanese population and in HCCs in the Japanese and Caucasian populations [3,4]. The different types of mutation in the same gene in Japanese patients and those of other racial backgrounds for colorectal and small intestinal tumors may reflect dietary or environmental differences or different genetic backgrounds.

Conclusions

Interstitial deletions or missense mutations involving exon 3, including critical serine/threonine residues in Japanese and Caucasian populations, respectively, may be less frequent than alterations of the *APC* gene, but they may be an early event in colorectal tumorigenesis equivalent to *APC* gene alterations. The Wnt/Wingless signal transduction pathway may be activated during early hepatic carcinogenesis.

References

1. Iwao K, Nakamori S, Kameyama M, et al (1998) Activation of the β-catenin gene by interstitial deletions involving exon 3 in primary colorectal carcinomas without adenomatous polyposis coli mutations. Cancer Res 58:1021–1026
2. Sparks AB, Morin PJ, Vogelstein B, et al (1998) Mutational analysis of the APC/β-catenin/Tcf pathway in colorectal cancer. Cancer Res 58:1130–1134
3. Miyoshi Y, Iwao K, Nagasawa Y, et al (1998) Activation of the β-catenin gene in primary hepatocellular carcinomas by somatic alterations involving exon 3. Cancer Res 58:2524–2527
4. Satoh S, Daigo Y, Furukawa Y, et al (2000) Axin 1 mutations in hepatocellular carcinomas, and growth suppression in cancer cells by virus-mediated transfer of axin 1. Nat Genet 24:245–250
5. Murata M, Iwao K, Miyoshi Y, et al (2000) Molecular and biological analysis of carcinoma of small intestine: β-catenin gene mutation by interstitial deletion involving exon 3 and replication error phenotype. Am J Gastroenterol 95:1576–1580

Growth Inhibition of Hepatoma Cells by Type 1 Interferons: Modification by Mutations in the Interferon Regulatory Factor-1 Gene

Hidetsugu Saito*, Shinichiro Tada, Kanji Wakabayashi, Tamako Takagi, Nobuhiro Nakamoto, Satoshi Kurita, and Hiromasa Ishii

Summary. Interferon regulatory factor-1 is an important transcription factor in the interferon system. We have demonstrated that the growth inhibitory effect of type 1 interferons on human hepatoma cells correlates with levels of transcription of the interferon regulatory factor-1 gene. In this study we investigated whether mutations in this gene cause different responses to type 1 interferons. DNA from several human hepatoma cell lines was investigated, and nucleotide sequences of the interferon regulatory factor-1 gene were determined. Several point mutations were detected in intron 8 of the gene, and one was found to cause deletion of BamHI cleavage sites. We found several point mutations in the upstream region of the interferon regulatory factor-1 exon 1, and the luciferase promoter assay demonstrated that these mutations modified its promoter activity. These results suggest that polymorphisms of the interferon regulatory factor-1 gene partially contribute to determining the response of cancer cells to growth inhibitory effect of type 1 interferons.

Key words. Interferon-α/β, Polymorphism, Interferon regulatory factor, Transcription factor

Introduction

An antiproliferative effect of interferon-α (IFNα) has been demonstrated in various types of cells in vitro, but the mechanism of growth inhibition is not fully understood. IFNα inhibits cell cycle progression of hepatoma cells, but it was demonstrated that its growth inhibitory effect varies among cell lines regardless of the expression levels of IFNα receptor 2 on the cell surface [1]. This study indicates that the growth inhibition levels do not depend on the expression levels of the receptor, and different efficiency levels of the signal transduction pathways of IFNα are postulated.

Department of Internal Medicine, School of Medicine, Keio University, 35 Shinanomachi, Shinjuku-ku, Tokyo 160-8582, Japan
* e-mail: hsaito@mc.med.keio.ac.jp

We reported the antiproliferative effect of the type I IFNs on several human hepatoma cell lines [2]. These lines could be divided into two types based on high or low sensitivity to IFN-induced growth suppression. The degree of growth inhibition of cells seemed to depend on their level of $p21^{WAF-1}$ induction, and these levels paralleled the *IRF-1* transcription levels. *IRF-1* gene rearrangement by BamHI digestion was found in some lines, but no significant nucleotide differences were detected in their whole cDNA. These results suggest that *IRF-1* gene abnormalities would modify its transcription levels and be associated with growth suppression rates. On the other hand, nucleotide polymorphisms are the most common form of human genetic variation and may contribute to the sensitivity of the person to various medicines [3]. The promoter of the human *IRF-1* gene is rich in GC and contains various transcription factor binding domains, such as CpG islands, GC boxes, putative nuclear factor κB (NF-κB) binding sites, and many positive regulatory domains for IFNs [4]. These observations suggest a relation between nucleotide polymorphisms and change in the IRF-1 transcription levels by IFN stimulation. We investigated nucleotide polymorphisms of the *IRF-1* gene in human hepatoma cell lines.

Materials and Methods

Cell Lines and IRF-1 *Gene Rearrangement by BamHI Digestion*

We investigated HLE, HLF, HepG2, Chang cells, HCC-T, HCC-M, and PLC/PRF/5 cell lines; the latter two were used as DNA sources for the *IRF-1* promoter. These cell lines showed different sensitivities to the growth inhibition of IFNα in the previous study [2].

DNA was extracted according to the procedure described previously [5]. Because DNA rearrangement of the *IRF-1* gene as detected by BamHI digestion was observed but no contributing mutation was detected in the cDNA sequence in our previous study [2], we investigated nine intron DNAs in this study. Because sequences in the *IRF-1* introns may be more variable than in the exons, primers were designed in the exons of the gene, using database GenBank No. L05072. Nine pairs of primers were synthesized as described previously [6]. The polymerase chain reaction (PCR) was performed according to the method described previously [7] using Gene Amp PCR System 2400 (Perkin-Elmer, Norwalk, CT, USA).

IRF-1 *Promoter*

The human *IRF-1* promoter was amplified by PCR. The PCR primers were designed from the database (GenBank No. X53095) to amplify 669 bp of the *IRF-1* promoter (nucleotide position at −492 to +177). The PCR product was purified and ligated to pGL3/XhoI-MluI (Promega, Madison, WI, USA). DNA sequencing was performed using the sequence primers in the genome of plasmid vector, followed by comparison with the database (GenBank). We determined the *IRF-1* promoter sequences of DNAs from HCC-M and PLC/PRF/5.

Luciferase reporter assays were performed using the Dual-Luciferase Reporter Assay System (Promega) and two promoter regions obtained from HCC-M and PLC/PRF/5 cells. We used FUGENE6 transfection reagent (Clontech, Palo Alto, CA, USA). Sampling was carried out 24 or 48h after the transfection. pRL-TK vector (Promega) was used as a control that contains a herpes simplex virus thymidine kinase promoter in the upstream region of the *Renilla* (*Renilla reniformis*) luciferase gene. The *IRF-1* promoter regions from both HCC-M and PLC/PRF/5 were cloned into a pGL3-Enhancer vector (Promega); and *IRF-1*-promoter–luciferase reporter constructs were obtained.

In some experiments, the PCR products were directly sequenced using an ABI BigDye Terminator Cycle Sequencing Ready Reaction Kit and an ABI PRISM 377XL DNA Sequencer (PE Applied Biosystems). The nucleotide sequence of the PCR product was analyzed using affiliated software in the DNA sequencer (Sequence Analysis 3.3, Basecaller SemiAdaptive, and Sequence Navigator 1.0.1; PE Biosystems) and FASTA or TFASTA as described previously [5].

Results

Point Mutations in the Intron 8 of the IRF-1 *Gene*

The PCR products of the introns of the *IRF-1* gene from the three human hepatoma lines showed no difference in size, suggesting an absence of deletions, insertions, or translocations in nine introns of the *IRF-1* gene. We digested the PCR products with BamHI and examined modifications of three specific BamHI sites in the *IRF-1* genome. Finally, in intron 8 the primer set generates a 1238-bp fragment, and BamHI digestion results in 404-bp and 834-bp fragments; however, the BamHI site could not be found in DNA from HCC-T and HCC-M, which shows that the DNA rearrangement demonstrated in our previous study was caused by deletion of BamHI sites in the genomes of HCC-T and HCC-M.

The PCR products from intron 8 in the cell lines were directly sequenced. The mutation at position 5445 (GenBank L05078) caused a GGATCC to GGATCT change that deleted the BamHI site in this region in HCC-M and HCC-T cells. PLC/PRF/5 had the same nucleotide sequence as that in the GenBank database (L05072).

IRF-1 *Promoter*

A point mutation in cell lines HCC-M and PLC/PRF/5 was found at one site. No point mutation was found in the reported GC boxes, NF-κB binding sites, AARKGA hexamers, or GAAANN motifs. We found other three-point mutations in the genome of PLC/PRF/5.

The luciferase reporter assay was performed before and 4h after the addition of IFNα and IFNβ (1000 IU/ml each) using either HCC-M or PLC/PRF/5. Although the normalized inducibility was different between experiments, the promoter activities were increased by both IFNα and IFNβ. Those activities were always higher in the PLC/PRF/5 cells, and those obtained with the PLC/PRF/5 promoter were always higher.

Discussion

A member of the cyclin-dependent kinase inhibitors, the *p21*$^{WAF-1}$ gene is regulated in response to DNA damage by both *IRF-1* and *p53* [8]. Others and we have demonstrated a *p53*-independent increase of *p21*$^{WAF-1}$ in response either to growth factor stimuli or exposure to differentiation-inducing agents [9,10]. Several *IRF-1*-binding sites have been found in the *p21*$^{WAF-1}$ promoter [8]. Moreover, one study directly demonstrated that the *p21*$^{WAF-1}$ gene is transactivated by *IRF-1* [11]. We demonstrated that growth inhibitory effects of IFNα partly depend on levels of expression of *p21*$^{WAF-1}$, which themselves depend on *IRF-1* transcription levels [2]. Thus, transcription seemed to vary among cell lines. We hypothesized that polymorphisms in the *IRF-1* gene contributed to interindividual differences in the response to type I IFNs and to the DNA rearrangement in the BamHI digestion site shown in the previous study [2]. We investigated variation of the BamHI sites in the *IRF-1* gene, and the nucleotide at position 5445*C was found to change to T, which resulted in the disappearance of the BamHI site in intron 8. We then screened the promoter of the *IRF-1* gene in search of common genomic variants with effects on transcription activity. We identified several point mutations in the *IRF-1* promoter. There are GC boxes within the CpG island of the *IRF-1* promoter [4]. Sp1 binds to elements containing a GC box and facilitates transcription [12], so the *IRF-1* gene is constitutively expressed. There are also κB motifs in this promoter, indicating that a number of agents can activate this gene [13]. However, we found no mutations in these known sites. These data suggest that novel transcription factors may bind to the site. Another possibility is that polymorphisms could change the conformation of this promoter region, which then changes the binding capacity of various transcription factors.

Conclusion

We found several nucleotide polymorphisms in the *IRF-1* gene. One of the mutations induces a DNA rearrangement of this gene by BamHI digestion. The polymorphisms in the upstream region of this gene modified its own promoter activity. These results demonstrated the possibility that nucleotide polymorphisms of the *IRF-1* gene cause intercellular variation of sensitivity to type I IFNs.

References

1. Yano H, Iemura A, Haramaki M, et al (1999) Interferon alfa receptor expression and growth inhibition by interferon alfa in human liver cancer cell lines. Hepatology 29:1708–1717
2. Tada S, Saito H, Tsunematsu S, et al (1998) Interferon regulatory factor-1 gene abnormality and loss of growth inhibitory effect of interferon-alpha in human hepatoma cell lines. Int J Oncol 13:1207–1216
3. Marth GT, Korf I, Yandell MD, et al (1999) A general approach to single-nucleotide polymorphism discovery. Nat Genet 23:452–456
4. Sims SH, Cha Y, Romine MF, et al (1993) A novel interferon-inducible domain: structural and functional analysis of the human interferon regulatory factor 1 gene promoter. Mol Cell Biol 13:690–702

5. Saito H, Tada S, Ebinuma H, et al (1996) Cloning of variable regions of an antibody that reacts with the soluble fraction of human liver cells and its possible value in chronic liver disease. Hepatology 23:1498–1506
6. Ebinuma H, Saito H, Saito Y, et al (1999) Antisense oligodeoxynucleotide against c-*myc* mRNA induces differentiation of human hepatocellular carcinoma cells. Int J Oncol 15:991–999
7. Shigematsu T, Miura S, Hirokawa M, et al (1998) Endothelins promote egg albumin-induced intestinal anaphylaxis in rats. Gastroenterology 115:348–356
8. Tanaka N, Ishihara M, Lamphier MS, et al (1996) Cooperation of the tumour suppressors *IRF-1* and *p53* in response to DNA damage. Nature 382:816–818
9. Zeng YX, el-Deiry WS (1996) Regulation of *p21* WAF1/CIP1 expression by *p53*-independent pathways. Oncogene 12:1557–1564
10. Saito H, Ebinuma H, Takahashi M, et al (1998) Loss of butyrate-induced apoptosis in human hepatoma cell lines HCC-M and HCC-T having substantial Bcl-2 expression. Hepatology 27:1233–1240
11. Coccia EM, Del Russo N, Stellacci E, et al (1999) Activation and repression of the 2-5A synthetase and *p21* gene promoters by IRF-1 and IRF-2. Oncogene 18:2129–2137
12. Kadonaga JT, Jones KA, Tjian R (1986) Promoter-specific activation of RNA polymerase II transcription by Sp1. Trends Biochem Sci 11:20–23
13. Baeuerle PA (1991) The inducible transcriptional activator NF-κB: regulation by distinct protein subunits. Biochim Biophys Acta 1072:63–80

Growth Inhibition of Pancreatic Cancer Cell Lines by Ligand Activation of Nuclear Hormone Receptors Through Up-Expression of WAF1/CIP1/p21

SHIGEYUKI KAWA* and KENDO KIYOSAWA

Summary. The aim of this study was to assess whether ligand activation of nuclear hormone receptors inhibits the growth of pancreatic cancer cells and to clarify the underling mechanisms with a special focus on restriction point control of the late G_1 phase of the cell cycle. Nine pancreatic cancer cell lines were used to study the effects of vitamin D and A analogs on cell growth by MTT assay, on cell cycle by flow cytometry, and on cell cycle-regulating factors of late G_1 phase by Western and Northern blotting and the CDK2 kinase assay. 1,25-Dihydroxyvitamin D_3 (calcitriol, 1,25D_3), 22-oxa-1,25-dihydroxyvitamin D_3 (22-oxa-calcitriol, OCT), and the vitamin A analog mofarotene showed a potent dose-response effect on growth inhibition of pancreatic cancer cell lines, and a vitamin D effect was seen selectively. All *trans*-retinoic acid, 9-*cis*-retinoic acid, and 13-*cis*-retinoic acid showed only slight inhibition at high concentrations. The growth inhibition was linked to the G_1 phase cell cycle arrest through the up-expression of *p21* mRNA and protein simultaneously with the inhibition of CDK2 kinase activity and the hypophosphorylation of Rb protein. In conclusion, 1,25D_3, OCT, and mofaroten have growth inhibitory effects on pancreatic cancer cell lines through the up-expression of *p21*, suggesting that ligand activation of nuclear hormone receptors is a new molecular target for effective therapy against pancreatic cancer.

Key words. Pancreatic cancer, Vitamin D, Vitamin A, 22-Oxa-calcitriol, *p21*

Introduction

Conventional chemotherapy for adenocarcinoma of the pancreas has not resulted in a significant survival benefit, stimulating the search for a new molecular target for effective therapy. Nuclear hormone receptors are transcription factors that transcript various genes acting in cell cycle control. Induction of differentiation through ligand

---

Second Department of Internal Medicine, Shinshu University School of Medicine, 3-1-1 Asahi, Matsumoto, Nagano 390-8621, Japan
* e-mail: skawapc@hsp.md.shinshu-u.ac.jp

activation of nuclear hormone receptors is a promising approach, as shown by the use of all *trans*-retinoic acid (ATRA) for the treatment of acute promyelocytic leukemia [1]. It may provide a novel target for preventing and treating other human cancers, including pancreatic cancer. Using growth assay systems of pancreatic cancer cell lines, we investigated the antiproliferative effects of vitamin D and A analogs, which activate corresponding nuclear hormone receptors, with a special focus on restriction point control of the late G_1 phase of the cell cycle [2–4].

Materials and Methods

Ligands

1,25-Dihydroxyvitamin D_3 (calcitriol, 1,25D_3) and 22-oxa-1,25-dihydroxyvitamin D_3 (22-oxa-calcitriol, OCT) were purchased from Philip Duphar Co. (Amsterdam, The Netherlands) and were kindly provided by Chugai Pharmaceutical Co. (Tokyo, Japan), respectively. Mofarotene was kindly provided by Hoffmann-La Roche (Basel, Switzerland) and ATRA , 9-*cis*-retinoic acid (9*cis*RA) and 13-*cis*-retinoic acid (13*cis*RA) were purchased from Sigma (St. Louis, MO, USA). The stock solution was prepared in dimethylsulfoxide (DMSO), and the final concentration of DMSO in the culture medium did not exceed 0.1%.

Effects of Ligands on the Growth of Pancreatic Cancer Cell Lines

Eight established pancreatic cancer cell lines (AsPC-1, BxPC-3, Capan-1, Capan-2, Hs 700T, Hs 766T, MIA PaCa-2, PANC-1) were obtained from the American Type Culture Collection (Rockville, MD, USA). SUP-1 was established from the pleural effusion of a patient with pancreatic cancer in our laboratory [2]. We assayed the viable cell number by the MTT [3-(4,5-dimetylthiazol-2-yl)-2,5-diphenyltetrazolium bromide; Sigma] method as described previously [2–5]. MTT absorbance was determined on days when cells with vehicle came close to confluence. Eight wells were used for each treatment, and experiments were repeated twice. The cytotoxicity of each ligands was examined by the trypan blue exclusion test.

Flow Cytometry

Cell lines were allowed to grow to 30% confluence. They were then treated with either vehicle or ligand for 4 days, harvested, and stained with a DNA staining solution containing propidium iodide and RNAse. The cells were analyzed with a FACScan flow cytometer equipped with an argon laser (488 nm; Becton Dickinson Immunocytometry System, Mountain View, CA, USA).

Immunoblotting

Immunoblotting was performed as described previously [2–4]. Briefly, protein extracts were separated by sodium dodecyl sulfate (SDS)-polyacrylamide gel electrophoresis (PAGE) and then transferred to supported nitrocellulose membranes

(GIBCO BRL, Gaithersburg, MD, USA) with a plate electrode apparatus (Idea Scientific, Minneapolis, MN, USA). The filters were blocked with nonfat milk followed by incubation with mouse monoclonal antibodies to *p21* (Clone 70, Transduction Laboratories, KY, USA) and Rb protein (G3–245, Pharmigen, CA, USA). Filters were then incubated with horseradish peroxidase-conjugated second antibody. Bound antibody was detected with an enhanced chemiluminescence system (Amersham, Bucks, England) and exposed to X-ray films. The experiments were repeated twice.

CDK2 Kinase Assay

Protein extracts were incubated with anti-CDK2 antibody (M2, Santa Cruz), and precipitated by the addition of protein G agarose (Calbiochem, La Jolla, CA, USA). Kinase activity of the immunopellets was assayed with the use of histone H1 and [γ-^{32}P]ATP as substrate. After electrophoresis with SDS-PAGE the gel was imaged by imaging plate autoradiography (BAS 2000; Fuji Photo Film, Tokyo, Japan).

RNA Analysis

Total RNA was extracted from pancreatic cancer cells with ISOGEN (Nippon Gene, Toyama, Japan). Following quantitation, the total RNA was electrophoresed through formaldehyde/agarose gels. The RNA was blotted to a Hybond-N nylon membrane (Amersham Pharmacia Biotech), cross-linked, hybridized, and washed. Labeling of the *p21* DNA fragment (kindly supplied by T. Sakai, Kyoto Prefectual University of Medicine) was done by random priming using the BcaBest Labeling Kit (Takara, Tokyo, Japan) and [α-^{32}P]dCTP. Filters were imaged by imaging plate autoradiography (BAS 2000).

Results

Effects of Ligands on the Proliferation of Each Cell Line

Marked dose-dependent antiproliferative effects of 1,25D_3 and OCT were observed in three of the nine cell lines tested, and those of mofarotene were observed in all cell lines with little cytotoxicity. ATRA, 13*cis*RA, and 9*cis*RA were less potent; and none suppressed the proliferation of any cell line to less than 50% of the control (Fig. 1). Furthermore, 9*cis*RA showed no synergistic effect on the growth inhibition induced by 1,25D_3, OCT, or ATRA (data not shown).

Cell Cycle Analysis

Cell cycle analysis of responsive cells showed a substantial increase in the fraction of cells in G_1 phase after treatment compared with the G_1 fraction of the control groups. This result indicated that these agents induced G_1 phase arrest of the cell cycle (data not shown).

Effects on G_1 Restriction Point Regulating Agents

Western blotting analysis of a representative cell line, BxPC-3, after OCT treatment showed marked induction of p21 protein. In proportion to the p21 change, it

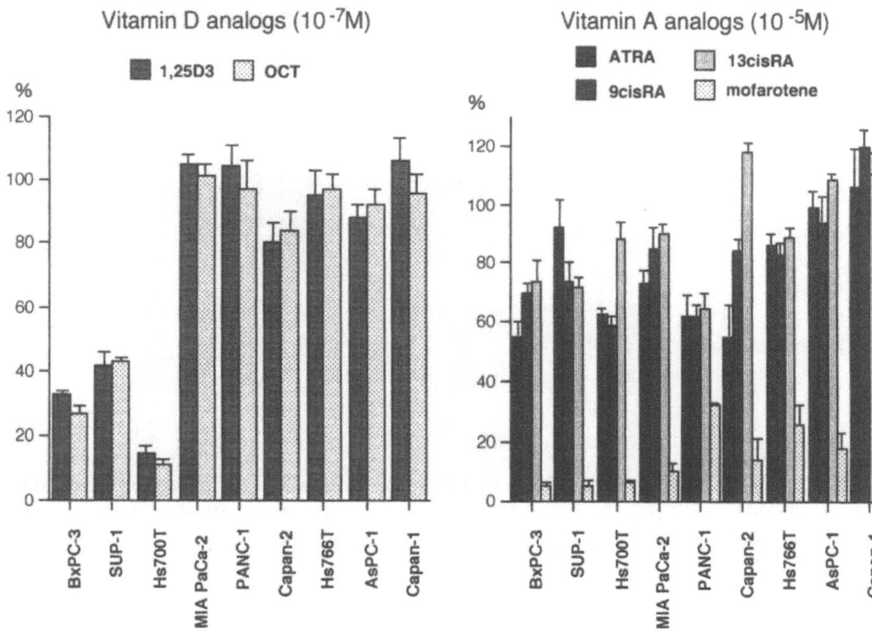

FIG. 1. Effect of vitamin D and A analogs on the growth of nine pancreatic cancer cell lines at concentrations of 10^{-7} M and 10^{-5} M, respectively. The mean value ± SD of eight wells determined by MTT assay are indicated as percentage of the control for each cell line. *1,25D3*, 1,25-dihydroxyvitamin D_3 (calcitriol); *OCT*, 22-oxa-1,25-dihydroxyvitamin D_3 (22-oxa-calctriol); *ATRA*, all-*trans*-retinoic acid; *9cisRA*, 9-*cis*-retinoic acid; *13cisRA*, 13-*cis*-retinoic acid

decreased CDK2 kinase activity and increased the hypophosphorylated forms of Rb protein (Fig. 2). In accordance with the changes in p21 protein, Northern blotting analysis showed a considerable increase in p21 mRNA levels (data not shown). The same results were obtained in other responsive cell lines.

Discussion

The present study revealed that vitamin D analogs markedly inhibited the growth of three of the nine pancreatic cancer cell lines, and that mofarotene is the most potent antiproliferative agent among the vitamin A analogs examined, with little cytotoxicity. Other retinoids such as ATRA, 13*cis*RA, and 9*cis*RA showed only slight inhibition at the high concentrations.

The growth inhibition induced by OCT and 1,25D_3 was selective, so it is important to clarify the factors contributing to this selectivity before clinical use. Various effects of vitamin D analogs were reported to depend on quantitative or qualitative differences in vitamin D receptor (VDR). Accordingly, we examined the presence of VDR protein and the differences of VDR among the cell lines tested. Scatchard analysis showed that cell lines responsive to OCT and 1,25D_3 had abundant functional VDR.

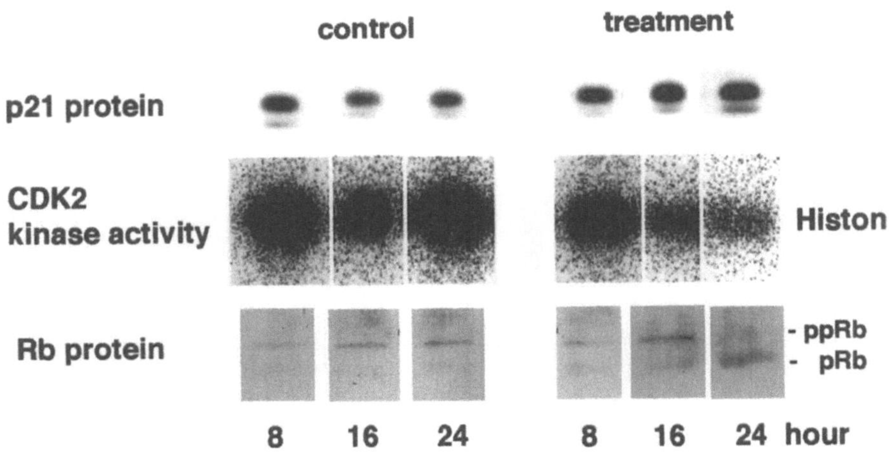

FIG. 2. Changes in the p21 protein level, CDK2 kinase activity, and the phosphorylation state of Rb (retinoblastoma) protein of BxPC3 cells after OCT (22-oxa-calcitriol) treatment. *ppRb*, phosphorylated Rb protein; *pRb*, hypophosphorylated Rb protein

However, some OCT and 1,25D$_3$ nonresponsive cell lines also showed sufficient amounts of functional VDR with no structural abnormality, suggesting that other factors also regulate the selectivity of the effects of vitamin D analogs [2].

VDR and RAR forms a heterodimeric complex with the retinoid X receptor (RXR), which binds to specific recognition sites on DNA and, upon binding of ligands for each receptor, regulates transcription of various genes. In this context the RXR ligand 9*cis*RA possibly increases the inhibitory effects of 1,25D$_3$, OCT, and ATRA. However, the present study showed that 9*cis*RA exerted no synergistc effects on the growth inhibition by these agents.

The growth inhibitory effect of these agents was linked to G$_1$ phase cell cycle arrest, suggesting a contribution of cell cycle regulating factors that act at a restriction point of late G$_1$. To proceed from G$_1$ phase to S phase, G$_1$ phase-associated cyclin–CDK complexes act to phosphorylate Rb protein; then the transcription factor E2F is released, resulting in expression of various genes whose products mediate DNA synthesis [6]. Levels of G$_1$ cyclin–CDK activities exceeding the threshold of inhibition set for cyclin-dependent kinase inhibitors, such as p21, are required to proceed from G$_1$ phase to S phase [7,8], indicating a major role for CDK inhibitors in the negative regulation of the cell cycle and in the signal pathway of nuclear hormone receptors. The present study showed that these agents induced up-expression of p21 protein and mRNA simultaneously with the inhibition of CDK2 kinase activity and hypophosphorylation of Rb protein. Accordingly, p21 may play a major role in exiting from the cell cycle and in maintenance of the irreversible growth arrest.

In conclusion, the present study showed that ligand activation of nuclear hormone receptors induces growth inhibition of pancreatic cancer cells through up-expression of p21. This finding suggests a new molecular target for effective therapy against pancreatic cancer.

Acknowledgments. This work was supported in part by Grants-in-Aid for Scientific Research from the Ministry of Education, Science, Sports, and Culture Japan (10670461, 12670471).

References

1. Huang ME, Ye YC, Chen S, et al (1988) Use of all-trans retinoic acid in the treatment of acute promyelocytic leukemia. Blood 72:567–572
2. Kawa S, Yoshizawa K, Tokoo M, et al (1996) Inhibitory effect of 22-oxa-1,25-dihydoroxyvitamin D_3 on the proliferation of pancreatic cancer cell lines. Gastroenterology 110:1605–1613
3. Kawa S, Nikaido T, Aoki Y, et al (1997) Vitamin D analogues up-regulate p21 and p27 during growth inhibition of pancreatic cancer cell lines. Br J Cancer 76:884–889
4. Kawa S, Nikaido T, Aoki Y, et al (1997) Arotinoid mofarotene (RO40-8757) up-regulate p21 and p27 during growth inhibition of pancreatic cancer cell lines. Int J Cancer 72: 906–911
5. Carmichael J, De Graff WG, Gazdar AF, et al (1987) Evaluation of a tetrazolium-based semiautomated colorimetric assay: assessment of chemosensitivity testing. Cancer Res 47:936–942
6. Chellapa SP, Hiebert S, Mudryj M, et al (1991) The E2F transcription factor is a cellular target for the Rb protein. Cell 65:1053–1061
7. Peter M, Herskowitz I (1994) Joining the complex: cyclin-dependent kinase inhibitory proteins and cell cycle. Cell 79:181–184
8. Peters G (1994) Stifled by inhibitors. Nature 371:204–205

Part 7
The Role of Antigen-Presenting Cells in Pathophysiology

Immunopathological Features of Granuloma Formation in the Intestinal Mucosa of Patients with Crohn's Disease

Takayuki Matsumoto[1,*], Shiro Nakamura[1], Jun-ichi Hara[1], Yoshio Jinno[1], Yoshinori Sawa[1], Nobuhide Oshitani[1], Kazuhide Higuchi[1], Tetsuo Arakawa[1], Yukio Nishiguchi[2], Kousei Hirakawa[2], Haruo Otani[3], and Hiroshi Nagura[3]

Summary. Crohn's disease is a long-lasting intractable inflammatory disorder of the large or small intestine with unknown etiology. Investigations suggest that combined genetic and environmental factors such as infectious agents or intraluminal antigens play important roles in the pathogenesis of the disease. Among them, we have proved that impaired immune responses in noncaseating granuloma, which has been thought to be an important histopathologic feature of the disease, play a crucial role in initiating candidate pathognomonic antigens. Immunohistochemical analysis of infiltrated cells around a granuloma revealed that class II major histocompatibility complex molecules and co-stimulatory molecules such as CD80/86 were up-regulated in the granuloma cells of macrophage lineage origin. Such granuloma cells often made close contact with CD28-positive T cells with either CD4 or CD8. These granulomas were often located in the luminal spaces, of which endothelial cells coating the lumen did not express vascular endothelial cell markers such as CD36 or von Willebrand factor. Electron microscopy showed that those cells were lymphatic endothelial cells. These results strongly suggest that noncaseating granulomas of Crohn's disease are formed close to lymphatic vessels, and antigenic stimuli through the lymphatic system may be important in the pathogenesis of Crohn's disease.

Key words. Crohn's disease, Granuloma, Antigen-presenting cells, Mesenteric lymph node, T cells

Introduction

Crohn's disease is a long-lasting chronic inflammatory disorder involving the whole gastrointestinal tract. Observations have revealed that Crohn's disease is closely

[1] Department of Gastroenterology, [2] Department of Surgery I, Osaka City University Medical School, 1-4-3 Asahi-machi, Abeno-ku, Osaka 545-8585, Japan
[3] Department of Pathology, Tohoku University School of Medicine, Sendai, Japan
* e-mail: matsut@med.osaka-cu.ac.jp

related to the combined abnormalities in genetic factors, environmental factors, and immunologic responses [1]. Among the immune responses in Crohn's disease, impaired function of macrophage lineage cells have been reported by a number of investigators [2]. For example, it was reported that abnormal phagocytic activities and oxygen radical production were related to disease activities and were not observed in patients with ulcerative colitis. It has been thought that noncaseating granuloma, one of the important pathologic features of Crohn's disease, is produced by impaired activation of macrophages by certain bacterial stimuli such as L-form bacteria or *Mycobacterium paratuberculosis* [3,4]. Wakefield et al. [5] reported that measles virus infection caused granulomatous vasculitis. Although the idea was supported by epidemiological data [6], there are a number of reports that failed to identify measles virus or measles virus DNA in intestinal tissue of Crohn's disease [7]. The purpose of this study is to clarify immunologic role of granulomas in Crohn's disease.

Methods

Biopsy or surgical specimens obtained from patients with inflammatory bowel disease were promptly fixed with periodated lysine and 2% paraformaldehyde (PLP) and were offered for immunostaining as previously reported [8]. Surface markers for immunocompetent cells and cytokines were analyzed by the indirect immunoperoxidase method [9]. A repertoire of infiltrated lamina propria T cells was analyzed by the reverse transcriptase-polymerase chain reaction (RT-PCR) method [10].

Results and Discussion

Location of Granuloma Formation in Crohn's Disease

Granulomas in the intestinal wall of patients with Crohn's disease are often surrounded by an endothelial cell monolayer. To evaluate the vasculature system relating to granuloma, we have determined the relation between granuloma and vascular or lymphatic vessels using immunohistocehmical procedures on PLP-fixed frozen sections as previously reported. Vascular endothelial cells were visualized by anti-von Willebrand factor antibody or anti-CD36 antibody.

Lymphatic vessels were increased in Crohn's disease, and dilated lymphatic vessels containing aggregated lymphocytes and macrophages were observed. Wakefield et al. [7]. showed that the granuloma was a kind of granulomatous vasculitis; and epidemiological data revealed that measles or vaccination for measles had a positive relation with the incidence of Crohn's disease in western Europe. However, most of the recent reports have failed to demonstrate measles virus antigen or DNA in the involved tissue of Crohn's disease.

Endothelial cells surrounding the granuloma were thought to be lymphatic vessels. Such features were common to granulomas located in the submucosal layer, proper muscle layer, subserosal layer, or mesenteric lymph nodes, which suggests that granuloma formation is closely related to the lymphatic system and proceeds to the mesenteric lymph node from the mucosal layer as an entrance for antigenic substances [11].

TABLE 1. Phenotypic features of infiltrating macrophage lineage cells in granulomas and intestinal inflammatory lesions in patients with Crohn's disease

Condition	S100p	CD68	CD80	CD86	CD56	HLA-DR
Control	–	+++	–	+	++	++
Granuloma	–	+++	W$^+$	+++	+++	+++
Intestinal inflammation	–	+++	–	+	++	++

–, negative; W$^+$, weakly positive; +, mildly positive; ++, moderately positive; +++, strongly positive; S-100p, S-100 protein

Granuloma Cells and Antigen Presentation

Although dysfunction of macrophages, such as impaired synthesis of oxygen radicals, has been thought to be an important factor in granuloma formation, we have proved that active antigen presentation does occur in noncaseating granulama. We demonstrated that multinucleated giant cells and epithelioid cells, which are major components of granulomas, strongly expressed the HLA-DR antigens CD80 and CD86. CD80 and CD86 are important co-stimulatory molecules on antigen-presenting cells and are indispensable for activating CD3-pulsed T cells by binding CD28 molecules on T cells. Most T cells surrounding granulomas, in which CD4 cells outnumbered CD8 cells, express CD28. By immunoelectron microscopy, we have identified that CD80/86 molecules were mainly localized on the side of the cell membranes, which were in close contact with CD28-positive lymphocytes, supporting the idea that antigen-specific T cell activation occurs in granulomas of Crohn's disease. These features of granuloma cells were common when the granulomas were located in lymphatic vessels, and CD80/86-positive cells were localized adjacent to lymphatic endothelium (Table 1).

Th1 Activation Around Granuloma

Immunological research has revealed that T cell activation is directed by the effects of cytokines, and CD4 cells are divided into two groups, T-helper lymphocytes, Th1 and Th2, according to the cytokine production patterns [12,13]. Th1 cells mainly produce interleukins (IL-2, IL-12) and interferon-γ (IFNγ), which stimulate cellular immune responses. In contrast, Th1 cells produce IL-4, IL-5, and IL-10, which stimulate the humoral immune response.

Our data on cytokine production in granulomas showed that granuloma cells, especially multinucleated giant cells and epithelioid cells, mainly produced IL-12 but not IL-4 or IL-10. Lymphocytes in or around granulomas produced IL-2 and IFNγ but not IL-4. In contrast, in the actively inflamed mucosa of ulcerative colitis, increased number of Th2 cells producing IL-4 and IL-10 were predominant. These data suggest that strong activation of Th1 cells in which CD4 cells predominate occurs in granulomas. Specific antigens may infiltrate into the intestinal mucosa via the lymphatic system and proceed to mesenteric lymph nodes. In that process, macrophages and T cells were stimulated in relation to lymphatic vessels and produce granulomas. These antigens may be related to disease-specific properties. Therefore, further analysis of the antigens and immune responses are important for clarifying the immunopathogenesis of Crohn's disease (Table 2).

TABLE 2. Tissue distribution of cytokine-bearing cells in intestinal tissue of patients with Crohn's disease

Condition	IL-2	IFNγ	IL-12	IL-4	IL-10	IL-8
Control	±	+	+	+	±	±
Intestinal inflammation	++	+	+	++	+	+++
Granuloma	+	++	+++	–	–	+

IL, interleukin; IFN, interferon

Repertoire of T Cells in Lamina Propria

In Crohn's disease lamina propria T cells of mainly CD4 lineage showed skewed expression in the T cell receptor Vβ repertoire. This result suggests that lamina propria T cells in Crohn's disease are activated by a limited variety of antigens probably originating in the intestinal lumen [14,15].

Conclusions

In Crohn's disease a limited variety of disease-specific antigens may exert specific immune responses characterized by noncaseating granuloma formation. Such responses may proceed through the lymphatic system in the intestinal wall.

References

1. Koutroubakis I, Pena AS (1997) Genetics of inflammatory bowel disease. In: Allan RN, Rhodes JM, Hanauer SB, et al (eds) Inflammatory bowel disease, 3rd edn. Churchill Livingstone, New York, 1997, pp 13–26
2. Ward M (1977) The pathogenesis of Crohn's disease. Lancet 2:903–905
3. Chiodini RJ, van Kruiningen HJ, Merkal RS (1984) Characteristics of unclassified *Mycobacterium* species isolated from patients with Crohn's disease. J Clin Microbiol 20:966–971
4. Fidler HM, Thurrell W, Johnson NM, et al (1994) Specific detection of *Mycobacterium paratuberculosis* DNA associated with granulomatous tissue in Crohn's disease. Gut 35:506–510
5. Wakefield AJ, Sankey EA, Dhillon AP, et al (1991) Granulomatous vasculitis in Crohn's disease. Gastroenterology 100:1279–1287
6. Baxter T, Radford J (1995) Measles vaccination as a risk factor for inflammatory bowel disease. Lancet 345:1363–1364
7. Iizuka M, Nakagomi O, Chiba M, et al (1995) Absence of measles virus in Crohn's disease. Lancet 345:199
8. Matsumoto T, Kitano A, Nakamura S, et al (1989) Possible role of vascular endothelial cells in immune responses in colonic mucosa examined immunocytochemically in subjects with and without ulcerative colitis. Clin Exp Immunol 78:424–430
9. Hara J, Ohtani H, Matsumoto T, et al (1997) Expression of costimulatory molecules B7-1 and B7-2 in macrophages and granulomas of Crohn's disease: demonstration of cell-to-cell contact with T lymphocytes. Lab Invest 77:175–184
10. Prindiville T, Cantrell M, Matsumoto T, et al (1996) Analysis of function, specificity and T cell receptor expression of cloned mucosal T cell lines in Crohn's disease. J Autoimmunity 9:193–204

11. Nakamura S, Ohtani H, Watanabe Y, et al (1993) In situ expression of the cell adhesion molecules in inflammatory bowel disease: evidence of immunologic activation of vascular endothelial cells. Lab Invest 69:77–85
12. Kakazu T, Hara J, Matsumoto T, et al (1999) Type 1 T helper cell predominance in granulomas of Crohn's disease. Am J Gastroenterol 94:2149–2155
13. Yamamura M, Uemura K, Deans RJ, et al (1991) Defining protective responses to pathogens: cytokine profiles in leprosy lesions. Science 254:277–279
14. Gulwani-Akolkar B, Akolkar PN, Minassian A, et al (1996) Selective expansion of specific T cell receptors in the inflamed colon of Crohn's disease. J Clin Invest 98:1344–1354
15. Sartor RB (1998) Postoperative recurrence of Crohn's disease: the enemy is within the fecal stream. Gastroenterology 114:398–407

Helicobacter pylori and *N*-Methyl-*N′*-nitro-*N*-nitrosoguanidine Induction of Dendritic Cell Infiltration of the Pyloric Mucosa of Mongolian Gerbils

MASASHI OKA[1,*], CHIE FURIHATA[2], MASAO ICHINOSE[1], NAOHISA YAHAGI[1], YASUHITO SHIMIZU[1], HIDENORI KURAKATA[1], AYAKO TATEISHI-NIIHATA[1], MITSUHIRO FUJISHIRO[1], YOSHIYUKI SAKAKI[3], and MASAO OMATA[1]

Summary. The dendritic cell is not only an antigen-presenting cell, it is immunologically resistant to stomach carcinogenesis induced by the carcinogen *N*-methyl-*N′*-nitro-*N*-nitrosoguanidine (MNNG). We have demonstrated that the mRNA expression of major histocompatibility complex (MHC) class II-associated invariant chain (Ii), which is produced in mature dendritic cells, is markedly enhanced by treatment with MNNG, and it was more enhanced in a carcinogen-resistant strain (Buffalo) than a sensitive strain (ACI). This suggests that the dendritic cell may play a key role in carcinogenic resistance. *Helicobacter pylori* is supposed to be a promoter of gastric cancer, and its infection causes massive dendritic cell infiltration. We have demonstrated that interferon-γ (IFNγ) may be an important player in resistance to carcinogenesis based on *H. pylori*-infected mongolian gerbil experiments. A group of 80 mongolian gerbils were divided into 16 groups and were treated with or without *H. pylori* and MNNG. Their pyloric mucosa mRNA was extracted for the reverse transcriptase-polymerase chain reaction. IFNγ mRNA expression was enhanced by MNNG treatment and *H. pylori* infection and was similar to that of Ii. On the other hand, the pattern of OX-62 (a dendritic cell marker expressed in mature or immature cells) was rarely enhanced by MNNG, and it was not like the Ii pattern. The different patterns for Ii and OX-62 suggest that INFγ, which is manufactured by MNNG-treated epithelial cells and is a stimulator of dendritic cell maturation, may play a key role in resistance to carcinogenesis.

Key words. Gastric carcinogenesis, *Helicobacter pylori*, Dendritic cell, Mongolian gerbil, *N*-Methyl-*N′*-nitro-*N*-nitrosoguanidine (MNNG)

---

[1] Department of Gastroenterology, Faculty of Medicine, The University of Tokyo, 7-3-1 Hongo, Bunkyo-ku, Tokyo 113-0033, Japan
[2] Faculty of Science, Aoyama-gakuin University, Atsugi, Kanagawa, Japan
[3] Human Genome Center, Institute of Medical Science, The University of Tokyo, Tokyo, Japan
* e-mail: moka@ims.u-tokyo.ac.jp

Introduction

Gastric cancer is one of the most common malignant diseases among Asian people, but its etiology is not fully known. Some chemicals are reported to cause stomach cancers in rats or other animals [1]. Low-dose carcinogens [e.g., drinking water with *N*-methyl-*N′*-nitro-*N*-nitrosoguanidine (MNNG) 100 g/l or more] is capable of causing gastric cancer [2]. *Helicobacter pylori* is also thought to be associated with gastrointestinal cancer; it is certainly a promoter agent with MNNG treatment in mongolian gerbils [3,4].

On the other hand, in rats the sensitivity to carcinogens is different among strains [5]. The dendritic cell is one of the candidates that can protect against gastric carcinogenesis. It is reported that the more infiltration of dendritic cells there is in the stomach or lymph nodes with cancer the better is the prognosis [6–8]. We have reported that MNNG treatment can cause dendritic cell infiltration [9]. We also reported that there was more dendritic cell infiltration in the pyloric mucosa in a less sensitive strain (Buffalo rats) than in a more sensitive strain (ACI rats) after treatment with MNNG [10]. The results suggest that the dendritic cell defends against stomach carcinogenesis. In this study we intended to clarify whether dendritic cells play an anticancer role in mongolian gerbils with *H. pylori* infection.

Materials and Methods

Animals

Eighty 7-week-old male mongolian gerbils (*Meriones unguiculatu*, MGS/Sea; Seac Yoshitomi, Fukuoka, Japan) were divided into 16 groups (Fig. 1). The gerbils in groups 1 to 4 were observed 3 weeks. Group 1 and 2 gerbils were treated with MNNG 100 mg/l (Tokyo Kasei Kogyo, Tokyo, Japan) in their drinking water for 2 weeks; groups 3 and 4 were treated with distilled water as control. Groups 1 and 3 were administered *H. pylori* 0.8 ml (~1.0×10^8 CFU/ml) (ATCC 43504; American Type Culture Collection, Rockville, MD, USA). The gerbils in groups 9 to 12 were observed 5 weeks. Group 9 and 10 gerbils were treated with MNNG 100 mg/l in drinking water for 4 weeks, and groups 11 and 12 were treated with water. Groups 9 and 11 were adminstered *H. pylori* during the first week. Groups 5 to 8 were observed 11 weeks. Group 5 and 6 gerbils were treated with MNNG 100 mg/l for 5 weeks and 300 mg/l for 5 weeks. Group 5 and 7 gerbils were administered *H. pylori* during the 11th week. Groups 13 to 16 were observed 15 weeks . Group 13 and 14 gerbils were treated with MNNG 100 mg/l for 5 weeks and 300 mg/l for 5 weeks. Group 13 and 15 gerbils were administered *H. pylori* during the 11th week. Their pyloric mucosae were removed surgically and frozen to be tested later by reverse transcriptase-polymerase chain reaction (RT-PCR).

RT-PCR

Each pyloric mucosa was dissolved with Trizol (GIBCO/BRL), and the total RNA was extracted by the AGPC method. Total RNA 5 μg was reverse-transcribed into cDNAs by Superscript (GIBCO/BRL) reverse transcriptase.

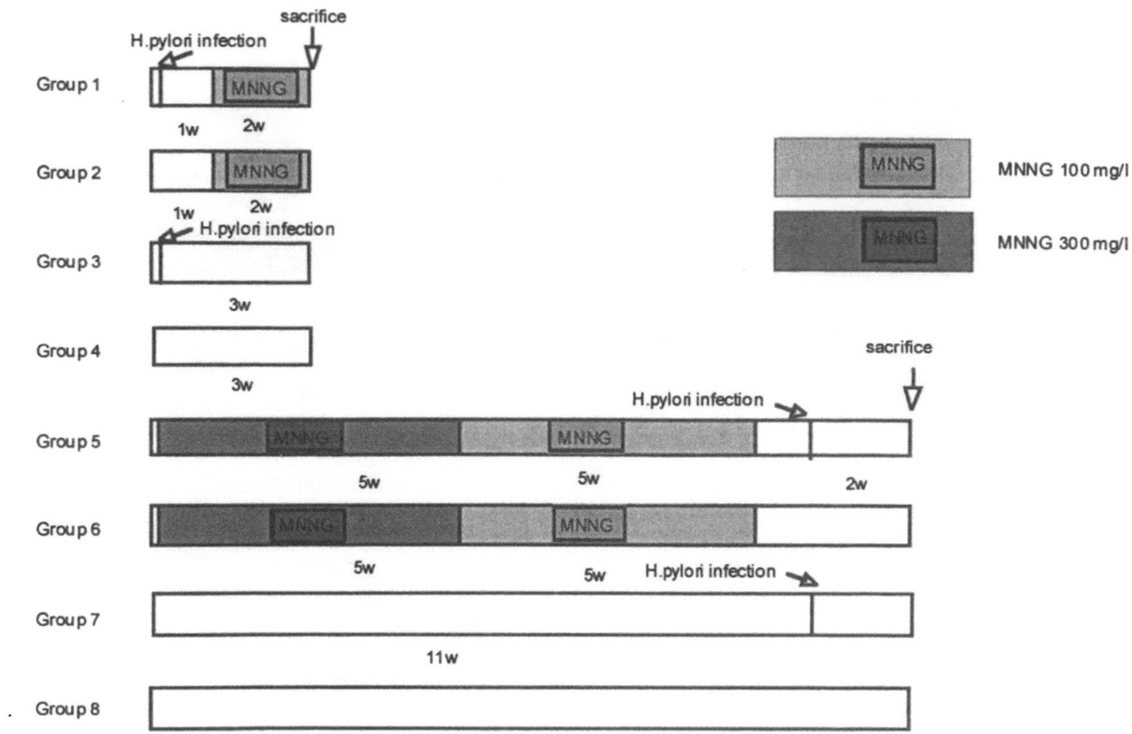

FIG. 1. Protocol for the study. *w*, weeks; *MNNG*, *N*-methyl-*N'*-nitro-*N*-nitrosoguanidine

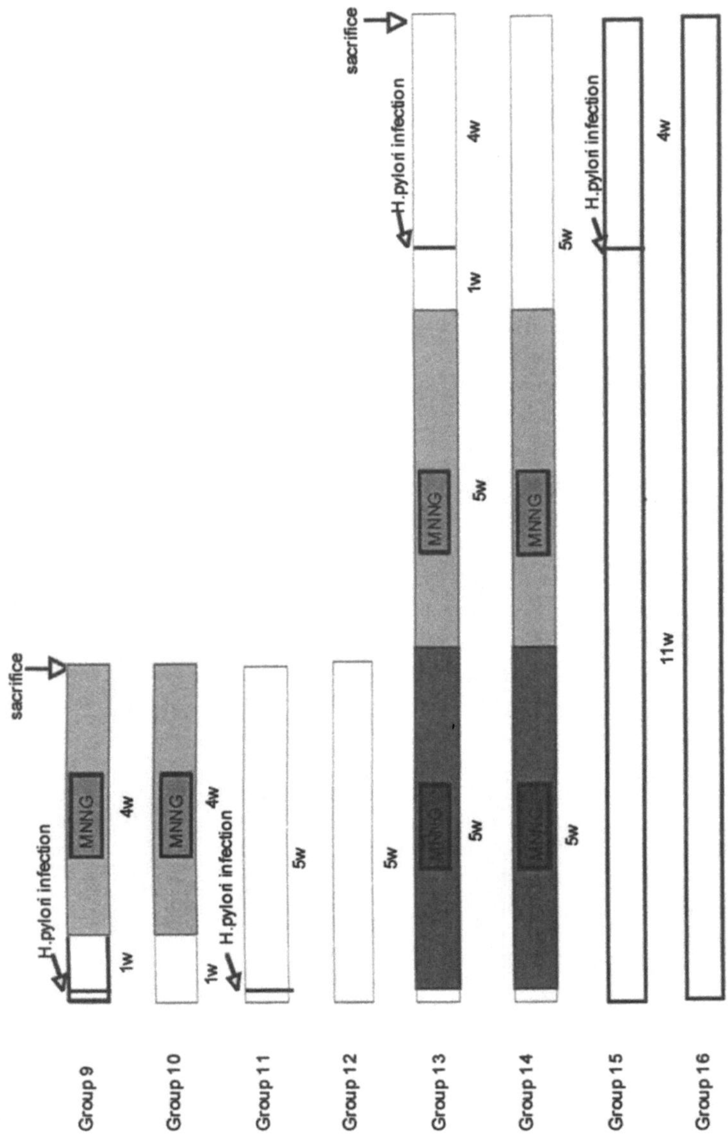

FIG. 1. *Continued*

Specific primers for major histocompatibility complex (MHC) class II-associated invariant chain (Ii) and OX-62 (a specific surface marker of dendritic cells) of the mongolian gerbil were used for PCR amplification of their cDNAs. Specific primers of *H. pylori* urease A were also used for PCR to analyze the *H. pylori* infection. The primers were described as follows.

Gerbil Ii 5′primer:	TGTACCAGCAGCAGGGCCGG
Gerbil Ii 3′primer:	CTCAGTTCAAACAAGAGCCACTG
Gerbil OX-62 5′ primer:	GTTACTAAGACTGCCTCAGCCATG
Gerbil OX-62 3′ primer:	CTGTGCCTTCCATATAGATGATGC
H. pylori urease A 5′primer:	GTTAGATAAGTTGATGCTCCACTACG
H. pylori urease A 3′ primer:	GTCTGCTTGTCTATCAACCAATGC

The amplified cDNAs were electrophoresed through 5% polyaerylamide gel electrophoresis (PAGE) with Tris-glycine buffer and stained by SYBR Green I. The density of the bands were analyzed by FluorImager (Molecular Dynamics,CA, USA).

Results

The results of PCR are shown in Figs. 2 and 3. The amount of amplified cDNA in group 8 of each PCR group is adjusted to 1.0 as a control, and other bands are adjusted at the same ratio.

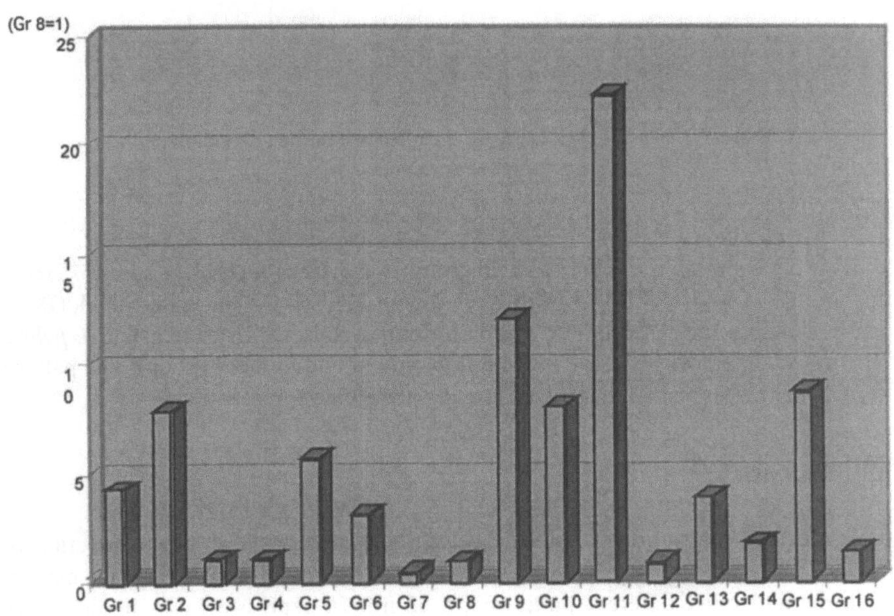

FIG. 2. Major histocompatibility complex (MHC) class II associated invariant chain (Ii) expression in the mongolian gerbil. *Gr*, group

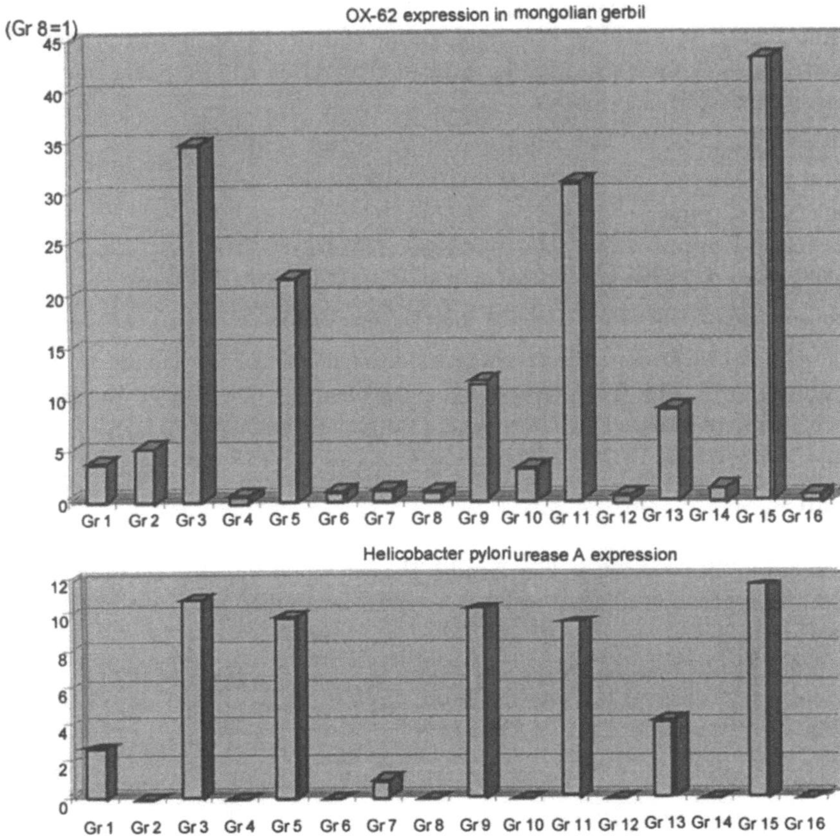

FIG. 3. OX-62 and *Helicobacter pylori* urease A expression in the mongolian gerbil

Ii mRNA expression was increased in groups 1, 2, 5, 6, 9, 10, 11, 13, 14, and 15. Except for groups 11 and 15, all had been treated with MNNG. On the other hand, OX-62 expression was increased in odd number group gerbils, which were given *H. pylori*. The mRNA of *H. pylori* urease A was found only in odd number groups. The pattern for OX-62 was similar to the pattern for *H. pylori* urease A.

Discussion

Dendritic cell infiltration is found in gerbils that underwent *H. pylori* infection or MNNG treatment, but there is a difference between them. OX-62 and Ii mRNA expression demonstrated different patterns: OX-62 mRNA expression was similar to *H. pylori* urease A expression. OX-62 is a specific marker of dendritic cells. Its expression is supposed to be associated with the extent of dendritic cell infiltration. On the other hand, Ii mRNA expression was increased mostly in the MNNG-treated group. Ii is supposed to be expressed in mature dendritic cells. The discrepancy between OX-62 and Ii expression can be explained by the hypothesis that mature dendritic cells with Ii expression are stimulated by MNNG treatment.

Groups 11 and 15 are the only exception: Both OX-62 and Ii mRNAs were increased despite no treatment with MNNG. In groups 11 and 15, a heavy *H. pylori* infection is observed, which may have caused significant dendritic cell infiltration. It can be said that Ii-positive dendritic cells are stimulated not only by MNNG but also by *H. pylori* infection. The Ii/OX-62 density ratio, however, is relatively low in group 11.

Conclusions

The dendritic cell is supposed to be associated with the defense against gastric carcinogenesis. Especially, Ii-positive dendritic cells are stimulated by MNNG, which may play a key role in defending against carcinogenesis.

References

1. Sugimura T, Fujimura S (1967) Tumor production in glandular stomach of rat by *N*-methyl-*N'*-nitro-*N*-nitrosoguanidine. Nature 216:943–944
2. Oka M, Ichinose M, Yahagi N, et al (1996) Induction of the genes for hepatocyte growth factor and keratinocyte growth factor in the pyloric mucosa of rat stomach by *N*-methyl-*N'*-nitro-*N*-nitrosoguanidine (MNNG) and sodium chloride(NaCl). In: Recent advances in gastroenterological carcinogenesis. I. Monduzzi Editore (Bologna), pp 643–646
3. Maruta F, Ikeno T, Ishida K, et al (1998) *Helicobacter pylori* infection enhances *N*-methyl-*N*-nitrosourea-induced stomach carcinogenesis in the Mongolian gerbil. Cancer Res 58:2067–2069
4. Shimizu N, Ikehara Y, Inada K, et al (2000) Eradication diminishes enhancing effects of *Helicobacter pylori* infection on glandular stomach carcinogenesis in Mongolian gerbils. Cancer Res 60:1512–1514
5. Bralow SP, Gruenstein M, Meranze DR (1973) Host resistance to gastric adenocarcinomatosis in three strains of rats injesting *N*-methyl-*N'*-nitro-*N*-nitrosoguanidine. Oncology 27:168–180
6. Tsujitani S, Furukawa T, Tamada R, et al (1987) Langerhans cells and prognosis in patients with gastric carcinoma. Cancer 59:501–505
7. Tsujitani S, Kakeji Y, Watanabe A, et al (1990) Infiltration of dendritic cells in relation to tumor invasion and lymph node metastasis in human gastric cancer. Cancer 66:2012–2016
8. Tsujitani S, Oka A, Kondo A, et al (1995) Infiltration of dendritic cells into regional lymph nodes in gastric cancer. Cancer 75:1478–1483
9. Oka M, Furihata C, Kitoh K, et al (1998) Involvement of dendritic cell response to resistance of stomach carcinogenesis caused by *N*-methyl-*N'*-nitro-*N*-nitrosoguanidine in rats. Cancer Res 58:4107–4112
10. Furihata C, Oka M, Yamamoto M, et al (1997) Differentially expressed MHC class II-associated invariant chain in rat stomach pyloric mucosa with *N*-methyl-*N'*-nitro-*N*-nitrosoguanidine exposure. Cancer Res 57:1416–1418

Cytotoxic Effect of Bone Marrow-Derived Dendritic Cells

Hiromune Shimamura*, Fuyuhiko Motoi, Jun-ichiro Yamauchi, Kazuhiko Shibuya, Makoto Sunamura, Kazunori Takeda, and Seiki Matsuno

Summary. Some reports suggest that cancer patients have a better prognosis when dendritic cells (DCs) infiltrate their tumors. Although the role of these DCs is not fully understood, we focused on a potential effector function of DCs and examined whether DCs could directly mediate tumor cell cytotoxicity. Murine DCs were propagated from bone marrow stem cells using granulocyte/monocyte colony-stimulating factor and interleukin-4 for 7 days and were sorted by a magnetic-activated cell sorter system. Purified $CD11c^+$ DCs were shown to be cytotoxic against murine tumor cells such as MCA205 fibrosarcoma. The annexin V staining assay showed that MCA205 underwent apoptosis when incubated with DCs for 4h. This cytotoxic effect was not blocked by an anti-Fas ligand antibody but was partially abrogated by the Ca^{2+} chelator EGTA/$MgCl_2$. These data suggest that DCs are directly cytotoxic to some kinds of tumor cell, and this effect is mediated via both calcium-dependent and calcium-independent pathways.

Key words. Dendritic cells, Cytotoxicity, Apoptosis, Tumor cells, Calcium

Introduction

Dendritic cells (DCs) are the most potent professional antigen-presenting cells (APC) in the immune system [1]. In the context of cancer immunology, DCs may play a pivotal role in a self-defense system against tumor cells. Indeed, some reports suggest that cancer patients have a better prognosis when DCs infiltrate their tumors [2]. Although, little is known about these tumor-infiltrating DCs, studies have evoked one possibility for their role: a direct cytotoxic effect. Both lymphoid and myeloid DCs were shown to induce apoptosis in activated T cells via Fas/Fas ligand interaction in the mouse system [3]. Having the ability to induce apoptosis in tumor cells could be of great advantage to DCs infiltrated in tumor tissues in that apoptotic cells or apoptotic bodies are thought to be a good source of antigen for DCs [4]. Here we show that

Department of Gastroenterological Surgery, Tohoku University Graduate School of Medicine, 1-1 Seiryo-machi, Aoba-ku, Sendai 980-8574, Japan
* e-mail: hshima-thk@umin.ac.jp

murine bone marrow-derived DCs can directly induce apoptosis in autologous tumor cells via calcium-dependent and calcium-independent pathways.

DCs and Direct Induction of Apoptosis in Tumor Cells

Dendritic cells were propagated from murine bone marrow stem cells using granulocyte/macrophage colony-stimulating factor (GM-CSF) and interleukin-4 (IL-4). $CD11c^+$ DCs were sorted with the magnetic-activated cell sorter (MACS) system and were used as effector cells in a cytotoxicity assay against target murine tumors (MCA205 fibrosarcoma, MC38 colon adenocarcinoma, TS/A mammary adenocarcinoma, P815 mastocytoma). When radioisotope-labeled tumor cells were incubated with DCs for 6h, they were shown to be killed with DNA fragmentation (Fig. 1a). Because effector DCs showed the best cytotoxicity against MCA205, we used this cell line in another assay. MCA205 was incubated with DCs for 4h, and DCs were removed by MACS. The tumor cells were eluted, stained with annexin V and propidium iodide (PI), and analyzed by flow cytometry. Fluorescence-activated cell sorting (FACS) analysis revealed that some population of MCA205 was annexin V-positive and PI-negative (i.e., apoptotic) (Fig. 1b). Taken together, it was shown that DCs could directly induce apoptosis in tumor cells.

Cytotoxic Effect of DCs: Mediation via Ca-Dependent and Ca-Independent Pathways

The mechanism of DCs' cytotoxicity remains unclear. Although MCA205 was functioning Fas receptor-positive (data not shown), the anti-Fas ligand antibody failed to block DCs' cytocidal effect (Fig. 2a). If EGTA/$MgCl_2$, a calcium chelator, was added to the assay, the antitumor cytotoxicity of DCs was significantly, but not completely, blocked (Fig. 2b). According to this assay, DCs might be able to kill tumor cells through both calcium-dependent and calcium–independent pathways.

Discussion

The present study reveals an antitumor cytotoxic effect of murine bone marrow-derived DCs against murine tumor cells. What kind of tumor cells DCs can kill remains unclear. DCs may use an immunogloblin-like receptor that contains immunoreceptor tyrosine-based inhibition/activation motifs (ITIM/ITAM) for the decision about tumor killing [5]. When DCs encounter tumor cells expressing inappropriate major histocompatibility complex (MHC)-antigen-peptide complexes, DCs might decide to kill and actually induce apoptosis in the tumors. To show that DCs phagocytose such apoptotic tumor cells and induce a specific antitumor effect, further investigations are needed. This new profile of DCs as effector cells provides hints that may help unveil DCs' physiology. When DCs are applied to cancer therapy, their cytotoxic capacity should be taken into account.

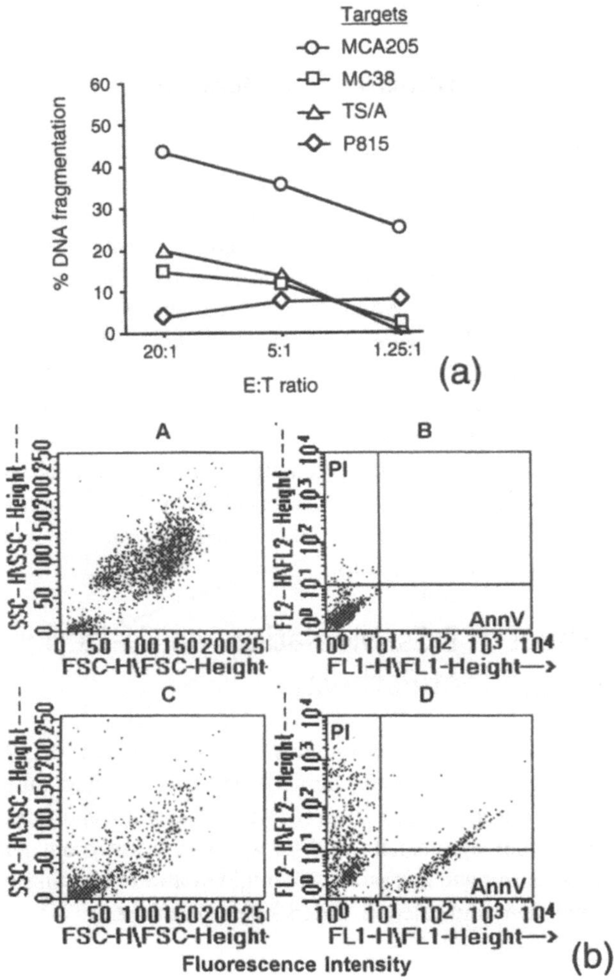

FIG. 1. DCs are directly cytotoxic against murine tumor cells. **a** Four kinds of tumor cells—MCA205 (*open circles*), MC38 (*open squares*), TS/A (*open triangles*), and P815 (*open diamonds*)—were used as target cells in an 18-h cytotoxicity assay. **b** MCA205 was eluted using MACS after incubation with medium only (*A, B*) or DCs (E:T ratio 10:1) (*C, D*) for 4h, stained with annexin V (Ann V) and propidium iodide (PI), and analyzed by flow cytometry

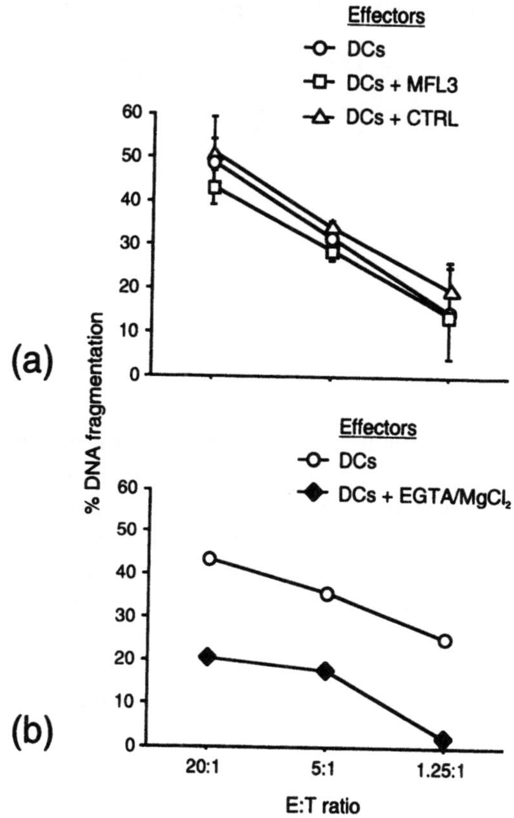

FIG. 2. DCs' effector function might be mediated via Ca-dependent, and Ca-independent pathways. **a** To block Fas/FasL interaction, either anti-FasL monoclonal antibodies (mAb) (MFL3, *open squares*), isotype-matched control mAb (CTRL, *open triangles*), or HBSS (no mAb, *open circles*) was added in an 18-h killing assay. **b** EGTA/$MgCl_2$ (*closed diamonds*) was used to chelate calcium in an 18-h killing assay

References

1. Banchereau J, Steinman RM (1998) Dendritic cells and the control of immunity. Nature 392:245
2. Tsujitani S, Kakeji Y, Watanabe A, et al (1990) Infiltration of dendritic cells in relation to tumor invasion and lymph node metastasis in human gastric cancer. Cancer 66:2012
3. Suss G, Shortman K (1996) A subclass of dendritic cells kills CD4 T cells via Fas/FasL-induced apoptosis. J Exp Med 183:1789
4. Albert ML, Sauter B, Bhardwaj N (1998) Dendritic cells acquire antigen from apoptotic cells and induce class I-restricted CTLs. Nature 392:86
5. Cella M, Døhring C, Samaridis J, et al (1997) A novel inhibitory receptor (ILT3) expressed on monocytes, macrophages, and dendritic cells involved in antigen processing. J Exp Med 185:1743

Autoimmune Mechanisms of Cancer-Associated Paraneoplastic Syndromes: A Review

Toshirou Nishida*

Summary. Paraneoplastic syndromes are organ disorders without direct tumor involvement. Some are syndromes trigged by autoimmunity induced by tumors. Neoplasia-induced immunity plays an important role in suppression of tumor progression but may cause paraneoplastic syndromes. Autoimmune paraneoplastic syndromes of the nervous and mucocutaneous systems are characterized by T cell-mediated autoantibody production. Cytotoxic T cells appear to be involved, although details of the mechanism remain unknown.

Key words. Paraneoplastic pemphigus, Autoantibody, Malignancy, Immunity

Introduction

Paraneoplastic syndromes represent organ dysfunction occurring at a site remote from the primary tumor and its metastasis. Most paraneoplastic syndromes occur in relation to specific tumors, and the presence of mediators is postulated. It is estimated that paraneoplastic syndromes occur in 7%–10% of patients with malignancy. The criteria include (1) association of the specific syndrome with a specific growing tumor; (2) dysfunctional organ not involved in tumor; (3) both conditions following a parallel course; and (4) factors causing the syndrome present in the blood and tumor [1]. Some paraneoplastic syndromes are caused by substances secreted from tumors, for example, ectopic adrenocorticotropic hormone (ACTH) secretion by small-cell lung carcinoma causes ectopic Cushing syndrome. Others occur by autoimmune mechanisms: Lambert-Eaton syndrome with small-cell lung carcinoma is caused by antibodies against the P/Q subtype of voltage-gated calcium channel (VGCC). This chapter reviews the association of neoplasia and autoimmunity and the mechanisms of paraneoplastic syndromes.

Department of Surgery (E1), Osaka University Graduate School of Medicine, 2-2 Yamadaoka, Suita, Osaka 565-0871, Japan
* e-mail: toshin@surg1.med.osaka-u.ac.jp

Relation Between Autoimmunity and Cancer

There appears to be a close relation between autoimmunity and malignancy [2]. An increased incidence of cancers has been observed among patients with autoimmune diseases. Alternatively, autoimmune conditions were found in patients with cancers. Indeed, various antibodies have been detected in sera of patients with malignancies even in the absence of overt autoimmune manifestations. For example, antinuclear antibodies (ANAs) are found in 13%–27% of cancer patients. Although mechanisms of neoplasia-induced autoimmunity are not known, it may play an important role in the prevention of tumor progression. Because tumor-induced immunity usually manifests as an autoimmune disorder, this autoimmunity may attack not only to tumor cells but also to host cells, resulting in paraneoplastic syndromes. When breast cancer expresses Yo proteins that are not expressed in the normal mammary gland but normally expressed in the cerebellum, antibodies against the Yo proteins induced by breast cancer may attack the Purkinje cells and cause cerebellar degeneration. One study showed that patients with small-cell lung cancer who have anti-Hu antibodies have a better prognosis than those who do not harbor such antibodies [3]. Others, however, noted that the presence of ANAs in the serum of patients with breast cancer was associated with a high risk of recurrence or metastasis [2]. Thus, the clinical and prognostic importance of autoimmunity and autoantibodies in cancer remains unknown. Futhermore, the mechanisms of neoplasm-induced autoantibody production and the interaction of autoantibodies with target cells in paraneoplastic syndromes are still open questions.

Autoimmune Paraneoplastic Syndromes

Most well-characterized autoimmune paraneoplastic syndromes are disorders of the nervous and mucocutaneous systems [3,4]. Some are listed in Table 1. For example, paraneoplastic cerebellar degeneration is associated with ovarian or breast cancer. Autoantibodies against the Yo proteins (cdr34, cdr62-1, cdr62-2) are postulated to be causative, as described above. Patients with paraneoplastic cerebellar degeneration show selective deletion of cerebellar Purkinje cells, and polyclonal immunoglobulin G (IgG) anti-Yo antibodies are found in both the cerebrospinal fluid and serum of patients. Paraneoplastic sensory neuropathy is found in some patients with small-cell lung cancer. The Hu antigen (35- to 40-kDa proteins), which refers to a family of nuclear proteins normally expressed in neurons but not in other cell types, is found in small-cell lung cancer, neuroblastoma, and less commonly sarcoma and prostatic cancer. The anti-Hu antibody is a marker of subacute sensory neuropathy and paraneoplastic encephalomyelitis.

The other important group of paraneoplastic syndromes show mucocutaneous manifestations. Pemphigus refers to a group of autoimmune mucocutaneous blistering diseases. There are several subgroups of pemphigus (e.g., pemphigus vulgaris, pemphigus foliaceus, paraneoplastic pemphigus) characterized by autoantibodies against desmoglein 3 (130-kDa protein), desmoglein 1 (160-kDa protein), and 250-, 230-, 210-, 190-, and 170-kDa proteins, respectively [4]. From 5% to 54% of patients

TABLE 1. Some well-characterized autoimmune paraneoplastic syndromes

Suspected antigen or mechanism	Syndrome	Typical cancers
Neural system		
Yo	Cerebellar degeneration	Breast cancer, ovarian cancer
Hu	Sensory neuropathy Encephalomyelitis	Lung cancer, neuroblastoma
Ri	Opsoclonus	Lung cancer, ovarian cancer
Tr	Cerebellar degeneration	Hodgkin's lymphoma
Amphiphysin	Stiff-man syndrome	Breast cancer, lung cancer
VGCC (P/Q type)	Lambert-Eaton syndrome	Lung cancer
VGKC	Neuromyotonia	Lung cancer, lymphoma
Acetylcholine receptor	Myasthenia gravis	Thymoma
Recoverin	Cancer-associated retinopathy, blindness	Lung cancer, melanoma
Glutamate receptor	Cerebellar ataxia	Hodgkin's lymphoma
Mucocutaneous system		
Desmoglein 3	Pemphigus vulgaris	Lymphoreticular tumors
Desmoglein 1	Pemphigus foliaceus	Lymphoreticular tumors
250, 230, 210, 190, 170 kDa	Paraneoplastic pemphigus	Lymphoreticular tumors
Insulin receptor	Acanthosis nigricans	Gastric cancer
Monoclonal light chain	Amyloidosis, acquired ichthyosis	Multiple myeloma, Hodgkin's lymphoma, sarcoma, breast cancer
Others		
Rh, LW, glycophorin, Pr, Wr, etc.	Hemolytic anemia	Lymphoma, leukemia
GP IIb/IIIa, GP Ib/IV	Thrombocytopenia	Lymphoproliferative diseases
NA1, NA2, CD11a, CD11b	Neutropenia	Lymphoproliferative diseases
Smooth muscle antigens?	Gastroparesis or intestinal pseudoobstruction	Carcinoid, thymoma, lung cancer

VGCC, voltage-gated calcium channel; VGKC, voltage-gated potassium channel

with pemphigus have occult or overt cancers: predominantly thymic tumors or lymphoreticular neoplasms followed by breast cancer and skin cancer.

Among the pemphigus groups, paraneoplastic pemphigus shows a practically 100% association with neoplasms. Paraneoplastic pemphigus was first reported by Anhalt et al. [5], with nearly 60 cases reported to date. This mucocutaneous disease occurs predominantly in middle-aged patients with lymphoreticular tumors and shows an unfavorable course because of associated tumors, immune suppression, and respiratory failure due to autoimmune mechanisms. Thus, paraneoplastic pemphigus is considered a neoplasia-induced autoimmune disease. We recently reported two cases of paraneoplastic pemphigus—myasthenia gravis and interdigitating reticulum cell sarcoma—at the 86th annual meeting of the Japanese Society of Gastroenterology. The patients had various autoantibodies, including ANA, and antibodies against acetylcholine receptor and desmoplakins. The tumors, interdigitating reticulum cell sarcomas, are considered neoplasia of the dendritic cells or antigen-presenting cells; and they expressed major histocompatibility complex (MHC) class II antigen and desmoplakin antigen, suggesting a possibility of antigen presentation by tumor cells and the possible involvement of T cell-mediated mechanisms in autoantibody production.

Pathogenesis of Paraneoplastic Syndromes

Most paraneoplastic syndromes appear to be mediated by autoantibodies or cytotoxic T cell-mediated mechanisms. Antibody-mediated mechanisms are characterized by Lambert-Eaton syndrome with anti-VGCC antibodies and by myasthenia gravis with anti-acetylcholine receptor antibodies. The above described cases suggested that antibody production was induced by antigen presentation of tumor cells through HLA class II-restricted T cell-mediated mechanisms. Removal of these antibodies by plasmapheresis may result in clinical improvement. Another mechanism, which is cytotoxic T cell (CTL)-mediated, is postulated in the anti-Hu syndrome. The CTL responses are restricted by HLA class I molecules, and plasmapheresis appears ineffective in this case. The other possibility is antibody production by tumor cells, as represented by multiple myeloma. However, detail mechanisms of paraneoplastic symptoms and neoplasia-induced autoimmunity are still not known.

In summary, autoimmune conditions induced by malignancies and paraneoplastic syndromes are not rare in patients with cancer. Neoplasia-induced autoimmunity plays an important role in tumor progression and paraneoplastic manifestations.

References

1. Cohen PR, Kurzrock R (1997) Mucocutaneous paraneoplastic syndromes. Semin Oncol 24:334–359
2. Tomer Y, Sherer Y, Shoenfeld Y (1998) Autoantibodies, autoimmunity and cancer. Oncol Rep 5:753–761
3. Posner JB, Dalmau J (1997) Paraneoplastic syndromes. Curr Opin Immunol 9:723–729
4. Nousari HC, Anhalt G (1999) Pemphigus and bullous pemphigoid. Lancet 354:667–672
5. Anhalt GJ, Kim S-C, Stabley JR, et al (1990) Paraneoplastic pemphigus: an autoimmune mucocutaneous disease associated with neoplasia. N Engl J Med 323:1729–1735

Antitumor Activity Against Gastrointestinal and Hepatocellular Carcinoma Induced by Immunization with Fusion of Dendritic and Carcinoma Cells in Mice

SADAMU HOMMA[1,2,*], TOSHIO IINUMA[1,2], GOTARO TODA[1], TSUNEYA OHNO[2], and DONALD KUFE[3]

Summary. Cancer immunotherapy targeting specific tumor-associated antigens (TAAs) is now being attempted. Dendritic cells (DCs) are potent antigen-presenting cells that play an important role in initiating and inducing antitumor immunity. DCs are used in cell therapy to present and prime TAAs to naive T cells for inducing antigen-specific antitumor immunity. Specific TAAs of gastrointestinal carcinomas (GICs) and hepatocellular carcinomas (HCCs) have not been identified. Immunization with fusion of DCs and cancer cells induce potent antitumor immunity against cancers whose TAA has not been identified. Immunotherapy with fusion of patients' DCs and cancer cells might be used to treat GICs and HCCs. We present results of basic studies of immunotherapy using DC/cancer cell fusions against GIC and HCC.

Key words. Dendritic cell, Cell fusion, Gastrointestinal carcinoma, Hepatocellular carcinoma, Cancer immunotherapy

Induction of Antitumor Immunity by Dendritic Cells

Identification of tumor-associated antigens (TAAs) has suggested that cancer might be treated by means of antigen-specific antitumor immunity [1]. Dendritic cells (DCs) are potent antigen-presenting cells that are essential for inducing the primary immune response [2]. These cells present and prime antigens, both "nonself" and "self" (e.g., TAAs), to naive T cells and play a key role in generating antitumor immunity [3,4]. Immunization of mice with DCs pulsed with tumor lysate or antigenic peptides eluted from cancer cells induces cytotoxic T lymphocytes against tumor cells in mice [5,6]. DCs transfected with genomic DNA coding the cloned TAA can induce specific T cell responses against the antigen [7].

[1] Division of Gastroenterology and Hepatology, Department of Internal Medicine, [2] Department of Oncology, Institute of DNA Medicine, Jikei University School of Medicine, 3-25-8 Nishi-shimbashi, Minato-ku, Tokyo 105-8461, Japan
[3] Dana-Farber Cancer Institute, Harvard Medical School, 44 Binney Street, Boston, MA 02115, USA
* e-mail: sahya@Jikei.ac.jp

Large numbers of human DCs can be collected by culturing peripheral blood mononuclear cells with granulocyte/macrophage colony-stimulating factor (GM-CSF) and interleukin-4 (IL-4) [8]. The level of function of DCs depends on their stage of maturation. Immature DCs can engulf exogenous antigens much better than can mature DCs, whereas mature DCs present antigens more effectively than do immature DCs [2]. Furthermore, DCs derived from patients with advanced cancer show lower antigen-presentation ability. Thus, assessing the functional properties of DCs is important for their use in immunotherapy.

Fusion of DCs and Cancer Cells: Efficient Induction of Specific Antitumor Immunity

Fusion of DCs and cancer cells can present antigens as genuine internal antigens. Furthermore, these fusions might be able to present and prime unidentified, poorly immunogenic multiple TAAs to naive T cells because whole cancer cells are used as immunogens (Fig. 1). In this setting, escape of cancer cells from immunological pressure by losing one specific target antigen might be avoided.

In our laboratory, fusions of DCs and cancer cells were generated by treatment of both cell types with 50% polyethyleneglycol. Figure 2 is a scanning electron micrograph of fusions of murine DCs and murine hepatoma cells. Splenocytes from mice immunized with these fusions showed specific cytotoxic activity against fusion partner cancer cells [9,10]. Fusion cell-immunized mice rejected inoculation with cancer cells, but treatment of the immunized mice with antibodies against CD8 and CD4 abolished this effect [9]. Established pulmonary metastases of murine colon cancer cells (MC38) were efficiently treated by immunization with DC/MC38 fusions [9]. However, solid tumors established by subcutaneous inoculation of BNL hepatoma cells in BALB/c mice were resistant to fusion immunotherapy. Combined treatment with the fusions and IL-12 inhibited the growth of BNL tumors in four of seven mice [10].

Immunization with DC/cancer cell fusions had preventive and therapeutic effects against gastrointestinal tumors in *APC* gene mutant mice. Mutation of the *APC* gene leads to familial polyposis coli and sequential development of colon cancers and is also observed in sporadic colon cancers [11,12]. In mice with mutations of codon 1309 of the *APC* gene, tumors begin to develop throughout the gastrointestinal tract 3 weeks after birth. Immunization with fusions of DCs and tumor cells and treatment with IL-12 at 6 weeks after birth significantly reduced tumor development in these mice. Immunization with fusions alone had somewhat weaker antitumor activity, but treatment with IL-12 alone had no significant antitumor effect.

Cancer Immunotherapy with Fusion of DCs and Cancer Cells

Cancer immunotherapy should be performed on the basis of the profile of "individual" cancer antigens, and cancer immunotherapy should be individualized for each patient in accordance with the multiplicity of TAAs. Cancer immunotherapy with

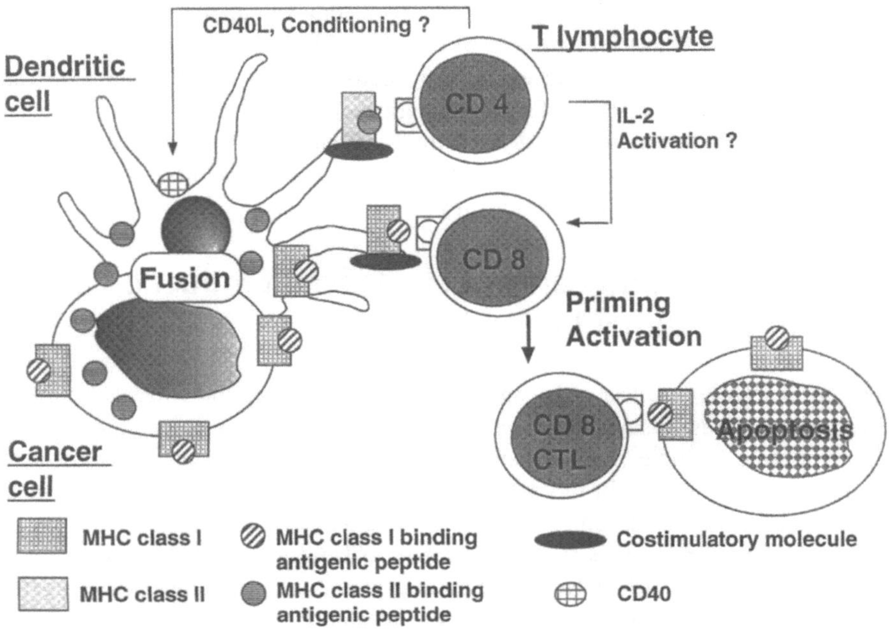

FIG. 1. Fusions (fusion cells) of dendritic cell and cancer cell present antigenic peptides of cancer antigens to naive T lymphocytes (both $CD4^+$ and $CD8^+$). Primed $CD8^+$ cytotoxic T lymphocytes (CTLs) recognize antigenic epitope of the cancer antigen complexed with major histocompatibility complex (*MHC*) class I molecules on the surface of cancer cell. Cancer cells undergo apoptosis by cytotoxic activity of the CTLs. Primed and activated $CD4^+$ helper-T lymphocytes might produce cytokines that activate $CD8^+$ CTLs and stimulate the function of fusions by CD40-CD40L system (conditioning)

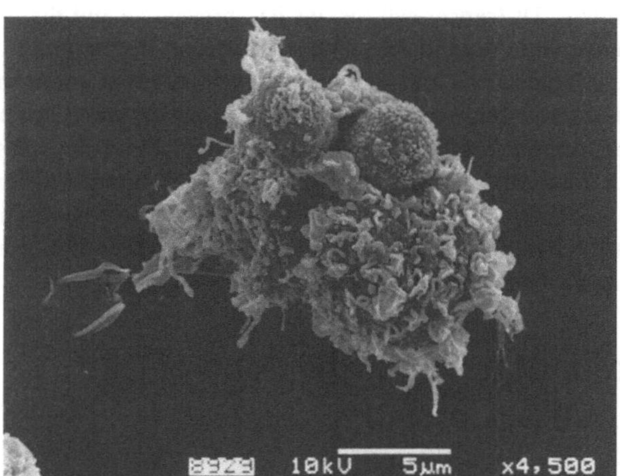

FIG. 2. Scanning electron micrograph of fusions of murine dendritic cell and murine hepatoma cell. Lymphocytes were attached to the surface of the fusion cell

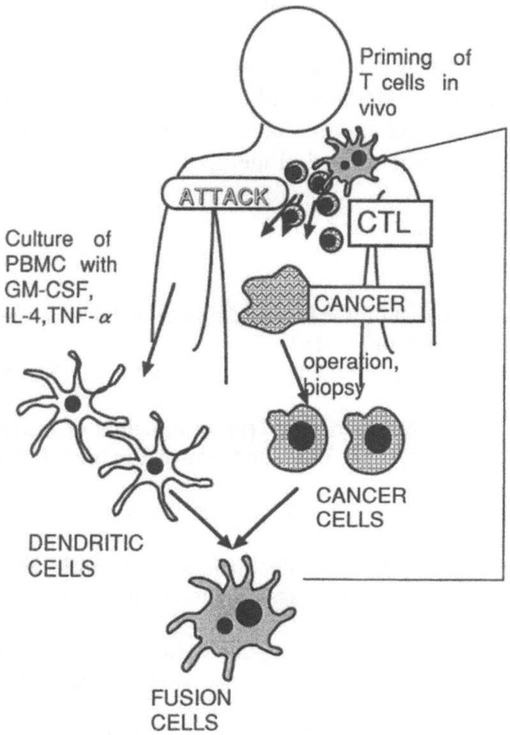

FIG. 3. Immunotherapy using dendritic cell/cancer cell fusions. Dendritic cells are obtained from progenitor cells in patients' peripheral blood mononuclear cells (*PBMCs*) by cultivation of PBMCs with granulocyte/macrophage stimulating factor (*GM-CSF*), interleukin-4 (*IL-4*), and tumor necrosis factor-α (*TNF*-α). Cancer cells obtained by surgical treatment or biopsy are irradiated and fused with autologous dendritic cells (DCs) by polyethyleneglycol treatment. Fusion cells are inoculated subcutaneously to the patient whose DCs and cancer cells are utilized to generate fusion cells; they migrate to lymph nodes and prime T lymphocytes, leading to induction of specific antitumor immunity

fusion of patients' own DCs and cancer cells may induce antitumor immunity based on the recognition of known, shared TAAs and of individually unique TAAs. Possibly, gastrointestinal carcinomas (GICs) and hepatocellular carcinomas (HCCs), whose specific TAAs have not been identified, might be efficiently treated with this immunotherapy.

Figure 3 shows an immunotherapy protocol using DC/cancer cell fusions. Viable cancer cells are collected from patients at surgery or with biopsy. Cancerous tissue is treated with digestive enzymes, and isolated cancer cells are cultured and stored. DCs obtained by culturing the patient's peripheral blood mononuclear cells with GM-CSF and IL-4 are fused with cancer cells. Before cell fusion, cancer cells are irradiated to prevent growth after inoculation. Fusions of DCs and cancer cells are suspended in saline and injected intradermally. Because antigens are primed by DCs in secondary lymphoid tissues, such as subcutaneous lymph nodes, intravenous administration of the fusions might be less effective than intradermal or subcutaneous administration. Primed T cells that can recognize TAAs and kill the cancer cells expressing them may be generated by immunization with fusions.

Supportive administration of cytokines may be needed to activate primed T cells and increase the susceptibility of cancer cells to T cells through such mechanisms as increased expression of major histocompatibility complex (MHC) molecules. An excellent therapeutic effect has been achieved against renal cell carcinoma by immunization with fusions of allogeneic DCs and autologous cancer cells [13].

In renal cell carcinoma allogeneic DCs may provide a more active immunological response, leading to enhanced production of cytokines; and the antigenic peptides of TAAs complexed with patients' MHC molecules are presented to T cells by functional co-stimulation of allogeneic DCs. Various immunological methods might be used to enhance the effects of fusion immunotherapy.

References

1. Rosenburg SA (1997) Cancer vaccines based on the identification of genes encoding cancer regression antigens. Immunol Today 18:175–182
2. Banchereau J, Steinman M (1998) Dendritic cells and the control on immunity. Nature 392:245–252
3. Grabbe S, Beissert S, Schwarz T, et al (1995) Dendritic cells as initiators of tumor immune responses: a possible strategy for tumor immunotherapy? Immunol Today 16:117–121
4. Shurin MR (1996) Dendritic cells presenting tumor antigen. Cancer Immunol Immunother 43:158–164
5. Paglia P, Chiodoni C, Rodolfo M, et al (1996) Murine dendritic cells loaded in vitro with soluble protein prime cytotoxic T lymphocytes against tumor antigen in vivo. J Exp Med 183:317–322
6. Celluzzi CM, Mayordomo JI, Storkus WJ, et al (1996) Peptide-pulsed dendritic cells induce antigen-specific CTL-mediated protective tumor immunity. J Exp Med 183:283–287
7. Butterfield LH, Jilani S, Chakraborty NG, et al (1998) Generation of melanoma-specific cytotoxic T lymphocytes by dendritic cells transduced with a MART-1 adenovirus. J Immmunol 161:5607–5613
8. Romani N, Grner S, Brang D, et al (1994) Proliferating dendritic cell progenitors in human blood. J Exp Med 180:83–93
9. Gong J, Chen D, Kashiwaba M, et al (1997) Induction of antitumor activity by immunization with fusions of dendritic and carcinoma cells. Nat Med 3:558–561
10. Homma S, Irie M, Toda G, et al (1999) Dendritic cell/cancer cell fusions CTL and antibody against cancer cells. In: Proceedings of 58th annual meeting of the Japanese Cancer Association, p 634
11. Kinzler KW, Nilbert MC, Su L-K, et al (1991) Identification of FAP locus gene from chromosome 5q21. Science 253:661–665
12. Nishisho I, Nakamura Y, Miyoshi Y, et al (1991) Mutation of chromosome 5q21 gene in FAP and colorectal cancer patients. Science 253:665–669
13. Kugler A, Stuhler G, Walden P, et al (2000) Regression of human metastatic renal cell carcinoma after vaccination with tumor cell-dendritic cell hybrids. Nat Med 6:332–336

Part 8
The Pathophysiology of Inflammatory Bowel Disease

Essential Role for Interleukin-6 in the Pathogenesis of Crohn's Disease

HIROAKI ITO[1,*] and TADAMITSU KISHIMOTO[2]

Summary. To investigate the role for interleukin-6 (IL-6) signaling in the pathogenesis of Crohn's disease (CD), we introduced anti-IL-6 receptor monoclonal antibody (anti-IL-6R mAb) to T-helpher type 1 (Th1) cell-mediated murine colitis and showed complete abrogation of intestinal inflammation by the treatment. Further examination revealed decreased colonic expression of intercellular adhesion molecule (ICAM-1) and vascular adhesion molecule (VCAM-1), marked reduction of interferon-γ, tumor necrosis factor-α, IL-1β, and inducible nitric oxide synthase mRNA, and increased TUNEL-positive apoptotic cells in the mice treated with anti-IL-6R mAb. These results show that IL-6 signaling plays an important role in the pathogenesis of intestinal inflammation by promoting leukocyte migration and inhibiting apoptosis of T cells; they also suggest a therapeutic potential of anti-IL-6R mAb for human CD.

Key words. Interleukin-6, Crohn's disease, Monoclonal antibody, Adhesion molecule, Apoptosis

Introduction

Proinflammatory cytokines have been demonstrated to play a crucial role in the pathogenesis of Crohn's disease (CD). Among those cytokines interleukin-6 (IL-6) must be especially important because increased serum concentration of C-reactive protein and fibrinogen, marked thrombocytosis, and loss of body weight are well explained by increased levels of IL-6. In a previous study we demonstrated transmural expression of IL-6 mRNA in the intestine of CD patients by in situ hybridization. The expression was most striking in subserosal vascular endothelium. Moreover, IL-6 can stimulate even receptor-negative cells to show a wide variety of bioactivities when complexed to the soluble form of IL-6 receptor. Therefore, to investigate the role for IL-6 signaling in CD pathogenesis, we introduced anti-IL-6 receptor monoclonal anti-

[1] Department of Molecular Medicine (C4), Osaka University Medical School, 2-2 Yamadaoka, Suita, Osaka 565-0871, Japan
[2] Osaka University, 2-2 Yamadaoka, Suita, Osaka 565-0871, Japan
* e-mail: hiroito@imed3.med.osaka-u.ac.jp

body (anti-IL-6R mAb) to murine wasting disease, T-helper type 1 (Th1) cell-mediated colitis [1].

Materials and Methods

Colitis was induced in CB17-SCID mice given CD45RB^{high} CD4^{+} T cells from normal Balb/c mice (both from Charles River Breeding Laboratories, Shiga, Japan). For cell preparation, CD4^{+} T cells were enriched from single-cell suspension of Balb/c splenocytes by the MACS magnetic separation system (Miltenyi Biotec, Auburn, CA, USA); then enriched CD4^{+} T cells were labeled with anti-CD4-PE (PharMingen, San Diego, CA, USA) and anti-CD45RB-FITC (PharMingen) and sorted on a FACS Vantage (Becton Dickinson, Sunnyvale, CA, USA). Anti-IL-6R mAb 2 mg [rat immunoglobulin G1 (IgG1), Chugai Pharmaceutical, Gotemba, Japan] or control rat IgG was administered intraperitoneally soon after T cell transfer, followed by weekly injection (1 mg). Body weight was monitored weekly. Colons were removed at 8 weeks, and colitis was graded histologically as 0 (minimal) to 3 (severe). Expansion of CD4^{+} cells were evaluated by fluorescence-activated cell sorter (FACS) and immunohistochemistry. Expression of intercellular (ICAM-1) and vascular (VCAM-1) adhesion molecules were analyzed by immunohistochemistry (anti-ICAM-1; Leico Technologies, St. Louis, MO, USA; anti-VCAM-1, Immunotech, Marseille, France). Apoptotic cells were demonstrated by the TUNEL method. Colonic expression of cytokine and inducible nitric oxide synthase (iNOS) were determined by reverse transcriptase polymerase chain reaction (RT-PCR).

Results

Mice treated with anti-IL-6R mAb showed normal growth, whereas controls lost weight. The average body weight at 8 weeks was as follows: mAb-treated mice 108.9% $\pm$ 1.9% and mice given control rat IgG 93.3% $\pm$ 5.0% of their initial body weight. The average colitis score was 0.6 $\pm$ 0.2 for mAb-treated mice and 1.8 $\pm$ 0.6 for controls. As shown in Fig. 1, colonic expression of ICAM-1 and VCAM-1, especially VCAM-1 in the vascular endothelium, was strongly suppressed by anti-IL-6R mAb treatment. Interferon-γ (IFN-γ), tumor necrosis factor-α (TNF-α), and IL-1β mRNA were markedly reduced; however, IL-10 and transforming growth factor-β (TGF-β) mRNA were detectable almost equally in both groups, whereas IL-4 was undetectable in either of the mice. Expression of iNOS mRNA, which was prominent in the mucosa of colitic mice, was also reduced by the treatment. Colonic and splenic CD4^{+} T cells were significantly decreased in mAb-treated mice. As shown in Fig. 2, increased TUNEL-positive apoptotic cells were observed in anti-IL-6R mAb-treated mice, and these cells were supposed to be CD4^{+} T cells from CD4 immunostaining.

Discussion

The data in this report provide evidence that IL-6 signaling plays a crucial role in the pathogenesis of Th1 cell-mediated wasting disease and colitis, a murine model of CD. Th1 cytokine IFN-γ is the major activator of macrophages, and activated macrophages

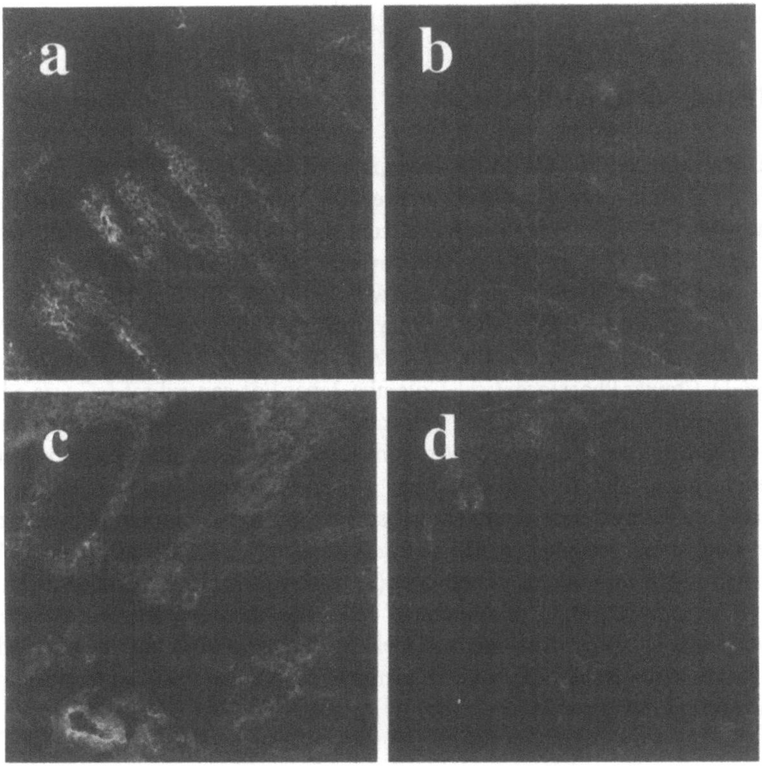

FIG. 1. Intercellular adhesion molecule-1 (ICAM-1) and vascular adhesion molecule-1 (VCAM-1) expression was suppressed by anti-interleukin-6 receptor (anti-IL-6R) monoclonal antibody (mAb). Colons from mice given rat immunoglobulin G (IgG) (**a**, **c**), mice treated with mAb (**b**, **d**) were stained by immunofluorescence for ICAM-1 (**a**, **b**) and VCAM-1 (**c**, **d**). ×200

produce proinflammatory cytokines, including IL-1, TNF-α, and IL-6. Furthermore, IL-6 is produced by various cells following IL-1 and TNFα stimulation. IL-6 is considered to play a central role in the regulation of inflammatory and immune reactions, and the requirement for IL-6 has been demonstrated for murine models of rheumatoid arthritis and multiple sclerosis. CD shares characteristics with these diseases in terms of activation of $CD4^+$ T cells and participation of proinflammatory cytokines. Proinflammatory cytokines are known to up-regulate a spectrum of cell adhesion molecules, including ICAM-1, VCAM-1, selectins, and integrins. In the study of human inflammatory bowel disease, ICAM-1^+ inflammatory infiltrates and venules were demonstrated to increase in parallel with the degree of inflammation [2]. In our study, there was enhanced expression of both ICAM-1 and VCAM-1 in the mice with wasting disease, and treatment with anti-IL-6R mAb significantly reduced the expression of both adhesion molecules. Reduction of expression was notable in small vessel walls and lamina propria infiltrates. Suppression of VCAM-1 by mAb treatment seemed more striking than suppression of ICAM-1 [3]. Recently insufficient T cell apoptosis

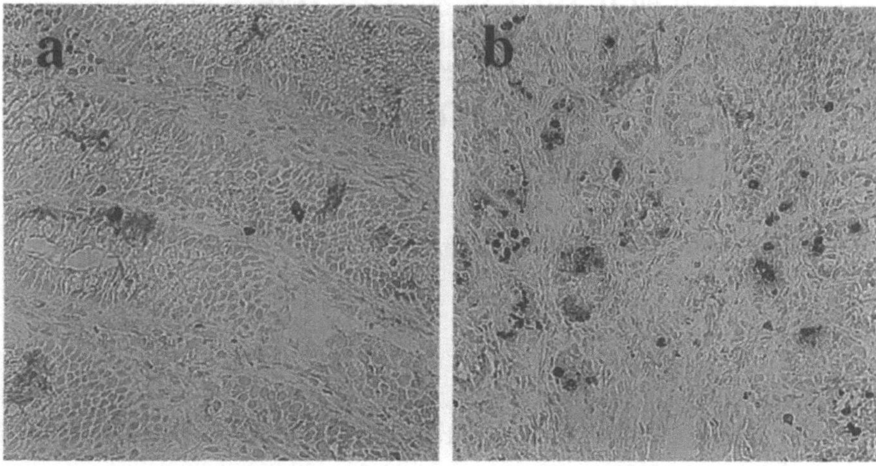

FIG. 2. Increased number of apoptotic cells were seen in the colon of mAb-treated mice. Colons from mice given rat IgG (**a**) and mAb-treated mice (**b**) were stained by the TUNEL method

in CD has been reported, which may result in inappropriate T cell accumulation contributing to chronic inflammation [4]. Our result of increased TUNEL-positive cells in mAb-treated mice showed a possible contribution of IL-6 in impaired apoptosis in those with chronic colitis.

Conclusions

The results presented here show that IL-6 actively participates in the pathogenesis of murine colitis by promoting leukocyte migration and inhibiting apoptosis of activated T cells. They suggest a therapeutic potential of anti-IL-6R mAb for human CD.

References

1. Powrie F, Leach MW, Mauze S, et al (1994) Inhibition of Th1 responses prevents inflammatory bowel disease in SCID mice reconstituted with CD45RB^{hi} CD4^{+} T cells. Immunity 1:553–562
2. Koizumi M, King N, Lobb R, et al (1992) Expression of vascular adhesion molecules in inflammatory bowel disease. Gastroenterology 103:840–847
3. Yamamoto M, Yoshizaki K, Kishimoto T, et al (2000) IL-6 is required for the development of Th1 cell-mediated murine colitis. J Immunol 164:4878–4882
4. Ina K, Itoh J, Fukushima K, et al (1999) Resistance of Crohn's disease T cells to multiple apoptotic signals is associated with a Bcl-2/Bax mucosal imbalance. J Immunol 163:1081–1090

Activation of Nuclear Factor κB in Dextran Sulfate Sodium-Induced Colitis in Mice and Their Inhibition by Phenyl *N-tert*-Butylnitrone

TOMOHISA TAKAGI[1,*], YUJI NAITO[1], TOSHIKAZU YOSHIKAWA[1], and YASHIGE KOTAKE[2]

Summary. Nuclear factor (NF)-κB is a transcriptional factor that regulates the activation of numerous genes in response to pathogens and proinflammatory cytokines; it is therefore pivotal in the initiation and perpetuation of chronic intestinal inflammation. This review discusses a series of studies that demonstrate NF-κB activation in the inflamed mucosa of animal models and patients with inflammatory bowel disease. There is increasing evidence that NF-κB is important in the pathophysiology of inflammatory bowel disease; therefore, therapeutic interventions aimed at limiting NF-κB activation and down-regulating production of inflammatory mediators could prove beneficial in decreasing host-derived tissue injury and colon dysfunction. A nitron-based free radical trapping agent, phenyl-*N-tert*-butylnitrone (PBN) has been shown to protect animals from various oxidative disorders and to inhibit the activation of NF-κB. Acute inflammation induced by dextran sulfate sodium (DSS) was significantly reduced by the injection of PBN. The elevation of inflammatory cytokines (IL-4, interleukin-4, interferon-γ, tumor necrosis factor-α) enhanced by DSS administration were also inhibited by PBN, accompanied with the inhibition of DNA-binding activity of NF-κB. These results indicate that NF-κB activation up-regulates the expression of inflammatory cytokines during the development of colitis, and PBN has antiinflammatory properties against DSS-induced colonic inflammation by inhibiting such up-regulation.

Key words. Inflammatory bowel disease, Crohn's disease, Ulcerative colitis, Dextran sulfate sodium, Nuclear factor κB, Phenyl *N-tert*-butylnitrone

---

[1] First Department of Medicine, Kyoto Prefectural University of Medicine, Kamigyo-ku, Kyoto 602-8566, Japan
[2] Free Radical Biology and Aging Reseach Program, Oklahoma Medical Research Foundation, OK 73104-5046, USA
* e-mail: takatomo@koto.kpu-m.ac.jp

Introduction

Inflammatory bowel disease, including Crohn's disease and ulcerative colitis, is characterized by increased expression of inflammatory cytokines, adhesion molecules, and inducible enzymes such as inducible nitric oxide synthase (iNOS) and cyclooxygenase 2. Expression of these genes by various environmental signals is primarily regulated by changing the transcription rate of the gene, a process controlled by sequence-specific DNA-binding proteins called transcriptional factors. Nuclear factor-κB (NF-κB), a family of transcriptional factors, is known to regulate a variety of genes controlling the cell cycle, immune function, and inflammatory processes [1]. Protective effects of an antisense oligonucleotide against the p65 subunit of NF-κB in an animal model of colitis [2] suggests that blockage of this transcriptional factor may represent a valuable therapeutic strategy for human inflammatory bowel disease.

NF-κB Activation Pathway

NF-κB is a dimer composed of 2 rel family members: NF-κB/p50 and Rel A/p65. Most of the NF-κB in unstimulated cells is regulated by association with one of many inhibitory molecules. NF-κB residues in the cytoplasm as an inactive complex bound to the inhibitor protein IkB. In response to a variety of stimuli, such as interleukin (IL)-1β, tumor necrosis factor (TNF)-α, lipopolysaccharide (LPS), or phorbol esters, IκB proteins are rapidly phosphorylated by the recently identified IκB kinase (IKK) complex (IKKα and IKKβ). IKK-induced phosphorylation of IκB occurs on residues Ser^{32} and Ser^{36} for IkBa and on Ser^{19} and Ser^{23} for IκBβ, which targets these inhibitory proteins for rapid polyubiquitination and degradation through the 28S proteasome, allowing active NF-κB to translocate to the nucleus. NF-κB translocation leads to expression of a large number of NF-κB-dependent genes, which are important mediators of immune and inflammatory responses, including TNFα, IL-1, IL-6, IL-8, IL-10, granulocyte/macrophage colony-stimulating factor (GM-CSF), inducible nitric oxide synthase, intercellular adhesion molecule 1 (ICAM-1), E-selectin, vascular cell adhesion molecule 1 (VCAM-1), and magic histocompatibility complex (MHC) class I and II molecules.

It is becoming clear that many of the clinically important antiinflammatory agents, including salicylates, glucocorticoids, and nitric oxide, share the ability to inhibit NF-κB-driven gene expression in leukocytes, macrophages, and endothelial cells. Thus, the NF-κB/IκBα regulatory pathway is a critical target for therapeutic intervention in pathological conditions, including inflammatory bowel disease.

NF-κB Activation in Inflammatory Bowel Disease

To investigate whether increased activation of NF-κB is important in inflammatory bowel disease, NF-κB activation has been determined by Western blot assessment for NF-κB p65 and electrophoretic mobility shift assay (EMSA) in nuclear extracts of colon biopsy samples as well as lamina propria mononuclear cells in patients with Crohn's disease or ulcerative colitis. Using a monoclonal antibody (a-p65 mAB), which recognizes an epitope on the p65 subunit that is masked by bound IκB, Rogler et al. [3] clearly demonstrated that activated NF-κB could be found in biopsy specimens from inflamed mucosa from the patients with inflammatory bowel disease, and that NF-κB activation was localized in macrophages and epithelial cells. Because a-p65 mAb recognizes p65 only if it is free of its inhibitor IκB, this antibody might serve as a simple tool for studying the transcriptional activity of NF-κB.

NF-κB Activation in Dextran Sulfate Sodium-Induced Colitis

Interleukin-2-deficient (IL-$2^{-/-}$) mice and dextran sulfate sodium (DSS)-treated animals have colitis with striking clinical and histologic similarity to ulcerative colitis in humans. Like patients with ulcerative colitis, these animals have increased activation of T and B cells, elevated immunoglobulin secretion, focal crypt lesions, mucosal and submucosal inflammation, and granulocyte infiltration. With IL-$2^{-/-}$ mice Yang et al. [4] clearly showed that nuclear NF-κB p65 and its inhibitor IκBα, but not IκBβ, were markedly elevated during the early phases of colitis and remained elevated throughout the course of the disease. Consistent with the activation of NF-κB, IL-1β and TNFα expression was increased. These data corroborate our observations obtained from DSS-induced colitis models [5]. The binding activity of NF-κB in nuclear extracts of mouse colonic tissue cells to its consensus oligonucleotide was analyzed by EMSA. Dramatically increased nuclear NF-κB DNA binding activity was observed in nuclear extracts from the colon of DSS-treated mice at 3, 5, 7, and 10 days but not in nuclear extracts from normal mucosa without DSS administration (Fig. 1). NF-κB can be activated by numerous stimuli including TNFα and interferon-γ (IFNγ), and gene expression of these cytokines is critically regulated by this transcriptional factor. Therefore, we examined the relation of these cytokines to NF-κB activation and the severity of the colitis. The mRNA expression for iNOS, TNFα, and IFNγ was increased over the levels of normal mice, which was consistent with the elevated NF-κB activation. The observation of increased mRNA expression of iNOS, TNFα, and IFNγ in the same inflammatory sites in which NF-κB were detected strongly suggests that NF-κB has transactivating activity in the intestinal mucosa.

Action of Phenyl *N-tert*-Butylnitrone

Phenyl *N-tert*-butylnitrone (PBN), originally developed as a free radical trapping agent, has a variety of pharmacological effects, including the prevention of death caused by endotoxin shock, antiaging, and an antidiabetic effect. These actions suggest that the effect of PBN is largely antiinflammatory. It has been demonstrated that NF-κB was clearly inhibited by PBN in lipopolysaccharide (LPS)/IFNγ-stimulated macrophages [6]. A 50% inhibitory concentration for NF-κB inhibition was estimated to be approximately 8 mM, which is consistent with that of iNOS mRNA inhibition [7], suggesting that NF-κB plays a major role in transcription of the iNOS gene. In addition, Sang et al. [8] demonstrated that PBN reduces LPS-induced cytokine expression including TNFα, IL-1β, IL-3, IL-4, IL-5, and IL-6; and it inhibits LPS-induced activa-

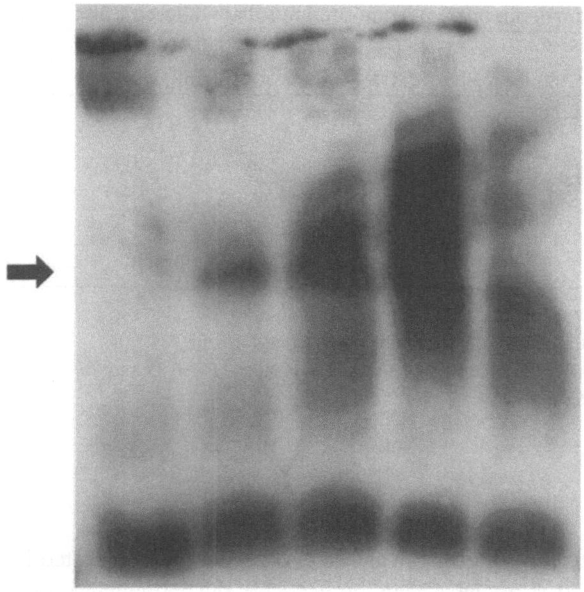

FIG. 1. Electrophoretic mobility shift assay for colonic mucosal NF-κB DNA binding activity in mice administered 8% dextran sulfate sodium

tion of NF-κB and AP-1 in vivo. Because activation of NF-κB is suggested to be redox-sensitive or free-radical-mediated, it is possible that PBN might prevent oxidative stress-associated injury through down-regulation or inhibition of transcriptional factor NF-κB.

Inhibition by PBN Against DSS Colitis

Mice exposed to 8% DSS developed symptoms of acute colitis, with diarrhea being observed first, followed by rectal bleeding and severe weight loss. The decreases in body weight and total length of the colon were significantly reversed by co-treatment with PBN at doses of 0.3, 3.0, and 30 mg/kg (Table 1) [5]. The increase in myeloperoxidase activity and thiobarbituric acid-reactive substances in the colonic mucosa after DSS administration was significantly inhibited by treatment with PBN in a dose-dependent manner. The colonic content of inflammatory cytokines (IL-4, IL-10, and IFN-γ) increased significantly 7 days after DSS administration. The increase in inflammatory cytokines in the colonic mucosa was significant inhibited by PBN at doses of 0.03, 0.1, and 0.3 mg/kg. Administration of DSS alone enhanced NF-κB DNA binding activity in inflamed colonic tissue, which was suppressed by PBN administration at a dose of 3.0 mg/kg. We also examined cytokine expression in the inflamed colonic tissues of DSS-treated mice. The mRNA expression of TNFα and IFNγ was increased

TABLE 1. Effects of phenyl *N-tert*-butylnitrone on body weight, total length of the colon, and intraluminal hemoblobin in 8% dextran sodium sulfate-induced colitis in mice

Condition	Weight gain (g/7 days)	Total length of the colon (cm)	Luminal hemoglobin (mg/cm)
No colitis	0.28 ± 0.17	11.43 ± 0.14	0.80 ± 0.19
DSS alone	−2.42 ± 0.21*	9.10 ± 0.37*	6.29 ± 1.12**
PBN co-administration			
0.3 mg/kg	−2.12 ± 0.46#	9.80 ± 0.26#	3.08 ± 1.21#
3.0 mg/kg	−1.34 ± 0.19#	10.25 ± 0.43#	2.21 ± 0.41#
30 mg/kg	−0.96 ± 0.21##	10.30 ± 0.20##	3.29 ± 0.73#

Values represent the mean + SEM for five to seven mice

DSS, dextran sodium sulfate; PBN, phenyl *N-tert*-butylnitrone

* $P < 0.01$ and ** $P < 0.005$ compared to untreated mice; # $P < 0.05$ and ## $P < 0.01$ compared to mice receiving only DSS

over that in the control group, which was consistent with elevated NF-κB activation. Both of these cytokines have been implicated in the pathogenesis of intestinal inflammation, and both are regulated by NF-κB.

Conclusions

The studies summarized above indicate that modulating the activation of NF-κB in intestinal cells, monocytes/macrophages, and endothelial cells is one of the mechanisms by which a number of antiinflammatory drugs inhibit inflammatory bowel disease. NF-κB increases colonic expression of the genes for proinflammatory cytokines, chemokines, enzymes, and adhesion molecules, leading to coordinated stimulation of the inflammatory response of the colon. Several therapeutic approaches successfully inhibit NF-κB DNA-binding activity, including treatment with antisense oligonucleotides to the p65 subunit and PBN. Understanding the action mechanisms of antiinflammatory drugs targeting the NF-κB pathway will greatly benefit treatment decisions and the development of novel strategies to treat inflammatory bowel disease.

References

1. Barnes PJ, Karin M (1997) Nuclear factor-κB: a pivotal transcriptional factor in chronic inflammatory disease. N Engl J Med 336:1066–1071
2. Neurath MF, Pettersson S, Meyer, Zum B, et al (1996) Local administration of antisense phosphorothioate oligonucleotides to the p65 subunit of NF-kappa B abrogates established experimental colitis in mice. Nat Med 2:998–1004
3. Rogler G, Brand K, Vogl D, et al (1998) Nuclear factor kappaB is activated in macrophages and epithelial cells of inflamed intestinal mucosa. Gastroenterology 115:357–369
4. Yang F, de Villiers WJ, Lee EY, et al (1999) Increased nuclear factor-kappaB activation in colitis of interleukin-2-deficient mice. J Lab Clin Med 134:378–385

5. Takagi T, Naito Y, Handa O, et al (2000) Expression of cytokines and activation of neutrophils in dextran sodium sulfate-induced colitis in mice and their inhibition by phenyl *N*-tert-butylnitrone. Gastroenterology 118:A578
6. Kotake Y, Sang H, Miyajima T, et al (1998) Inhibition of NF-kappaB, iNOS mRNA, COX2 mRNA, and COX catalytic activity by phenyl-*N-tert*-butylnitrone (PBN). Biochim Biophys Acta 1448:77–84
7. Miyajima T, Kotake Y (1997) Optimal time and dosage of phenyl *N-tert*-butyl nitrone (PBN) for the inhibition of nitric oxide synthase induction in mice. Free Radic Biol Med 22:463–470
8. Sang H, Wallis GL, Stewart CA, et al (1999) Expression of cytokines and activation of transcription factors in lipopolysaccharide-administered rats and their inhibition by phenyl *N-tert*-butylnitrone (PBN). Arch Biochem Biophys 363:341–348

Essential Roles for Th2-Type Responses in Chronic Intestinal Inflammation

TAEKO DOHI*

Summary. Potential involvement of T-helper (Th) 2-type responses in experimental murine models for inflammatory bowel diseases (IBDs) were investigated. Trinitrobenzene sulfonic acid (TNBS)-induced colitis was assessed in the Th1- or Th2-cytokine dominant condition using cytokine gene knockout mice and anti-cytokine monoclonal antibodies. Th1-type cytokine-dominant mice developed acute, focal, and transmural lesions. In contrast, Th2-type responses played a significant role in the diffuse atrophic changes in crypts and mucosal layer and in perpetuating disease. These findings will contribute to future immunological interventions in IBD.

Key words. Inflammatory bowel disease, T cells, Cytokines, Hapten-induced colitis, Gut-associated lymphoid tissue

Introduction

To maintain the homeostasis of the normal mucosal immune system in the intestinal tract, there is a delicate regulation system that balances between immunity to microbial pathogens and tolerance to food antigens and indigenous flora. The mucosal immune system can be divided into inductive sites and an effector region. The former are termed gut-associated lymphoreticular tissues (GALT) and include Peyer's patches, whereas the latter is a lamina propria characterized by more diffuse collections of lymphocytes and plasma cells. In the GALT, immune responses lead to up-regulation of antipathogenic responses (including antibody production and activation of cytotoxic cells) or to suppression of systemic immunity to ubiquitous luminal antigens.

Inflammatory bowel diseases (IBDs), Crohn's disease and ulcerative colitis, are chronic tissue destructive diseases in the intestine that have different pathological characteristics. Although their etiology is yet unknown, accumulating circumstantial evidence supports the notion that IBD is linked to failure of the mucosal immune

Department of Gastroenterology, Research Institute, International Medical Center of Japan, 1-21-1 Toyama, Shinjuku-ku, Tokyo 162-8655, Japan
* e-mail: dohi@ri.imcj.go.jp

system to attenuate immunity to luminal antigens [1]. It is generally recognized that excess Th1-type immune responses may have a significant role in Crohn's disease, whereas Th2-type responses are more involved in ulcerative colitis [2–4].

Various experimental murine models of IBD support a central role for T cells in chronic intestinal inflammation [5]. These models were characterized by disturbed cytokine balance, most notably excessive production of the Th1-cytokine interferon-γ (IFNγ). Colitis induced by rectal administration of the hapten 2,4,6-trinitrobenzene sulfonic acid (TNBS) was also first shown to be mediated by a Th1-type inflammation [6]. This model has the important advantage of employing normal mice with an intact immune system, thereby allowing systematic investigation of the exact roles of individual immunocompetent cells for the development of mucosal inflammation. We used the TNBS-induced colitis model to determine if mice that develop either predominant $CD4^+$ Th1- or Th2-type responses exhibit distinct inflammatory lesions.

Colitis in the Absence of IFNγ

To examine the possible significance of Th2-type responses, we first queried if colitis would develop in mice deficient in IFNγ production [7]. TNBS in 50% ethanol solution was intrarectally given to IFNγ gene knockout mice (IFN$\gamma^{-/-}$) or normal mice. Interestingly, IFN$\gamma^{-/-}$ mice developed weight loss, ulcers, crypt distortion, and loss of goblet cells to the same extent as did the control mice. Another major finding was enlarged lymphoid follicles in the colon (Fig. 1A). We found that these follicles are colonic patches (colonic GALT) by identifying M cells, T and B cell zones, and germinal centers. The enlargement of colonic patches in the inflamed colon was enhanced in IFN$\gamma^{-/-}$ mice. T cells prepared from colonic patches produced interleukins 4 and 5 (IL-4, IL-5) after restimulation with TNBS. Treatment with anti-IFNγ monoclonal antibody failed to prevent colitis, whereas anti-IL-4 monoclonal antibody ameliorated inflammatory changes of the crypts.

These results clearly show that intestinal tissue damage occurs in the absence of IFNγ. In this regard, Th2-type cytokine production takes place in the enlarged colonic patches, which are colonic inductive sites. Thus, chronic intestinal inflammation may occur in immunologically altered conditions where Th2-type responses are dominant.

Phenotypes of Colitis in the Th1- or Th2-Dominant Condition

Next we hypothesized that the Th1- or Th2-dominant condition causes distinct forms of colitis. To address this idea we compared TNBS colitis induced in IFNγ gene knockout mice (IFN$\gamma^{-/-}$), IL-12 gene knockout mice (IL-$12^{-/-}$), IL-4 gene knockout mice (IL-$4^{-/-}$), and background C57BL/6 mice [8].

First, we found that IL-$4^{-/-}$ mice showed greater sensitivity to TNBS; half of the mice survived the TNBS enema treatment, and most deaths occurred within 4 days after the first TNBS enema. With the same dose of TNBS, more than 90% of the IFN$\gamma^{-/-}$ and IL-$12^{-/-}$ mice survived. By histological analysis, IFN$\gamma^{-/-}$ and IL-$12^{-/-}$ mice all developed patterns of colitis characterized by distortion of crypts, loss of goblet cells, and mononuclear cell infiltration with fibrosis of the mucosal layer (Fig. 1B). In contrast,

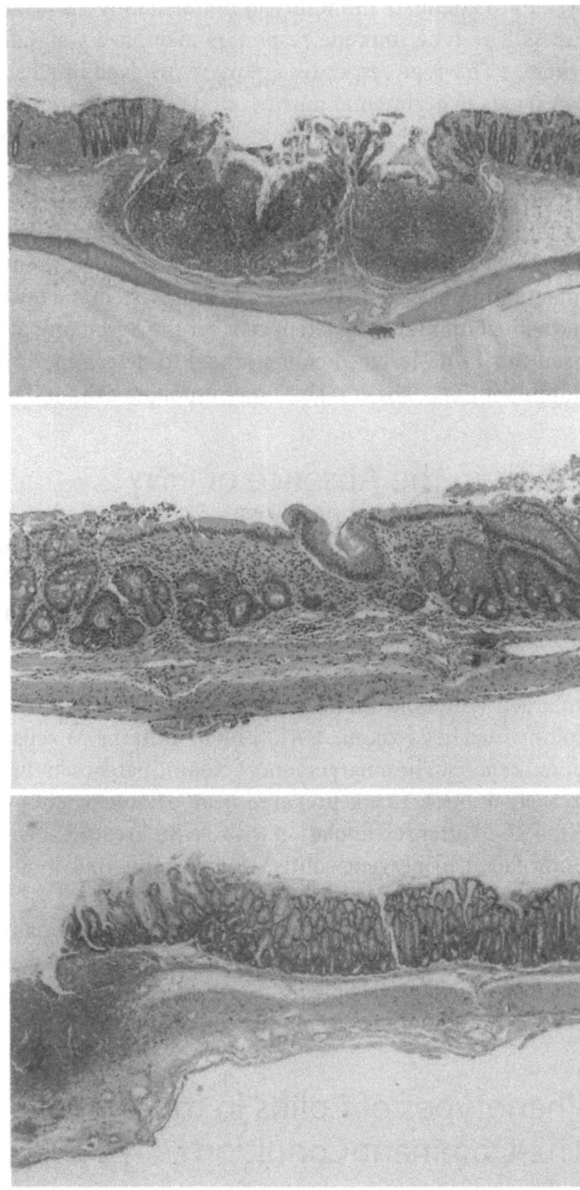
A B C

FIG. 1. Histological features of trinitrobenzene sulfonic acid (TNBS) colitis induced in cytokine knockout mice. Colonic tissues were fixed with acid alcohol, and paraffin-embedded sections were stained with hematoxylin and eosin. **A** Enlarged colonic patch with diffuse mucosal atrophic changes in interferon-$\gamma^{-/-}$ (IFN$\gamma^{-/-}$) mice. **B** Severe crypt distortion with mononuclear cell infiltration is observed in interleukin-$12^{-/-}$ (IL-$12^{-/-}$) mice. **C** IL-$4^{-/-}$ mice developed transmural ulcers, but adjacent crypts and goblet cells are almost intact. Original magnification: **A** and **C** ×10, **B** ×40

the higher mortality of IL-$4^{-/-}$ mice was due to penetrating ulcers; the survivors developed milder lesions, which were limited to focal acute ulceration. Colonic epithelial cells showed rather reactive hyperplasia with elongation of the crypts (Fig. 1C). Colonic $CD4^+$ T cells from IL-$4^{-/-}$ mice produced IFNγ and tumor neurosis factor (TNFα) during the early phase of colitis, whereas IFN$\gamma^{-/-}$ or IL-$12^{-/-}$ mice produced both IL-4 and IL-5 during the later stage. Serum levels of IFNγ increased sharply 2 days after the TNBS enema in control and IL-$4^{-/-}$ mice. IL-$12^{-/-}$ mice did not show this acute up-regulation of IFNγ. Based on these results we conclude that with TNBS colitis the Th1-like cytokine responses induce acute, fatal, transmural and focal ulcer types of lesions, and the Th2-like cytokine responses play a significant role in the diffuse atrophic changes limited to the crypts or the mucosal layer that occur during the late stages of this disease.

Conclusions

Our comparative study of experimental colitis illustrated that a single antigen can induce different types of inflammation depending on the dominance of the Th1 or the Th2 type responses. These results also provide new clues to the differential pathogenesis of Crohn's' disease and ulcerative colitis.

References

1. Brandtzaeg P, Haraldsen G, Rugtveit J (1997) Immunopathology of human inflammatory bowel disease. Springer Semin Immunopathol 18:555–589
2. Niessner M, Vold BA (1995) Altered Th1/Th2 cytokine profiles in the intestinal mucosa of patients with inflammatory bowel disease as assessed by quantitative reversed transcribed polymerase chain reaction (RT-PCR). Clin Exp Immunol 101:428–435
3. Fuss IJ, Neurath M, Boirivant M, et al (1996) Disparate $CD4^+$ lamina propria (LP) lymphokine secretion profiles in inflammatory bowel disease. J Immunol 157:1261–1270
4. Monteleone G, MacDonald TT, Wathen NC, et al (1999) Enhancing lamina propria Th1 cell responses with interleukin 12 produces severe tissue injury. Gastroenterology 117:1069–1077.
5. Elson CO, Sartor RB, Tennyson GS, et al (1995) Experimental models of inflammatory bowel disease. Gastroenterology 109:1344–1367
6. Neurath MF, Fuss I, Kelsall BL, et al (1995) Antibodies to interleukin-12 abrogate established experimental colitis in mice. J Exp Med 182:1281–1290
7. Dohi T, Fujihashi K, Rennert PD, et al (1999) Hapten-induced colitis is associated with colonic patch hypertrophy and T-helper type 2 responses. J Exp Med 189:1169–1179
8. Dohi T, Fujihashi K, Kiyono H, et al (2000) Mice deficient in Th1-type and Th2-type cytokines develop distinct forms of hapten-induced colitis. Gastroenterology 119:724–733

Induction of Colitis and Exocrinopathy in Nude Mice Induced by Immunocompetent Cell Transfer from Murine Retrovirus-Infected Mice

Kenji Suzuki[1,*], Yasuyuki Baba[1], Hidehisa Suriki[1], Hiroshi Kawachi[2], Fujio Shimizu[2], and Hitoshi Asakura[1]

Summary. LP-BM5 murine leukemia virus (MuLV) is known to induce murine acquired immunodeficiency syndrome (MAIDS). We have shown that Sjögren syndrome (SS)-like exocrinopathy can be induced in mice with MAIDS and that adoptive transfer of immunocompetent cells of MAIDS mice can induce inflammatory bowel disease (IBD)-like colitis, which we termed "MAIDS colitis," and exocrinopathy in recipient syngeneic nude mice. To identify which phenotype of cells in MAIDS induces colitis and exocrinopathy in our model, we analyzed adoptive transfer of separated cell fraction into nude mice. LP-BM5 MuLV was inoculated in 4-week-old C57BL/6 (B6) mice intraperitoneally. Eight weeks after infection, lymph node cells from the virus-infected mice were separated into three fractions using magnetic beads as follows: group1, whole lymph node cells; group2, $CD4^+$ T cells; group3, non-T, non-B ($Mac\text{-}1^+$) cells. Each fraction was transferred to B6 nude mice. Four to six weeks after cell transfer the mice were killed and their tissues analyzed histopathologically. All of the mice inoculated with MAIDS lymph node cells (group 1) exhibited colitis and systemic exocrinopathy, and they died within 6 weeks after cell transfer. Transfer of the $CD4^+$ fraction (group 2) induced exocrinopathy but not colitis. Transfer of the non-T, non-B ($Mac\text{-}1^+$) cell fraction (group 3) induced colitis but not exocrinopathy. $Mac\text{-}1^+$ macrophages and $CD4^+$ T cells of mice with MAIDS play a distinct role in the development of organ-specific autoimmune-like lesions (i.e., ulcerative colitis-like colitis and SS-like exocrinopathy, respectively).

Key words. LP-BM5, Murine AIDS, Ulcerative colitis, Sjögren syndrome, Exocrinopathy

---

[1] Third Department of Internal Medicine, [2] Department of Immunology, Institute of Nephrology, Niigata University School of Medicine, 1-757 Asahimachi-dori, Niigata 951-8122, Japan
* e-mail: kjsuzuki@med.niigata-u.ac.jp

Introduction

The LP-BM5 murine leukemia virus (MuLV) is a retrovirus that is known to induce profound immunodeficiency with splenomegaly and generalized lymphadenopathy in susceptible strains of mice such as the B6 mouse [1–3]. Virus-infected B6 mice show symptoms similar to those of human acquired immunodeficiency syndrome (AIDS), and therefore they have been studied as a murine model of AIDS [2]. We have reported previously that systemic exocrinopathy resembling Sjögren syndrome (SS) was induced in virus-infected mice [4], and that nude mice inoculated with lymph node cells or spleen cells from mice with murine AIDS (MAIDS) developed inflammatory bowel disease (IBD)-like colitis, which we termed MAIDS colitis, as well as SS-like exocrinopathy [5].

Histopathological analysis revealed that infiltration of inflammatory cells was limited to the mucosal and submucosal layers, and that mucosal erosion and hyperplasia of epithelial cells were also induced. These histological characteristics suggest that MAIDS colitis mimics ulcerative colitis (UC) rather than Crohn's disease (CD). Inflammatory cells infiltrating the colitis lesions of MAIDS colitis mice were shown to be mainly $CD4^+$ T cells and Mac-1^+ cells. As for SS-like exocrinopathy, $CD4^+$ T cells, Mac-1^+ cells, and $B220^+$ cells were detected in the exocrine gland lesions of mice with MAIDS. These results suggest that $CD4^+$ T cells and Mac-1^+ cells play a key role in the induction of organ-specific lesions in MAIDS mice. It remains unknown, however, which phenotype of cells (e.g., Mac-1^+ or $CD4^+$ cells) from MAIDS mice induce these lesions. Here, we analyzed adoptive transfer of separated fractions of MAIDS cells into nude mice to identify the phenotype of the MAIDS cells that could induce colitis and exocrinopathy.

Materials and Methods

Four-week-old female C57BL/6 (B6) mice were inoculated intraperitoneally with LP-BM5 MuLV. Eight weeks after infection, lymph node cells from the virus-infected mice were separated into three fractions using magnetic beads as follows: group 1, whole lymph node cells; group 2, $CD4^+$ T cells; group 3, non-T, non-B (Mac-1^+) cells. Each fraction was transferred to B6 nude mice. Four to six weeks after cell transfer the mice were killed. Tissue samples were taken from the colon, salivary glands, pancreas, and liver; and these samples were analyzed histopathologically using light microscopy.

Results

All of the mice inoculated with MAIDS lymph node cells (group 1) had diarrhea, rectal prolapse, and anal bleeding as well as systemic exocrinopathy; they died within 6 weeks after cell transfer. Histopathological analysis revealed the occurrence of UC-like colitis and systemic exocrinopathy in the salivary glands and pancreas. In nude mice given the $CD4^+$ fraction of MAIDS cells (group 2), systemic lymphadenopathy developed without diarrhea or intestinal bleeding; and the mice died within 6 weeks of the mice in group 1. In this group of mice, systemic exocrinopathy was induced, but colitis was not. Transfer of the non-T, non-B (Mac-1^+) cell fraction (group 3) induced systemic lymphadenopathy and diarrhea, rectal prolapse, and intestinal bleeding. In these mice only colitis was induced; there was no systemic exocrinopathy.

Discussion

We have clearly shown that adoptive transfer of Mac-1^+ cells of MAIDS mice can induce UC-like colitis but not exocrinopathy in recipient nude mice; in contrast, adoptive transfer of $CD4^+$ cells of MAIDS mice can induce exocrinopathy without colitis (Fig. 1). This is the first report, as far as we know, that different mouse cells populations induce different organ-specific autoimmune-like lesions.

Animal models of IBD that have been established so far are divided into two categories, such as the T-helper type 1 (Th1) and type 2 (Th2) cell models based on their cytokine production pattern of mucosal $CD4^+$ T-helper cells in the colon [6]. Interestingly, regardless of their skewing cytokine production pattern, these mice resemble each other remarkably in terms of the histopathology of their colitis. It is suggested that strong polarization of mucosal T cell responses along either pathway can result in IBD. In contrast, as reported previously, many interleukin-10 (IL-10) and interferon-γ (IFNγ)-expressing cells coexist in the inflamed colons of our mice with MAIDS colitis. IFNγ was mainly detected on Mac-1^+ cells, which we assume is the main effector of tissue destruction; and IL-10 was detected on both Mac-1^+ and $CD4^+$ cells (Fig. 2). In our preliminary study of biopsy specimens from patients with UC, some macrophages expressed IFNγ in the colon. We thus should reconsider the role of macrophages in the induction and progression in UC.

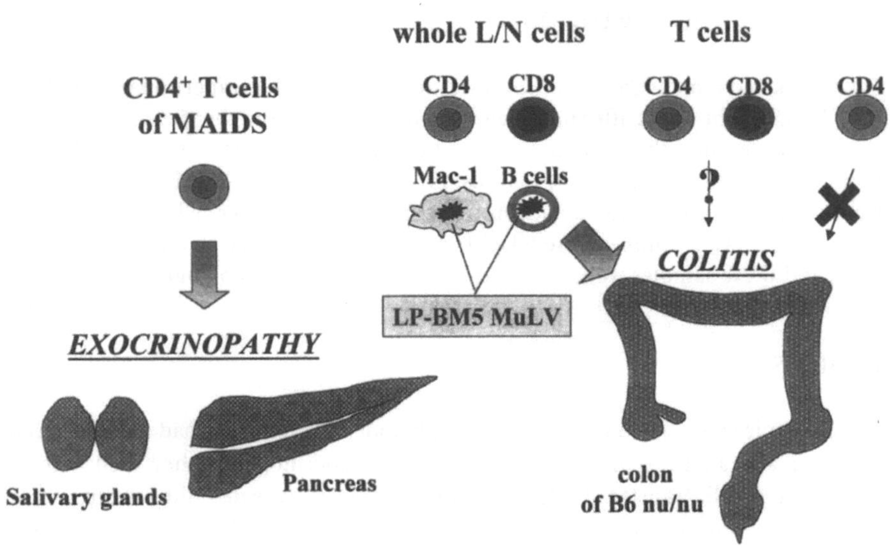

FIG. 1. Difference in the developmental mechanisms of Sjögren's syndrome-like exocrinopathy and colitis in mice with murine acquired immunodeficiency syndrome (MAIDS). *LP-BM5 MuLV*, LP-BM5 murine leukemia virus; *L/N*, lymph node

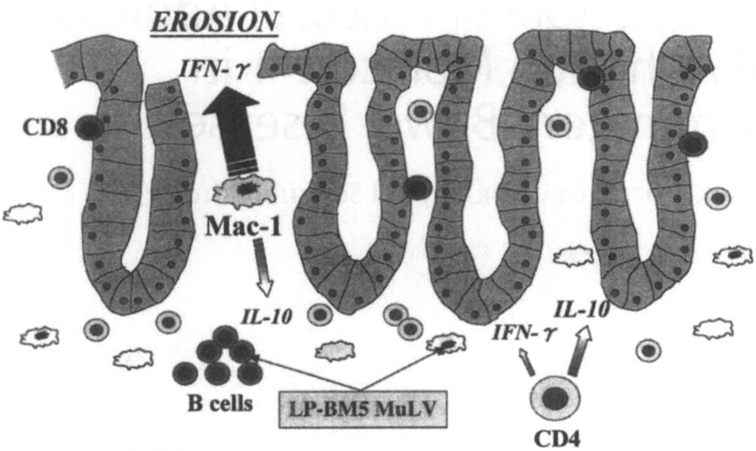

FIG. 2. Postulated mechanism of induction of MAIDS colitis. *IL-10*, interleukin-10; *IFN-γ*, interferon-γ

Recently it was shown that specific combinations of certain chemokines and their receptors play a key role in some organ-specific lesions. Murai et al. reported that $CCR5^+$ $CD8^+$ T cells specifically infiltrated the liver, inducing hepatic injury in graft versus host disease (GVHD) mice and that anti-CCR5R antibody treatment blocks infiltration of $CD8^+$ cells into the liver, thereby preventing the disease [7]. In future we should determine the chemokine expression patterns in each population of cells and each organ in mice with MAIDS colitis.

References

1. Mosier DE, Yetter RA, Morse HC III (1985) Retroviral induction of acute lymphoproliferative disease and profound immunosuppression in adult C57BL/6 mice. J Exp Med 161:766–784
2. Jolicoeur P (1991) Murine acquired immunodeficiency syndrome (MAIDS): an animal model to study the AIDS pathogenesis. FASEB J 5:2398–2405
3. Hitoshi Y, Okada Y, Sonoda E, et al (1993) Delayed progression of a murine retrovirus-induced acquired immunodeficiency syndrome in X-linked immunodeficient mice. J Exp Med 177:621–626
4. Suzuki K, Makino M, Okada Y, et al (1993) Exocrinopathy resembling Sjögren's syndrome induced by a murine retrovirus. Lab Invest 69:430–435
5. Suzuki K, Narita T, Yui R, et al (1997) Induction of intestinal lesions in nu/nu mice induced by transfer of lymphocytes from syngeneic mice infected with murine retrovirus. Gut 41:221–228
6. Fiocchi C (1993) Cytokines and animal models: a combined pathogenesis to inflammatory bowel disease pathogenesis. Gastroenterology 104:1202–1205
7. Murai M, Yoneyama H, Harada A, et al (1999) Active participation of $CCR5^+CD8^+$ T lymphocytes in the pathogenesis of liver injury in graft-versus-host disease. J Clin Invest 104:49–57

Potential Role of Mucosal Addressin Cell Adhesion Molecule-1 in Inflammatory Bowel Diseases

SHINGO KATO*, RYOTA HOKARI, and SOICHIRO MIURA

Summary. Mucosal addressin cell adhesion molecule-1 (MAdCAM-1) mediates recruitment of lymphocytes into the gut mucosa. Activated lymphocytes recirculate from blood to inflamed intestine by an interaction between α4β7-integrin and MAdCAM-1. Expression of MAdCAM-1 has been shown to be up-regulated at the inflammatory mucosa in murine experimental colitis and in human inflammatory bowel disease (IBD). Administration of anti-MAdCAM-1 antibody significantly reduced colonic injury and infiltration of β7-integrin-positive lymphocytes in experimental colitis. These evidence suggests the possibility that inhibition of excessive expression of MAdCAM-1 may be a useful tool for control of IBD.

Key words. MAdCAM-1 (mucosal addressin cell adhesion molecule-1), DSS (dextran sulfate sodium), β7-Integrin, Inflammatory bowel disease, Experimental colitis

Introduction

Mucosal addressin cell adhesion molecule-1 (MAdCAM-1) is largely involved in lymphocyte homing to mucosal lymphoid tissues such as Peyer's patches [1]. Expression of MAdCAM-1 has been reported to be up-regulated at the inflammatory site of human inflammatory bowel disease (IBD) and murine experimental colitis (Table 1) [2–7]. It is uncertain whether increased expression of MAdCAM-1 plays an important role in the progression of IBD. This review provides an overview of a potential role of MAdCAM-1 in human IBD and murine experimental colitis.

Human Inflammatory Bowel Disease

Increased expression of MAdCAM-1 in human IBD has been reported. Briskin et al. showed that MAdCAM-1 was constitutively expressed in venular endothelium of

Second Department of Internal Medicine, National Defense Medical College, 3-2 Namiki, Tokorozawa, Saitama 359-8513, Japan
* e-mail: kato@itsa.ucsf.edu

TABLE 1. MAdCAM-1 in human and experimental colitis

Human/animal model	Study	Year	Comment
Human IBD	Briskin [2]	1997	MAdCAM-1-positive vessels were increased (compared with normal tissues) at inflammatory foci associated with ulcerative colitis and Crohn's disease.
	Souza [3]	1999	Expression of α4β7/MAdCAM-1 and 0X40/0X40 ligand was increased only at sites of inflammation in patients with IBD.
Animal models			
IL-10-deficient mouse	Connor [4]	1999	Systemic administration of TNFα enhanced MAdCAM-1 expression in wild-type mice and IL-10 knockout mice.
IL-2 knockout mice	McDonald [5]	1997	There were increased numbers of MAdCAM-1-positive endothelial cells in IL-2 knockout mice.
SCID mice reconstituted with CD45RB high CD4 +T cells	Picarella [6]	1997	Anit-β7 and MAdCAM-1 monoclonal antibody blocked recruitment of lymphocytes to the colitic colon and reduced colitis.
TNBS colitis mice	Viney [7]	1997	Concordant increase in MAdCAM-1 expression was associated with increased cellular infiltrates in areas of intestinal inflammation.
DSS-induced colitis mice	Kato [8]	2000	Anti-MAdCAM-1 antibody significantly ameliorated DSS-induced colitis

MAdCAM-1, mucosal addressin cell adhesion molecule-1; IBD, inflammatory bowel disease; TNBS, trinitrobenzene sulfonic acid; DSS, dextran sulfate sodium; IL, interleukin; TNFα, tumor necrosis factor-α

lamina propria and the submucosa of normal intestine, and it was slightly increased at inflammatory foci associated with ulcerative colitis and Crohn's disease [2]. Expression of MAdCAM-1/α4β7 and OX40/OX40 ligand is increased in sites of mucosal inflammation in patients with IBD [3]. No evidence was found for increased MAdCAM-1 expression in the proximal intestine of patients with distal IBD. Increased MAdCAM-1 expression is therefore associated only with the sites of inflammation.

Experimental Colitis Models

It has been reported that the expression of MAdCAM-1 is up-regulated in some animal models of colitis, such as interleukin-10 (IL-10)-deficient mice [4], IL-2 knockout mice [5], SCID mice reconstituted with CD45RB high CD4 +T cells [6], and trinitrobenzene sulfonic acid (TNBS) colitis [7]. In these models expression of MAdCAM-1 was significantly increased in the inflamed colonic mucosa. Prophylactic effects of anti-

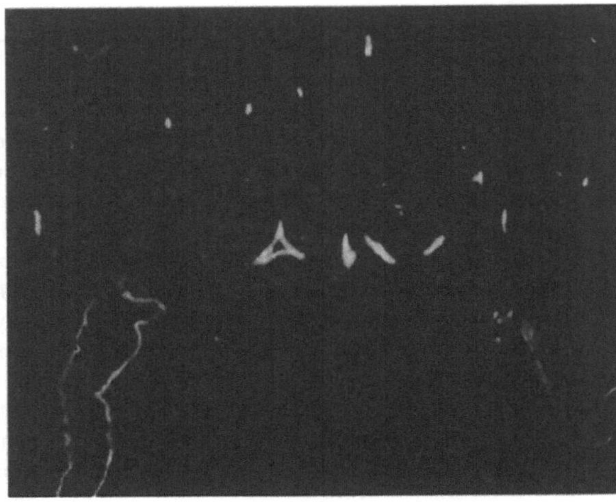

FIG. 1. Immunohistochemical study of mucosal addressin cell adhesion molecule-1 (MAdCAM-1) expression in the colonic mucosa of dextran sulfate sodium (DSS)-treated mice, demonstrating the increased MAdCAM-1 on vessels in the lamina propria and in the submucosal layer. (×200)

MAdCAM-1 antibody for SCID mice reconstituted with CD45RB high CD4 +T cell counts was previously demonstrated [6]. Recently we examined the prophylactic effect of anti-MAdCAM-1 antibody treatment on dextran sulfate sodium (DSS)-induced colitis [8]. Figure 1 shows the increased expression of MAdCAM-1 in the colonic mucosa of DSS-induced colitis. Expression of MAdCAM-1 had already been increased before there was an evident histological change and increase in lymphocyte infiltration. Daily intraperitoneal administration of anti-MAdCAM-1 monoclonal antibody significantly inhibited the progression of DSS-induced colitis.

MAdCAM-1 is induced on a murine intestinal endothelial cell line (bEND.3) by tumor necrosis factor-α (TNFα)- and IL-1-mediated nuclear factor κB (NF-κB) protein in vitro [9,10]. In this regard, in vivo expression of MAdCAM-1 was time-dependently increased in the colon of wild-type C57BL/6 mice by systemic administration of TNFα [4].

Conclusions

We mentioned that MAdCAM-1 expression was significantly increased in human IBD and experimental colitis. Because MAdCAM-1 is an adhesion molecule more unique to the gut mucosa than intercellular adhesion molecule-1, which is generally expressed outside the gastrointestinal tract as well, attenuation of MAdCAM-1 may be more specific therapy for colitis. This evidence suggests the possibility that inhibition of excessive expression of MAdCAM-1 may be a useful tool for the control of IBD.

References

1. Berlin C, Berg EL, Briskin MJ, et al (1993) α4β7 Integrin mediates lymphocyte binding to the mucosal vascular addressin MAdCAM-1. Cell 74:185–195
2. Briskin M, Winsor-Hines D, Shyjan A, et al (1997) Human mucosal addressin cell adhesion molecule-1 is preferentially expressed in intestinal tract and associated lymphoid tissue. Am J Pathol 151:97–110

3. Souza HS, Elia CC, Spencer J, et al (1999) Expression of lymphocyte endothelial receptor-ligand pairs, α4β7/MAdCAM-1 and OX40/OX40 ligand in the colon and jejunum of patients with inflammatory bowel disease. Gut 45:856–863
4. Connor EM, Eppihimer MJ, Morise Z, et al (1999) Expression of mucosal addressin cell adhesion molecule-1 (MAdCAM-1) in acute and chronic inflammation. J Leukoc Biol 65:349–355
5. McDonald SA, Palmen MJ, Van Ree EP, et al (1997) Characterization of the mucosal cell mediated immune response in IL-2 knockout mice before and after the onset of colitis. Immunology 91:73–80
6. Picarella D, Hurlbut P, Rottman J, et al (1997) Monoclonal antibodies specific for β7 integrin and mucosal addressin cell adhesion molecule-1 (MAdCAM-1) reduce inflammation in the colon of scid mice reconstituted with CD45RB high $CD4^+$ T cells. J Immunol 158:2099–2106
7. Viney JL, Jones S, Chiu HH, et al (1996) Mucosal addressin cell adhesion molecule-1; a structual and functional analysis demarcates the integrin binding motif. J Immunol 157:2488–2497
8. Kato S, Hokari R, Matsuzaki K, et al (2000) Amelioration of murine experimental colitis by inhibition of mucosal addressin cell adhesion morecule-1 (MAdCAM-1). J Pharmacol Exp Ther 295:183–189
9. Sikoruski EE, Hallmann R, Berg EL, et al (1993) The Peyer's patch high endothelial receptor for lymphocytes, the mucosal vascular addressin, is induced on a murine endothelial cell line by tumor necrosis factor-α and IL-1. J Immunol 151:5239–5250
10. Takeuchi M, Baichwal VR (1995) Induction of the gene encoding mucosal vascular addressin cell adhesion molecule-1 by tumor necrosis factor-α is mediated by NF-κB protein. Proc Natl Acad Sci USA 92:3561–3565

Anti-*Saccharmomyces cerevisiae* Antibody in Inflammatory Bowel Disease

Nobuhide Oshitani*, Kazuhide Higuchi, Takayuki Matsumoto, and Tetsuo Arakawa

Summary. Elevation of anti-*Saccharomyces cerevisiae* antibody (ASCA) in patients with Crohn's disease suggests involvement of this antigen in the pathophysiology of the disease. Elevation of immunoglobulin G (IgG) ASCA is related to the small bowel involvement in patients with Crohn's disease. Administration of mesalazine also affects the level of IgG ASCA. Complete elimination of dietary yeast, which is widely distributed in nature, is difficult unless total parenteral nutrition or a complete elemental diet can be tolerated, which are effective for treatment of patients with active Crohn's disease. *S. cerevisiae* is usually not virulent in humans, and altered immunological responses or cross-reactivity to human intestinal antigens may play roles in the pathogenesis of Crohn's disease.

Key words. Inflammatory bowel disease, Crohn's disease, ASCA, *Saccharomyces cerevisiae*, Bakers' yeast

Dietary antigens have been postulated to be pathogenetic factors in inflammatory bowel disease (IBD). Although several circulating antibodies to dietary and bacterial antigens have been investigated in patients with IBD, no specific antigens contributing to its pathogenesis have yet been identified. In 1988 Main et al. [1] first reported the specific increase in serum anti-*Saccharomyces cerevisiae* (bakers' yeast) antibody (ASCA) titers of both immunoglobulin G (IgG) and IgA classes in patients with Crohn's disease (CD). *S. cerevisiae* is widely found in nature in various plants, fruits, and soil. Humans have used this organism widely for centuries when brewing and baking and are exposed extensively to *S. cerevisiae* through daily foods.

S. cerevisiae antigen was heat-extracted from bakers' yeast and subsequently found to be an oligomannoside [2]. The IgG ASCA titer raised depends on the site of involvement of CD, and CD patients with small bowel involvement have higher IgG ASCA titers than those with only large bowel involvement. Age, sex, disease activity, and

Third Department of Internal Medicine, Osaka City University Medical School, 1-4-3 Asahi-mach, Abeno-ku, Osaka 545-8585, Japan
* e-mail: nobu@med.osaka-cu.ac.jp

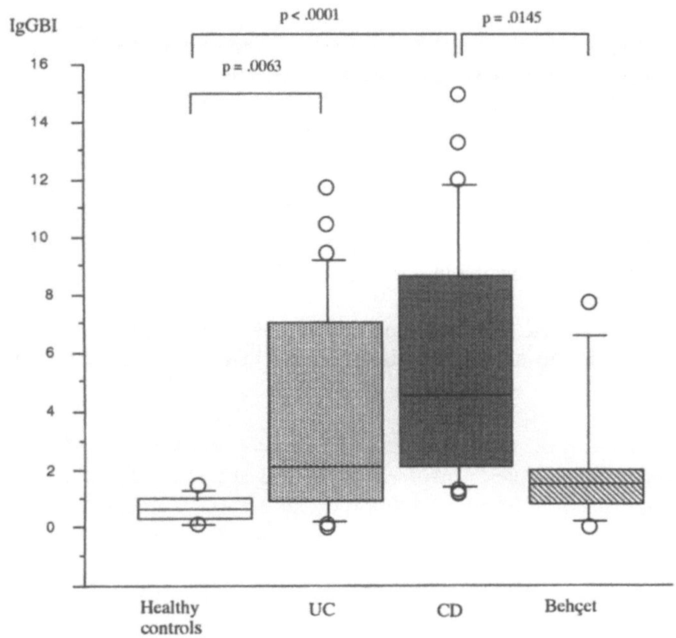

FIG. 1. Serum anti-*Saccharomyces cerevisiae* antibody (*ASCA*) titers were measured from 12 healthy volunteers, 29 patients with ulcerative colitis (*UC*), 30 patients with Crohn's disease (*CD*), and 7 patients with intestinal Behçet's disease using the enzyme-linked immunosorbent assay (ELISA) to which heat-extracted *S. cerevisiae* antigen was immobilized. *IgGBI*, immunoglobulin G binding index $= \dfrac{\text{A492nm (test serum)} - \text{A492nm (background)}}{\text{A492nm (reference negative)} - \text{A492nm (background)}}$

previous intestinal resection had no effect on IgG ASCA titers [3]. In our experience using commercially available bakers' yeast as antigen, patients with CD and those with ulcerative colitis had significantly higher IgG ASCA levels than did normal controls; moreover, patients with CD had significantly higher IgG ASCA levels than patients with Behçet's disease (Fig. 1). We found that age, gender, disease activity, and administration of corticosteroid did not significantly altered IgG ASCA titers. Patients with CD taking mesalazine had significantly lower IgG ASCA levels than those not taking it [4].

Because *S. cerevisiae* is widely distributed in the nature, it is difficult to completely eliminate it from the diet. A study of low-yeast diets suggested that exclusion of yeast from the diet helps maintain remission in patients with quiescent CD [5]. The beneficial effects of total parenteral nutrition or a complete elemental diet, by which complete yeast elimination diet can be achieved for patients with active CD, suggest that *S. cerevisiae* may play a role in the pathogenesis of CD. *S. cerevisiae* does not act as a pathogen in patients with CD, as it is a ubiquitous microorganism that is not virulent in uncompromised hosts. Altered immunoreactivity or cross-reactive antigens in human tissue might thus play roles in the pathogenesis of Crohn's disease.

References

1. Main J, McKenzie H, Yeaman GR, et al (1988) Antibody to *Saccharomyces cerevisiae* (bakers' yeast) in Crohn's disease. BMJ 297:1105–1106
2. Sendid B, Colombel JF, Jacquinot PM, et al (1996) Specific antibody response to oligomannosidic epitopes in Crohn's disease. Clin Diagn Lab Immunol 3:219–226
3. Giaffer MH, Clark A, Holdsworth CD (1992) Antibodies to *Saccharomyces cerevisiae* in patients with Crohn's disease and their possible pathogenic importance. Gut 33:1071–1075
4. Oshitani N, Hato F, Matsumoto T, et al (2001) Decreased anti-*Saccharomyces cerevisiae* antibody titer by mesalazine in patients with Crohn's disease. J Gastroenterol Hepatol 15:1400–1403
5. Barclay GR, McKenzie H, Pennington J, et al (1992) The effect of dietary yeast on the activity of stable chronic Crohn's disease. Scand J Gastroenterol 27:196–200

Reactive Oxygen Species and Colonic Epithelial Cell Apoptosis in Ulcerative Colitis

Atsushi Hayashi[1,*], Tetsuji Kitahora[1], and Hiromi Ono[2]

Summary. Ulcerative colitis (UC) is one of the inflammatory bowel diseases of unknown etiology characterized by its localization to the large intestine. According to pathological examination, which reveals mucosal inflammatory cell infiltration, goblet cell depletion, and distortion of crypt architecture, it is clear that the target of this disease is epithelial cells. Some reports note that epithelial cell damage is mediated by apoptotic cell death. The aim of this study was to elucidate the role of reactive oxygen species (ROS) in the induction of colonic epithelial cell apoptosis. Colonic biopsies from active and inactive lesions of UC patients and from normal tissues of patients with colon polyps were used. ROS production from the colonic tissues were measured using a chemiluminescence assay. Apoptotic cells were detected by the TUNEL technique. Superoxide dismutase (SOD), Fas, and Bcl-2 were detected by immunohistochemistry. ROS production was increased in active UC compared with inactive UC or normal mucosa. SOD was strongly expressed in the epithelial cells of active UC compared with inactive UC mucosa. The extent of TUNEL-positive epithelial cells was more extensive in active UC compared with inactive UC or nomal mucosa. There was a positive correlation between ROS production and the extent of TUNEL-positive cells. There was a tendency for Fas-positive cells to be fewer in active and inactive UC compared with normal mucosa, but there was no clear tendency for Bcl-2-positive cells. Based on these results, ROS rather than the Fas/Fas ligand system is suggested to have an important role in inducing epithelial cell apoptosis in UC.

Key words. Ulcerative colitis, Reactive oxygen species, Apoptosis, Polymorphonuclear cell, TUNEL

[1]Department of Gastroenterology, [2]Institute of Clinical Research, National Ohkura Hospital, 2-10-1 Ohkura, Setagaya-ku, Tokyo 157-8535, Japan
* e-mail: woods@sub-tky.hosp.go.jp

Introduction

Ulcerative colitis (UC) is one of the inflammatory bowel diseases of unknown etiology and affects only the large intestine. Pathological examination reveals mucosal inflammatory cell infiltration, goblet cell depletion, and distortion of crypt architecture. Although the initial events are unclear, the main target of this disease are epithelial cells. We reported that reactive oxygen species (ROS) generated from peripheral blood polymorphonuclear cells (PMNs) of UC patients were increased [1]. Others have reported that epithelial cell damage is mediated by apoptotic cell death [2,3].

In the present study, we measured ROS production in colonic tissues and evaluated the relation between mucosal ROS production and distribution of apoptotic cells, detected by TUNEL, in the colonic epithelial cells of UC patients. Furthermore, we examined Fas and Bcl-2 expression, which are well-known apoptosis-related markers, in the epithelial cells in UC to clarify the possible role of ROS in the induction of epithelial cell apoptosis in UC.

Materials and Methods

Materials

Colonic biopsy specimens were obtained from active or inactive (vascular pattern visible) lesions of UC patients. Colonic biopsy specimens were also obtained from the endoscopically normal mucosa of patients with colonic polyps. Some specimens were obtained from the normal mucosa of the resected colon of patients with colon cancer. In all cases the diagnosis was based on the clinical history and endoscopic and histopathological findings. Some specimens were used for chemiluminescence assays immediately after sampling. Other specimens were fixed in 4% paraformaldehyde, embedded in OCT compound, frozen, sectioned, and used for immunohistochemical observations.

Chemiluminescence Assay

A chemiluminescence (CL) analyzer (Biolumat; Berthold, Germany) was used to measure CL activity generated by biopsied specimens. Test vials containing a piece of biopsied colonic mucosa were initially warmed in an incubator at 37°C for 10 min. After adding 0.02 mg luminol (Sigma, St. Louis, MO, USA) to the vials, the CL activity generated by the samples was measured for 5 min. The CL activity counted for 2 s was recorded consecutively on a television monitor and saved in a computer for analysis. Statistical differences between subjects were analyzed by Student's *t*-test.

Immunohistochemistry

The indirect peroxidase-labeled antibody method was used. Sections were washed in phosphate-buffered saline at 4°C. Endogenous peroxidase activity was then inactivated by methanol containing 0.3% hydrogen peroxide (H_2O_2). For the first antibodies, rabbit anti-recombinant human superoxide dismutase (SOD), mouse anti-Fas (MBL, Nagoya, Japan), and mouse anti-human Bcl-2 (MBL) were used. For the second antibodies, peroxidase-labeled goat anti-rabbit immunoglobulin G (IgG) (MBL) and peroxidase-labeled anti-mouse IgG (Amersham, London, UK) were used. The sections were incubated in a solution containing 3,3′-diaminobenzidine 4-HCl (DAB) and H_2O_2 and were counterstained with methyl green. For Fas and Bcl-2 staining, grading of the number of stained epithelial cells was follows: (–), no positive cells; (+), a few positive cells scattered in the epithelial cells; (++), many positive cells in groups.

In Situ DNA End-Labeling (TUNEL)

TUNEL was carried out essentially as described elsewhere [4]. Grading the extent of TUNEL-positive epithelial cells was follows: grade 0, no TUNEL-positive cells; grade 1, TUNEL-positive cells only on the luminal surface; grade 2, TUNEL-positive cells into the upper half of the crypt; grade 3, TUNEL-positive cells in the lower half of the crypt.

Results

ROS Generated from the Biopsied Specimen

The CL activities generated by active UC lesions (358.1 ± 140.8 count/2 s/mg) ($n = 13$) were significantly increased compared with that generated by inactive UC lesions (14.0 ± 2.3) ($n = 11$) ($P < 0.01$) or normal mucosa of patients with colon polyps (9.1 ± 1.8) ($n = 5$) ($P < 0.01$).

SOD in Epithelial Cells

The SOD was stained in cytoplasm of epithelial cells. The intensity of staining was higher in active UC lesions than in inactive UC lesions (data not shown).

Localization of TUNEL-Positive Epithelial Cells

In active UC lesions the extent of TUNEL-positive cells was deeper into the crypt (grades 0/1/2/3 were 2:5:5:1) ($n = 13$) compared with inactive lesions (4:4:3:0, respectively) ($n = 11$). Furthermore, the extent in inactive lesions was deeper than in normal mucosa (1:4:0:0, respectively) ($n = 5$).

Figure 1 shows the relation between the extent of TUNEL-positive cells and CL activity. There was a positive correlation between them.

Fas and Bcl-2 Expression

Fas was stained on the surface of epithelial cells, and Bcl-2 was stained in the cytoplasm of epithelial cells. Figure 2 shows percentages of the grades of Fas and Bcl-2 staining in active UC, inactive UC, and normal mucosa. There were more Fas-negative samples in active and inactive UC lesions than in normal mucosa. There was no clear tendency for Bcl-2 staining.

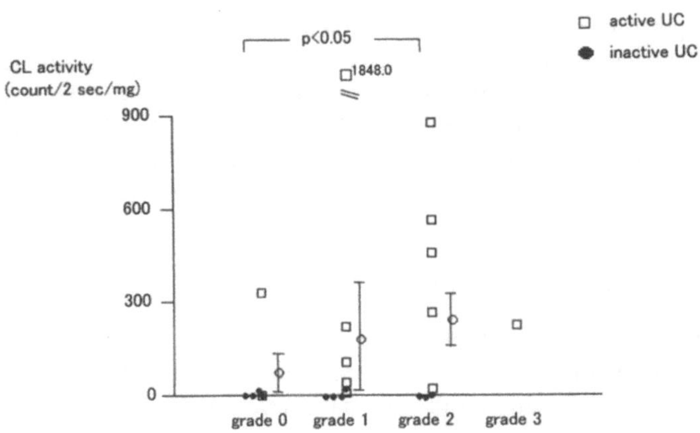

FIG. 1. Relation between the extent of TUNEL-positive cells and chemiluminescence (*CL*) activities generated from the colonic mucosa of ulcerative colitis (*UC*) and normal controls. There was a significant difference between CL activities at grade 0 and grade 2 ($P < 0.05$). *Bars*, SEM; *open circles*, mean values. See Materials and Methods for the grading

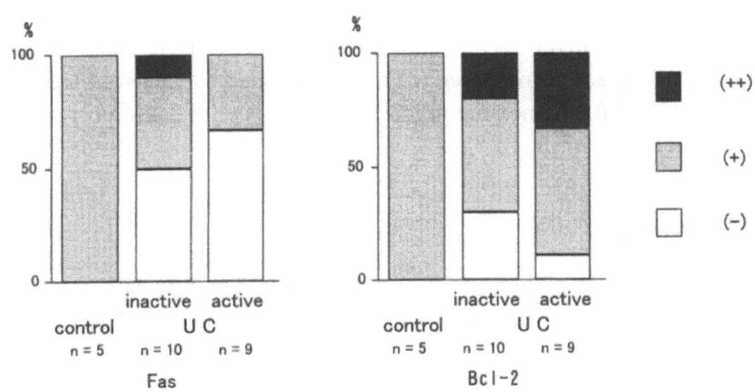

FIG. 2. Percent of the grades of Fas and Bcl-2 staining. Nearly half of the samples of active and inactive ulcerative colitis were Fas-negative (*open bars*). There was no clear tendency with Bcl-2 staining. See Materials and Methods for the grading

Discussion

Apoptotic cell death is believed to have an important pathological role in many disorders. Iwamoto et al. [2] reported that apoptotic colonic epithelial cells were observed not only on the luminal surface but also in crypts in active UC, and that these apoptotic cells were found mainly in Fas-positive cells. As a result, they concluded that epithelial cell damage in UC is due to apoptosis, and that this process is mediated by the Fas/Fas ligand system.

In the present study we also found more extensive (deep in the crypt) distribution of apoptotic cells in active UC mucosa than in inactive UC or normal mucosa, but there were no correlations between apoptosis and Fas or Bcl-2, which are well-known apoptosis-related markers. Instead, there was a positive correlation between apoptosis and the CL activity generated by colonic mucosa.

Although this is not direct evidence that ROS induces epithelial cell apoptosis in UC, it strongly suggests the causal relation between them. The facts that ROS is one of the apoptosis-inducing factors and that leukocyte apheresis is an effective therapy for UC support our hypothesis.

Immunohistochemical study revealed increased expression of SOD in epithelial cells in active UC. The induction of SOD is thought to be a result of the influence of ROS to epithelial cells. All of these facts suggest that ROS is at least one of the causes of epithelial cell apoptosis in UC. In our preliminary study there was a positive correlation between ROS production by colonic mucosa and mucosal PMN infiltration. Therefore PMNs were thought to be the major source of ROS.

In active and inactive UC there was a tendency for Fas-negative samples to dominate compared with normal mucosa. This observation seems not to be in accordance with the pathophysiology of UC being epithelial cell loss. There may be two explanations for this. One is that epithelial cell turnover is so rapid in UC that epithelial cells drop out before they express Fas antigens. Another is that epithelial cells down-regulate Fas antigens to protect themselves against the apoptotic signal of ROS.

In conclusion, the present study suggests that ROS generated by PMNs infiltrating active UC mucosa induce apoptotic cell death in the colonic epithelial cells. In this regard, therapy targeted to PMNs must be one of the most promising strategies for treating UC.

Acknowledgments. The rabbit anti-recombinant human superoxide dismutase was a gift of Prof. K. Watanabe, Tokai University, Isehara, Japan.

References

1. Suematsu M, Suzuki M, Kitahora T, et al (1987) Increased respiratory burst of leukocytes in inflammatory bowel diseases: the analysis of free radical generation by using chemiluminescence probe. J Clin Lab Immunol 24:125–128
2. Iwamoto M, Koji T, Makiyama K, et al (1996) Apoptosis of crypt epithelial cells in ulcerative colitis. J Pathol 180:152–159
3. Strater J, Wellisch I, Riedl S (1997) CD-95 (APO-1/Fas)-mediated apoptosis in colon epithelial cells: a possible role in ulcerative colitis. Gastroenterology 113:160–167
4. Gavrieli Y, Sherman Y, Ben-Sasson SA (1992) Identification of programmed cell death in situ via specific labelling of nuclear DNA fragmentation. J Cell Biol 119:493–501

Part 9
NSAID-Induced Gastric Lesions

Effect of Antiulcer Drugs for Treatment of Nonsteroidal Antiinflammatory Drug-Induced Ulcers

YUJI MIZOKAMI*, TAKAHISA SHIRAISHI, TOSHIYA OTSUBO, YOSHIYUKI KARIYA, HIROSHI NAKAMURA, KATSUHIKO NARUSHIMA, and TAKESHI MATSUOKA

Summary. It is difficult to heal ulcers during continuous administration of nonsteroidal autiinflammatory drugs (NSAIDs). We retrospectively studied 136 rheumatoid arthritis patients who were taking NSAIDs at least 3 months, and who could be followed within 12 weeks of being diagnosed with an ulcer using endoscopy. Among patients who had ulcers in the antrum (A region), healing rates were 46.7% (21/45), 46.7% (21/45), and 73.3% (11/15) in the famotidine (F) group, lansoprazole (L) group, and misoprostol (MP) group, respectively; the rate was higher in the MP group than in the F and L groups. On the other hand, for ulcers in the body (M region) there were no differences among the groups; healing rates were 94.1% (16/17), 86.7% (13/15), and 100% (1/1), respectively. To study the background regarding A region ulcers and cardia/body (C/M) region ulcers, we studied acid output and *Helicobacter pylori* (HP)-positive rates. There were no differences in acid output between the two groups. In the NSAID group, the HP-positive rate was significantly lower among A region ulcers (48.3%) than in C/M region ulcers (100%). A large-scale, multicenter study that also considers the role of HP is needed to establish the best treatment of NSAIDS-induced ulcers.

Key words. Nonsteroidal antiinflammatory drugs, Gastric ulcer, Ulcer site, Acid output, *Helicobacter pylori*

Introduction

It is difficult to heal ulcers during continuous administration of nonsteroidal antiinflammatory drugs (NSAIDs). We therefore studied the healing rate of NSAID-induced ulcers in patients with rheumatoid arthritis (RA), and report our findings here.

Department of Internal Medicine 5, Tokyo Medical University, Kasumigaura Hospital, 3-20-1 Chuo, Ami, Inashiki-gun, Ibaraki 300-0395, Japan
* e-mail: yuji-m@tokyo-med.ac.jp

TABLE 1. General characteristics of subjects

	Group F	Group L	Group MP
Number	65	55	16
Age (average years)	62.7	59.2	62.9
Sex (M/F)	15/50	8/47	3/13
Location of ulcer			
stomach	54	47	16
duodenum	5	8	0
stomach + duodenum	6	0	0

F, treated with famotidine; L, treated with lansoprazole; MP, treated with misoprostol

Subjects

We studied 136 RA patients who were receiving treatment at Tokyo Medical University Kasumigaura Hospital, and Kakogawa National Hospital, were taking NSAIDs at least 3 months, and could be followed within 12 weeks of being endoscopically diagnosed with an ulcer. They were treated with antiulcer drugs: 65 patients were treated with famotidine (F group), 55 with lansoprazole (L group), and 16 with misoprostol (MP group). There were no significant differences in age, gender, or site of ulcer among the F, L, and MP groups (Table 1).

Methods

In each group we studied the healing rate, acid output, and *Helicobacter pylori* (HP)-positive rate.

Healing Rates. We retrospectively studied the healing rates in the F group (8–12 weeks), L group (8 weeks), and MP group (8–12 weeks) by drug and ulcer site (C, cardia; M, body; A, antrum; D, duodenum) affected.

Acid Output. We measured the basal acid output (BAO), maximal acid output (MAO), and serum gastrin in 11 cases. We also studied acid output from the ulcer site.

HP-positive Rate. We evaluated positivity by either culture or rapid urease test and conducted a study from the ulcer sites in 38 patients in the NSAID-administered group and 65 patients in the control group (non-NSAID-administered group).

Results

Healing Rates by Drug. Based on the drug prescribed, the healing rates were 63.1% (41/65) in the F group, 63.6% (35/55) in the L group, and 75% (12/16) in the MP group. There were no differences among the groups.

Healing Rates by Ulcer Site. Among patients who had ulcers in the A region, healing rates were 46.7% (21/45), 46.7% (21/45), and 73.3% (11/15) in the F, L, and MP groups,

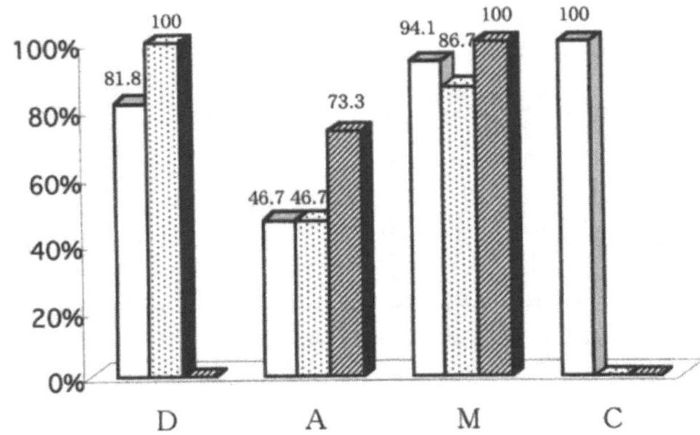

Fig. 1. Healing rates by ulcer site. *Open bars*, famotidine (F); *dotted bars*, lansoprazole (L); *hatched bars*, misoprostol (MP); *D*, duodenum; *A*, antrum; *M*, body; *C*, cardia

respectively. The rate was higher in the MP group than in the F and L groups. Among patients who had ulcers in the M region, there were no differences among the F, L, and MP groups. Healing rates were 94.1% (16/17), 86.7% (13/15), and 100% (1/1), respectively (Fig. 1).

Acid Output. BAO, MAO, and gastrin in the A region were 1.9 ± 0.4 mEq/l, 7.46 ± 1.15 mEq/l, and 129 ± 22.9 pg/ml, respectively; and in the C/M region they were 0.95 ± 0.35 mEq/l, 7.96 ± 1.0 mEq/l, and 127 ± 11.1 pg/ml, respectively. No differences were seen between the two groups.

HP-Positive Rates. Based on ulcer site, the HP-positive rate was significantly low among patients with A region ulcers in the NSAID group: HP-positive rates in the NSAID group were 48.3% (14/29) for A region ulcers and 100% (9/9) for C/M region ulcers. In the control group the HP-positive rates were 87.5% (14/16) for A region ulcers and 92% (45/49) for C/M region ulcers. There were no significant differences in the HP-positive rate based on ulcer site in the control group.

Discussion

During the treatment of NSAID-induced ulcers, if the NSAIDs can be discontinued there is no difference from ordinary ulcer healing [1]. However, it is difficult to discontinue NSAIDs, even if a gastric ulcer is diagnosed, owing to persistent arthralgia, as in RA patients. Walan et al. [2] reported that there were no differences in the gastric ulcer healing rates using omeprazole when NSAIDs were used or not used concomitantly; moreover, healing rates were low in the ranitidine group when NSAIDs were also used. There have thus been many reports of the effectiveness of proton pump inhibitors (PPIs) for treating NSAID-induced gastric ulcers. The efficacy of prostaglandins have been often reported. When Roth et al. [3] studied the rates of gastric and duodenal ulcer healing under conditions of continuous aspirin administration in RA patients, they found significantly higher healing rates with misoprostol than with placebo. Hawkey et al. [4] compared the healing rates using omeprazole and misoprostol. It was found that the healing rates for gastric and duodenal ulcers were better with omeprazole than with misoprostol. Our present study was retrospective; and although strict comparison was not possible. However, there were differences in the healing rates by ulcer site: Efficacy was higher in the MP group than in the F and L groups for ulcers in the A region. On the other hand, for ulcers in the C/M region there were no differences among the drugs.

To study the background regarding A region ulcers and C/M region ulcers, we studied acid output and HP-positive rates. For acid output there were no differences between the two groups. In the NSAID group, the HP-positive rate was significantly lower among A region ulcers (48.3%) than for C/M region ulcers (100%). Cyclooxygenase (COX-2), derived from an HP infection, is valuable in the healing of ulcers, so it is thought that HP infection promotes ulcer healing. In other words, could it be that in C/M region ulcers HP infection is high so the ulcer healing rate is high; and in A region ulcers HP infection is low so the ulcer healing rate is low? It has not been shown whether the primary selection of treatment should be PPIs or prostaglandins. To establish policies for treating NSAID-induced ulcers in Japan a large-scale, multicenter study that also considers the role of HP is needed.

References

1. Lancaster-Smith MJ, Jaderberg ME, Jackson DA (1991) Ranitidine in the treatment of non-steroidal anti-inflammatory drug associated gastric and duodenal ulcers. Gut 32:252–255
2. Walan A, Bader J, Classen M, et al (1989) Effect of omeprazole and ranitidine on ulcer healing and relapse rates in patients with benign gastric ulcer. N Engl J Med 320:69–75
3. Roth S, Agrawal N, Mahowald M, et al (1989) Misoprostol heals gastroduodenal injury in patients with rheumatoid arthritis receiving aspirin. Arch Intern Med149:775–779
4. Hawkey CJ, Karrasch JA, Szezepanski L, et al (1998) Omeprazole compared with misoprostol for ulcers associated with nonsteroidal antiinflammatory drugs. N Engl J Med 338:727–734

Role of Intravascular Neutrophils in the Pathogenesis of Aspirin-Induced Gastric Mucosal Injury

NORIMASA YOSHIDA* and TOSHIKAZU YOSHIKAWA

Summary. Gastric mucosal injury induced by nonsteroidal antiinflammatory drugs (NSAIDs) has been attributed to activated polymorphonuclear leukocytes (PMNs) that adhere to the postcapillary venules and subsequently migrate to the interstitium. Our objective was to determine whether intravascular PMNs or migrant PMNs were more important in the pathogenesis of aspirin-induced gastric mucosal injury. Myeloperoxidase (MPO) activity, an index of neutrophil accumulation, was significantly increased in the gastric mucosa of rats given oral aspirin (200 mg/kg) compared with that in normal rats not given aspirin. MPO activity was significantly decreased after perfusion of the blood vessels with physiological saline compared with the activity in rats without perfusion. When a PMN suspension with aspirin or sodium salicylate was perfused for 10 min over human umbilical vein endothelial cells (HUVECs) at a shear stress of 0–2.0 dynes/cm^2, aspirin but not salicylate promoted PMN adhesion to HUVECs at shear stresses less than 1.0 dyne/cm^2. An anti-CD18 monoclonal antibody completely inhibited aspirin-induced promotion of PMN adhesion. The number of cells that migrated underneath the HUVEC monolayers did not differ among aspirin-treated, salicylate-treated, and untreated PMNs. These results suggest that PMNs adhering to the blood vessels, but not PMNs migrating to the interstitium, are implicated in aspirin-induced gastric mucosal injury.

Key words. Neutrophils, Endothelial cells, Adhesion, Aspirin, Gastric mucosal injury

Introduction

Adherence of polymorphonuclear leukocytes (PMNs) to the endothelium and subsequent extravascular migration of these cells are characteristic steps in the process of inflammation. PMN–endothelial cell interactions are known to be mediated by adhesion molecules expressed on these two cell types [1]. Among the various adhesion

---

First Department of Internal Medicine, Kyoto Prefectural University of Medicine, Kawaramachi-Hirokoji, Kamigyo-ku, Kyoto 602-8566, Japan
* e-mail: nyoshida@koto.kpu-m.ac.jp

molecules, CD11b/CD18 (Mac-1) plays a central role in the adhesion of activated neutrophils to endothelial cells [2]. We previously reported that aspirin promoted neutrophil adherence to the endothelium via CD11/CD18-dependent interactions, with intercellular adhesion molecule-1 (ICAM-1) expressed on endothelial cells [3]. In addition, our investigations and those of others have demonstrated that monoclonal antibodies (mAbs) for CD11a, CD11b, CD18, and ICAM-1 can inhibit neutrophil accumulation in the gastric mucosa and gastric mucosal injury induced by administration of nonsteroidal antiinflammatory drugs (NSAIDs) [4–6]. These results suggest that adherent or migrating neutrophils (or both) may play an important role in NSAID-induced gastric mucosal injury. The objective of the present study was to determine whether adherence of PMNs to blood cells or extravascular migration of PMNs was more important in the pathogenesis of aspirin-induced gastric mucosal injury.

Materials and Methods

Myeloperoxidase Activity in Aspirin-Treated Gastric Mucosa

Gastric hemorrhagic lesions were induced by intragastric administration of aspirin (200 mg/kg) and 0.15 N HCl in a volume of 0.5 ml/100 g body weight, as reported previously [5,6]. At 3 h after administration of aspirin the animals were killed by exsanguination via the abdominal aorta under urethane anesthesia. In some rats the residual intravascular blood was completely washed out by perfusion with physiological saline via the abdominal aorta. The gastric mucosa was scraped off using two glass slides and was homogenized to measure myeloperoxidase (MPO) activity as an index of PMN accumulation. MPO activity was determined by a modification of the method of Krawisz et al. [7].

Preparation of Endothelial Cells and PMNs

Human umbilical vein endothelial cells (HUVECs) and PMNs were isolated from umbilical cords and the venous blood of healthy adults, respectively [8].

Flow Chamber System

We assessed the effect of shear stress on aspirin-induced PMN adherence to HUVEC monolayers. To produce well-defined shear stress, we used a flow chamber developed by Lawrence et al. [9]. The chamber consisted of a glass slide with a confluent HUVEC monolayer that was attached to a polycarbonate base, as described previously [10]. A PMN suspension (10^6 cells/ml) in Hanks' balanced salt solution (HBSS) and aspirin (300 μg/ml) or salicylate (300 μg/ml) were co-incubated for 30 min and then perfused through the flow chamber. PMNs that adhered to the endothelial cell monolayers appeared as phase-bright objects, whereas those migrating to the subendothelial space were flattened and appeared as phase-dark objects [11].

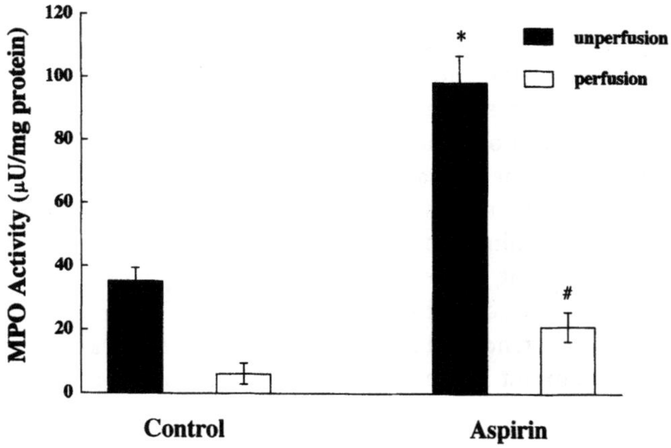

FIG. 1. Myeloperoxidase (*MPO*) activity in the gastric mucosa 3h after oral administration of aspirin. In some rats (unperfused group), the stomachs were removed after exsaguination via the abdominal aorta. In the other rats (perfused group), intravascular blood was completely washed out by perfusion with physiological saline via the abdominal aorta after exsanguination. Data are expressed as the mean ± SE. **P* < 0.01 vs. control rats without aspirin. #*P* < 0.01 vs. rats without perfusion

Results

MPO Activity in Gastric Mucosa

An index of neutrophil accumulation, MPO activity was significantly increased in the gastric mucosa of aspirin-treated rats compared with that in normal rats not given aspirin. MPO activity in the rats perfused with physiological saline was significantly decreased compared with that in rats without perfusion (Fig. 1).

PMN Adhesion and Migration Induced by Aspirin Under Flow Conditions

The PMN suspensions with aspirin or sodium salicylate were perfused over HUVECs for 10min at shear stresses of 0–2.0 dyn/cm^2. Salicylate had no influence on PMN adhesion under static or flow conditions, whereas aspirin promoted PMN adhesion to HUVECs at less than 1.0 dyne/cm^2 (Fig. 2). Anti-CD18 monoclonal antibody completely inhibited aspirin-induced PMN adhesion at low shear stresses (<0.5 dynes/cm^2). The number of cells that migrated underneath the HUVEC monolayers did not differ among aspirin-treated, salicylate-treated, and untreated PMNs.

Discussion

The present in vivo study suggests that aspirin-induced PMN accumulation in the gastric mucosa occurs mainly in the blood vessels and not extravascularly. These results are consistent with the report by the Asako et al. [12] that aspirin promotes

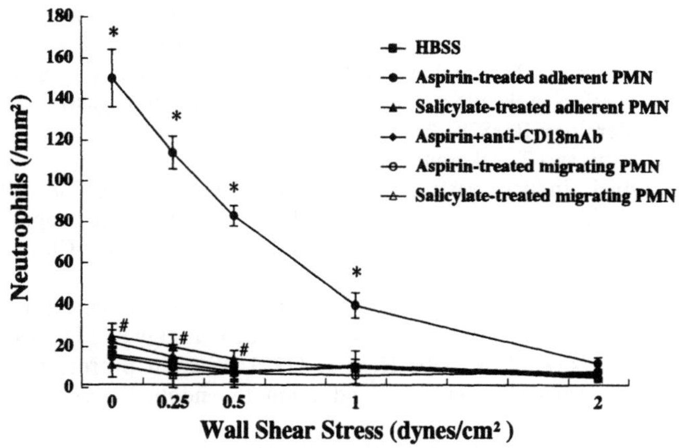

FIG. 2. Effect of shear stress on the interaction between polymorphonuclear leukocytes (*PMN*) and endothelial cells induced by aspirin or salicylate. PMNs preincubated with aspirin or salicylate were perfused at shear stresses of 0–2.0 dynes/cm^2 over endothelial cell monolayers. A monoclonal antibody (*mAb*) to CD18 was added to the PMN suspension. Ten minutes later the number of adherent or migrating PMNs was calculated. Data are expressed as the mean ± SE of five or six experiments. *HBSS*, Hanks' balanced salt solution. $^{*}P < 0.01$ vs. HBSS. $^{\#}P < 0.01$ vs. aspirin-treated PMN

PMN adhesion to rat postcapillary venules but does not affect PMN migration. Previously, we reported that reduction of neutrophil-endothelial cell adhesion by administration of anti-CD11b, anti-CD18, or anti-ICAM-1 mAbs had a protective effect against aspirin-induced gastric mucosal injury. Taken together, these results suggest that neutrophils adhering to and plugging the blood vessels, but not neutrophils migrating into the interstitium, are implicated in the pathogenesis of aspirin-induced gastric mucosal injury.

In addition, we investigated the effect of aspirin and shear stress on PMN adhesion and migration under flow conditions. We demonstrated that aspirin, but not salicylate, induced CD11/CD18-dependent PMN adherence to endothelial cells under static and low-flow conditions, as reported previously [3]. Aspirin did not influence PMN migration in the present in vitro study or the in vivo study of Asako et al. [12] using rat mesenteric postcapillary venules. Our previous study revealed that adherent PMNs stimulated by aspirin induced endothelial retraction and detachment by releasing neutrophil-derived elastase [13].

In summary, the present in vivo study and other in vitro studies suggest that intravascular PMNs, but not migrating PMNs, play an important role in aspirin-induced gastric mucosal injury by causing endothelial cell damage and microcirculatory disturbance.

References

1. Springer TA (1990) Adhesion receptors of the immune system. Nature 346:425–434
2. Carlos TM, Harlan JM (1990) Membrane proteins involved in phagocyte adherence to endothelium. Immunol Rev 114:5–28

3. Yoshida N, Takemura T, Granger DN, et al (1993) Molecular determinants of aspirin-induced neutrophil adherence to endothelial cells. Gastroenterology 105:715–724
4. Wallace JL, Arfors K-E, McKnight GW (1991) A monoclonal antibody against the CD18 leukocyte adhesion molecule prevents indomethacin-induced gastric damage in the rat. Gastroenterology 100:878–883
5. Yoshida N, Yoshikawa T, Nakamura Y, et al (1995) Role of neutrophil-mediated inflammation in aspirin-induced gastric mucosal injury. Dig Dis Sci 40:2300–2304
6. Yoshida N, Yoshikawa T, Nakamura Y, et al (1995) Role of neutrophil-endothelial cell interactions in gastric mucosal injury induced by aspirin. J Clin Gastroenterol 21:S73–S77
7. Krawisz JE, Sharon P, Stenson WF (1984) Quatitative assay for acute intestinal inflammation based on myeloperoxidase activity. Gastroenterology 87:1344–1350
8. Yoshida N, Yoshikawa T, Manabe H, et al (1999) Vitamin E protects against polymorphonuclear leukocyte-dependent adhesion to endothelial cells. J Leukoc Biol 65:757–763
9. Lawrence MB, McIntire LV, Eskin SG (1987) Effect of flow on polymorphonuclear leukocyte/endothelial cell adhesion. Blood 70:1284–1290
10. Yoshida N, Yoshikawa T, Nakamura Y, et al (1997) Interactions of neutrophils and endothelial cells under low flow conditions in vitro. Shock 8:125–130
11. Abbassi O, Kishimoto TK, McIntire LV, et al (1993) E-selectin supports neutrophil rolling in vitro under conditions of flow. J Clin Invest 92:2719–2730
12. Asako H, Kubes P, Wallace JL, et al (1992) Modulation of leukocyte adhesion in rat mesenteric venules by aspirin and salicylate. Gastroenterology 103:146–152
13. Yoshida N, Cepinskas G, Granger DN, et al (1995) Aspirin-induced, neutrophil mediated injury to vascular endothelium. Inflammation 19:297–312

Mucin Secretion Evoked by Prostaglandin E_2 in Guinea Pig Antral Mucous Cells: Role of EP1/EP4 Receptors

Atsuko Ohnishi[1], Chikao Shimamoto[1,*], Takashi Nakahari[2], Shoko Fujiwara[1], Yoshikatsu Nakahata[1], Kumiko Kojima[1], and Ken-ichi Katsu[1]

Summary. Effects of prostaglandin E_2 (PGE_2) on exocytosis in antral mucous cells isolated from guinea pigs were studied using video-microscopy. Stimulation with PGE_2 evoked a sustained increase in the frequency of exocytotic events, which was under regulation by both Ca^{2+} and cyclic adenosine monophosphate (cAMP) signals. An EP1 agonist (17-P-T-PGE_2) activated the Ca^{2+} signals and evoked only small increases in the frequency of exocytotic events, increasing the sensitivity of exocytosis to the cAMP signal. An EP4 agonist (ONO-AE1-329), which activated the cAMP signals and elicited a sustained increase in the frequency of exocytotic events, potentiated the frequency of exocytotic events regulated by the Ca^{2+} signals by increasing the sensitivity to the Ca^{2+}. In conclusion, PGE_2-evoked exocytotic events in antral mucous cells were regulated by interactions between EP1 and EP4 receptors.

Key words. Gastric mucin secretion, Exocytosis, Prostanoid EP type receptor, cAMP, Intracellular Ca^{2+} concentration

Introduction

The prostanoid EP type receptors (EP1, EP2, EP3, EP4) have been reported to be linked to different second messenger systems [1]. In this report, the regulation mechanisms of prostaglandin E_2 (PGE_2)-evoked exocytosis in antral mucous cells were studied using video-enhanced contrast (VEC) optical microscopy.

Materials and Methods

The solutions used (pH 7.4) were HEPES and HCO_3^--buffered solution, gassed with 95% O_2/5% CO_2 at 37°C as described previously [2]. Cell preparations and experimental procedures have been described elsewhere [2]. The exocytotic events, which

[1] Second Department of Internal Medicine, [2] Department of Physiology, Osaka Medical College, Takatsuki, Osaka 569-8686, Japan
* e-mail: in2021@poh.osaka-med.ac.jp

were detected by the rapid changes in light intensity of the granules, were counted in five or six cells every 30 s.

Results and Discussion

Stimulation with 1 μM PGE_2 caused sustained increases in the frequency of exocytotic events. These sustained increases evoked by 1 μM PGE_2 were reduced by approximately 50% in the absence of extracellular Ca^{2+}; and further addition of 50 μM H-89 (a protein kinase A inhibitor) eliminated the exocytotic events (Fig. 1A).

Addition of ONO-8713 (an EP1 receptor antagonist) decreased the frequency of exocytotic events evoked by 1 μM PGE_2 by approximately 50% (Fig. 1B). However, stimulation with 1 μM 17-P-T-PGE_2 (an EP1 receptor agonist) evoked only a small increase in the frequency of the exocytotic events (Fig. 1B). Thus, the EP1 receptor appears to be linked to the Ca^{2+} signal and to affect the frequency of exocytotic events during PGE_2 stimulation, although little Ca^{2+} mobilization was evoked by PGE_2.

Stimulation with 1 μM ONO-AE1-329 (an EP4 receptor agonist) evoked a sustained increase in the frequency of exocytotic events, which was about 20% of that evoked by 1 μM PGE_2 stimulation (Fig. 1C). The exocytotic responses evoked 1 μM ONO-AE1-329 were not affected in the absence of extracellular Ca^{2+} and were completely eliminated by addition of 50 μM H-89 in the absence of extracellular Ca^{2+}. Thus, stimulation with an EP4 receptor evoked an increase in the frequency of exocytotic events via activation of the cyclic adenosine monophosphate (cAMP) signal. These results indicate that exocytotic events evoked by PGE_2 were under regulation by both Ca^{2+} and cAMP signals.

Addition of 1 μM 17-P-T-PGE_2 potentiated the frequency of exocytotic events evoked by ONO-AE1-329 alone, and addition of both EP1 and EP4 agonists mimicked effects of PGE_2 stimulation on the frequency of exocytotic events. However, the effects of 17-P-T-PGE_2 were not detected in the absence of extracellular Ca^{2+} (Fig. 2A). The effects of 17-P-T-PGE_2 on forskolin (FK)-evoked exocytotic events were also examined (Fig. 2B,C). Stimulation with 10 μM FK evoked a sustained increase in the frequency of exocytotic events similar to ONO-AE1-329. Addition of 1 μM 17-P-T-PGE_2 also potentiated the frequency of exocytotic events evoked by FK. This effect of 1 μM 17-P-T-PGE_2 was not noted in the absence of extracellular Ca^{2+} (Fig. 2B).

Figure 2C shows the effects of 17-P-T-PGE_2 on the dose-response curve for FK in relation to the frequency of exocytotic events. The sustained frequencies of exocytotic events were plotted against the FK concentrations. The dose-response curve of FK ([inhibitory concentration of 50% (IC_{50})] 0.36 μM) was shifted to the low concentration side by the addition of 17-P-T-PGE_2 (IC_{50} 0.1 μM), whereas it shifted to the high concentration side in the absence of extracellular Ca^{2+} (IC_{50} 0.79 μM). These results indicate that stimulation with 17-P-T-PGE_2 increased the sensitivity of the exocytotic events to cAMP by activating the Ca^{2+} signal, although it alone did not evoked any increase in the frequency of exocytotic events. Increases in the frequency of exocytotic events activated by the cAMP signal were not explained by increases in the sensitivity to cAMP, which suggests that the cAMP signal also increases the sensitivity of exocy-

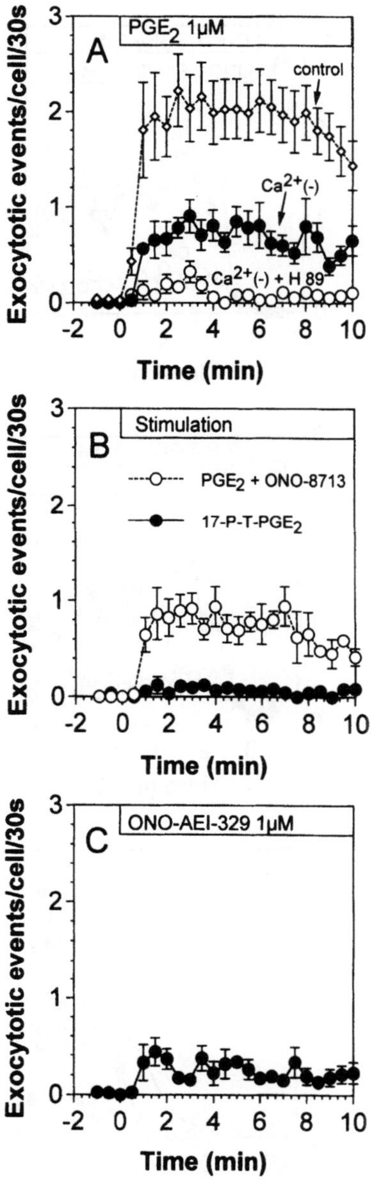

FIG. 1. **A** Effects of prostaglandin E_2 (PGE_2) on the frequency of exocytotic events in the presence (*diamonds*, $n = 24$) and the absence of Ca^{2+} (*filled circles*, $n = 6$). Addition of 50 μM H-89 eliminated the frequency of exocytotic events evoked by 1 μM PGE_2 in the absence of extracellular Ca^{2+} (*open circles*, $n = 4$). **B** Effects of EP1 agonist (1 μM 17-P-T-PGE_2, *filled circles*, $n = 6$) and EP1 antagonist (10 μM ONO-8713, *open circles*, $n = 6$) on PGE_2-evoked frequency of exocytotic events. **C** Effects of EP4 agonist (1 μM ONO-AE1-329) on the frequency of exocytotic events ($n = 6$)

totic responses to the Ca^{2+} signal. The interactions between cAMP and Ca^{2+} signals have been reported to regulate various cellular functions [3]. The PGE_2-stimulated exocytosis in antral mucous cells were also regulated by interactions between the Ca^{2+} and cAMP signals activated via the EP1 and EP4 receptors, respectively.

Acknowledgment. We thank Ono Pharmaceutical Company (Osaka, Japan) for giving us the opportunity to use EP1 receptor selective antagonist (ONO-8713) and EP4 receptor selective agonist (ONO-AE1-329).

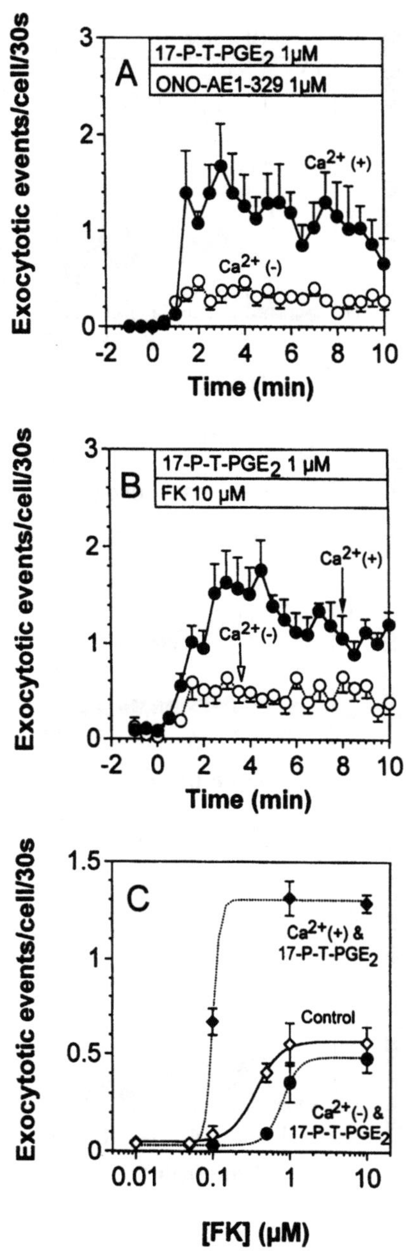

FIG. 2. **A** Stimulation with both EP1 agonist (1 μM 17-P-T-PGE_2) and EP4 agonists (1 μM ONO-AE1-329) in the presence of Ca^{2+} (*filled circles*) and the absence of Ca^{2+} (*open circles*). **B** Effects of on EP1 agonist (1 μM 17-P-T-PGE_2) on forskolin (*FK*)-evoked exocytotic events in the presence of Ca^{2+} (*filled circles*) and the absence of Ca^{2+} (*open circles*). **C** Effects of 1 μM 17-P-T-PGE_2 on the dose-response curve for forskolin (*FK*) in relation to the sustained frequency of exocytotic events

References

1. Coleman RA, Smith WL, Narumiya S (1994) VIII. International Union of Pharmacology: classification of prostanoid receptors: properties, distribution, and structure of the receptors and their subtypes. Pharmacol Rev 46:205–229
2. Fujiwara S, Shimamoto C, Katsu K, et al (1999) Isosmotic modulation of Ca^{2+}-regulated exocytosis in guinea-pig antral mucous cells: role of cell volume. J Physiol (Lond) 516:85–100
3. Nakahari T, Ito S, Yoshida H, et al (2000) Accumulation of cAMP evoked by acetylcholine stimulation in rat submandibular acinar cells: observation of exocytosis, fluid secretion and $[Ca^{2+}]_i$. Exp Physiol 85:159–169

Effects of Indomethacin and NS-398 on Acid-Induced E-Cadherin Surface Expression in Rat Gastric Epithelial Cells

Yasuhide Takezono*, Takashi Joh, Makoto Sasaki, Hiromi Kataoka, Kyouji Senou, Naotsuka Okayama, Yoshifumi Yokoyama, and Makoto Itoh

Summary. Previous studies indicated that gastric E-cadherin, an extracellular Ca^{2+}-dependent cell–cell adhesion molecule, was induced by acid exposure to maintain epithelial cell permeability. However, the effects of nonsteroidal antiinflammatory drugs (NSAIDs) on acid-induced E-cadherin expression in gastric epithelial cells are not known. In this study the effects of NSAIDs (indomethacin and NS-398) on surface expression of E-cadherin and epithelial permeability were investigated in rat gastric epithelial cells (RGM1). Rats not treated or treated with NSAIDs (10^{-7} M indomethacin, 10^{-5} M for NS-398) were exposed to solutions at different pH (pH 7.4–3.0) for 30 min. E-cadherin expression increased in an acidity-dependent manner, and gastric epithelial permeability was maintained. E-cadherin expression induced by acid exposure decreased after treatment with small doses of indomethacin, which did not damage to the cell, although gastric epithelial permeability increased. Treatment with NS-398, however, did not affect either E-cadherin expression or epithelial permeability. These findings suggest that expression of E-cadherin may play an important role in a gastric mucosal defense mechanism against acid exposure, and that cox-1 inhibitors such as indomethacin may break down this protective mechanism.

Key words. RGM1, NSAIDs, E-Cadherin, Permeability, Cell culture insert

Introduction

Epithelial (E)-cadherin, an extracellular Ca^{2+}-dependent cell–cell adhesion molecule, reportedly is expressed in normal epithelial and tumor cells of the gastrointestinal tract [1,2]. Previous studies indicated that gastric E-cadherin expression was induced by acid exposure to maintain epithelial cell permeability. The effects of nonsteroidal antiinflammatory drugs (NSAIDs) on acid-induced E-cadherin expression in gastric

First Department of Internal Medicine, Nagoya City University, 1 Kawasumi, Mizuho-cho, Mizuho-ku, Nagoya 467-8601, Japan
* e-mail: ytz@med.nagoya-cu.ac.jp

epithelial cells are not known. In this study the effects of indomethacin and the specific cox-2 inhibitor NS-398 on surface expression of E-cadherin and epithelial permeability were investigated in cultured rat gastric epithelial cells.

Materials and Methods

A rat gastric epithelial cell line (RGM1) [3] was cultured in Dulbecco's modified eagle medium (DMEM; GIBCO BRL, Grand Island, NY, USA) and F-12 nutrient mixture (GIBCO) (1:1) supplemented with 20% fetal bovine serum (FBS) (Bio Whittaker, Walkersville, MD, USA) and an antibiotic-antimycotic agent (GIBCO) at 37°C in a 5% CO_2 incubator.

The surface expression of E-cadherin was measured using a modified method of Khan et al. [4]. RGM1 was cultured in 24-well plates. After 30 min of treatment with (or without) NSAIDs (10^{-7} M indomethacin, 10^{-5} M NS-398), the cells were exposed to acidified (HCl) Hank's balanced salt solutions (HBSS) (pH 7.4–3.0) for 30 min at 37°C. The cells were then fixed with 0.2 ml of 1% paraformaldehyde in phosphate-buffered saline (PBS) for 10 min at room temperature. After washing three or four times with HBSS/PBS (1:1), the cells were incubated with an anti-E-cadherin antibody solution at 37°C for 30 min. After washing, the cells were incubated with a horseradish peroxidase-conjugated secondary antibody at 37°C for 30 min. The cells were washed four times, followed by incubation with 0.25 ml of 0.003% hydrogen peroxide and 3, 3′, 5, 5′-tetramethylbenzidine 0.1 mg/ml at 37°C for 60 min in the dark. The reaction was stopped by adding 75 μl of 8 N H_2SO_4. Absorbance at 450 nm of the samples were measured with a microplate reader.

For the epithelial permeability assay, RGM1 was seeded onto Boyden-type chambers consisting of polycarbonate micropore membranes (9 mm diameter, 8 μm pore size) mounted on plastic cylinders (cell culture insert; Becton Dickinson, Franklin Lakes, NJ, USA). The inserts were placed on 24-well plates; each well contained 1 ml of culture medium. The cells were then incubated for 3 or 4 days at 37°C in a 5% CO_2 incubator. The cells were exposed to NSAIDs (10^{-7} M indomethacin, 10^{-5} M NS-398) for 30 min and then exposed to the acidified HBSS (pH 7.4–3.0) for 30 min at 37°C. Immediately after acid exposure, 50 μl of 5 mM FITC-dextran was added to each insert, and the cells were incubated for 30 minutes at 37°C. Cell permeability was evaluated by measuring absorbances at 450 nm of solutions in both inserts and wells with a microplate reader; the results were expressed as absorbance ratios of well/insert + well.

All values are expressed as means ± SE. Data were analyzed using an one-way ANOVA with Fisher's test for multiple comparisons and the Student's *t*-test for a single comparison. Probability (*P*) values of <0.05 were considered significant.

Results

Exposure to acid significantly increased E-cadherin surface expression in a dose-dependent manner (Fig. 1a, open bars) but not epithelial permeability (Fig. 1b, open bars). Treatment with indomethacin decreased E-cadherin expression and canceled the E-cadherin expression induced by acid exposure (Fig. 1a, filled bars). In the

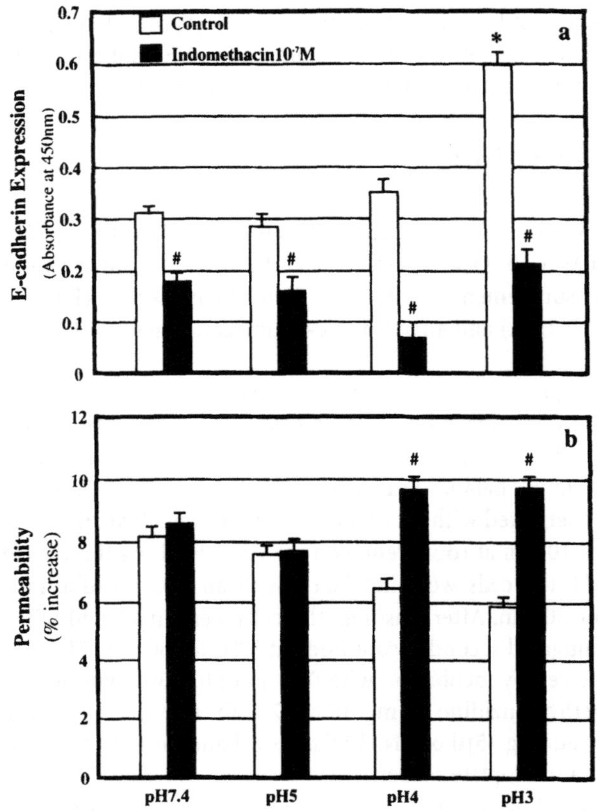

FIG. 1. Effects of indomethacin on E-cadherin surface expression and epithelial permeability during acid exposure. $^*P < 0.05$ vs. pH 7.4; $^\#P < 0.05$ vs. control

presence of indomethacin, acid exposure significantly increased epithelial permeability. NS-398 did not affect either E-cadherin expression or epithelial permeability (Fig. 2).

Discussion

For gastric epithelial cells, preservation of intercellular permeability is an important defense mechanism against gastric acid back-diffusion. Studies had shown that VE-cadherin plays an important role in maintaining vascular endothelial permeability [5], indicating that E-cadherin expressed in gastric epithelial cells might play a similar role in gastric mucosal permeability. The results shown in this study suggest that during acid exposure E-cadherin on RGM1 cells was significantly induced to maintain epithelial permeability, and that prostalgandin production may be essential for such E-cadherin expression and the preservation of permeability. The difference between the effects of indomethacin and NS-398 may be explained by cox-1 and cox-2 expression on the cells, which control the production of prostaglandins. Cox-1 expression might much higher than cox-2 expression on RGM1 cells.

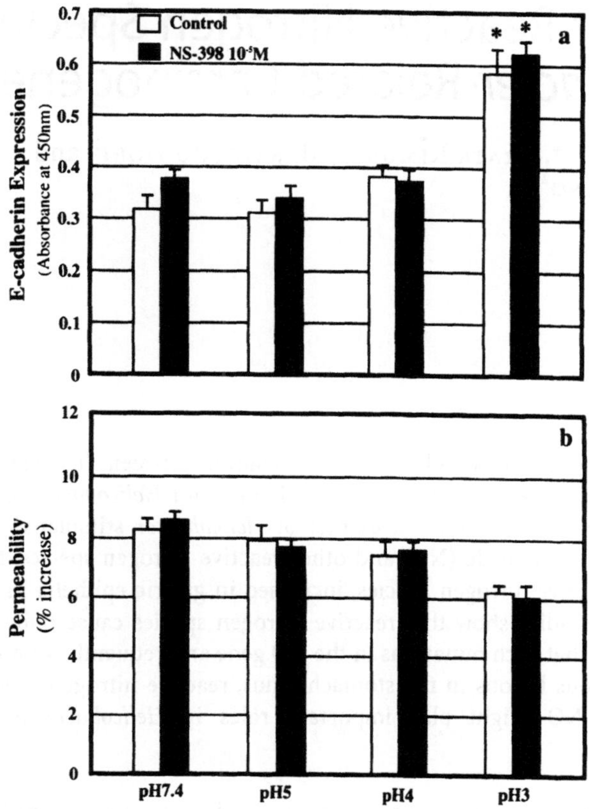

FIG. 2. Effects of NS-398 on E-cadherin surface expression and epithelial permeability during acid exposure. $^{*}P < 0.05$ vs. pH 7.4

In conclusion, surface expression of E-cadherin may play an important role in a gastric mucosal defense mechanism against acid, and cox-1 inhibitors such as indomethacin may break down this protective mechanism.

References

1. Mayer B, Johnson JP, Leitl F, et al (1993) E-cadherin expression in primary and metastatic gastric cancer: down-regulation correlates with cellular dedifferentiation and glandular disintegration. Cancer Res 53:1690–1695
2. Shino Y, Watanabe A, Yamada Y, et al (1995) Clinicopathologic evaluation of immunohistochemical E-cadherin expression in human gastric carcinomas. Cancer 76:2193–2201
3. Kobayashi I, Takei Y, Kawano S, et al (1996) RGM1, a cell line derived from normal gastric mucosa of rat. In Vitro Cell Dev Biol Anim 32:259–261
4. Khan BV, Parthasarathy SS, Alexander RV, et al (1995) Modified low density lipoprotein and its constituents augment cytokine-activated vascular cell adhesion molecule-1 gene expression in human vascular endothelial cells. J Clin Invest 95:1262–1270
5. Alexander JS, Jackson SA, Chaney E, et al (1998) The role of cadherin endocytosis in endothelial barrier regulation: involvement of protein kinase C and actin-cadherin interactions. Inflammation 22:419–433

Roles of Reactive Nitrogen Species in *Helicobacter*-Related Carcinogenesis

SHINGO TSUJI[1,*], ARATA KIMURA[1], MASATSUGU HORI[1], and SUNAO KAWANO[2]

Summary. Although data indicate an association between *Helicobacter* infection and gastric carcinogenesis, the precise mechanism for *Helicobacter*-related carcinogenesis are not yet clarified. An extract of *Helicobacter* stimulated inflammatory production of nitric oxide (NO) and other reactive nitrogen species. Nitrotyrosine, an adduct of active nitrogen species, increased in gastric epithelia in subjects with the infection. Studies show that reactive nitrogen species cause point mutations at CpG sites; and that such mutations in the *p53* gene are frequently found in cancerous and precancerous lesions in the stomach. Thus, reactive nitrogen species including inflammatory NO might play important roles in *Helicobacter*-induced gastric carcinogenesis.

Key words. Cancer, *Helicobacter pylori*, Nitric oxide, Nitrotyrosine, *p53*, Stomach

Introduction

Helicobacter pylori has been classified as a class I biological carcinogen by the World Health Organization and the International Agency for Research of Cancer [1] since 1994. The mechanism for *Helicobacter*-related carcinogenesis, however, has not yet clarified.

We and others have shown that *H. pylori* activates inflammatory cells to produce nitric oxide (NO) and consequent reactive nitrogen species [2,3]. NO [4] and its metabolites, particularly peroxynitrite [5], have mutagenic effects on cells. In this paper we briefly review possible roles of reactive nitrogen species in *H. pylori*-related gastric carcinogenesis.

[1]Department of Internal Medicine and Therapeutics, Osaka University Graduate School of Medicine, [2]Department of Clinical Laboratory Sciences, School of Allied Health Science, Osaka University Medical School, 2-2 Yamadaoka, Suita, Osaka 565-0871, Japan
* e-mail: tsuji@medone.med.osaka-u.ac.jp

H. pylori and Inflammatory NO

There are several sources for NO and NO-related compounds in the stomach (Fig. 1). Nitrite and nitroso compounds can be taken orally and release NO depending on the intragastric environment. Oral bacteria reduce salivary nitrate to nitrite, which forms nitroso compounds in acidic conditions in stomach. When peritoneal macrophages and neutrophils were incubated with *H. pylori* extract, significant production of nitrate and nitrite was observed [2]. This activity of the extract was significantly attenuated by heat treatment or protease digestion, indicating that the activity stimulating NO production was due to heat-labile and protease-sensitive factors at least in part [2].

The targets of these reactive nitrogen species in the stomach have not yet been clarified. Consequently, we observed localization of nitrotyrosine in gastric mucosa; nitrotyrosine is a biologic marker for endogenous exposure to reactive nitrogen species and for increased risks for carcinogenesis [5].

In subjects with *H. pylori* infection, nitrotyrosine immunoreactivity was detected in mucosal epithelial cells and inflammatory mononuclear cells including monocytes, macrophages, and components of extracellular matrix. In contrast, there was absence of nitrotyrosine immunoreactivity in other interstitial cells, such as vascular endothelial cells and myofibroblasts. In subjects without the infection, nitrotyrosine immunoreactivity was much less frequently observed in the stomach. These results indicate that NO and NO-related nitrating compounds exist and interact with epithelial and subepithelial inflammatory cells in the stomach in *Helicobacter*-infected subjects. Therefore, inflammatory cells appear to be one of the sources of reactive nitrogen species which nitrosate, nitrate, alkylate, and oxidate components in gastric epithelial cells and possibly cause nitration of tyrosine residues in gastric mucosa.

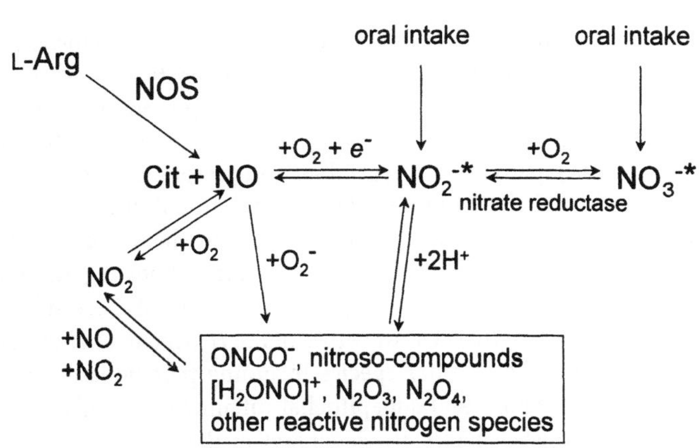

FIG. 1. Metabolic pathways for reactive nitrogen species in human stomach. Note that some nitrosocompounds may be taken orally with preserved foods. *Excreted through the kidney in urine

NO and Subsequent *p53* Mutations in Gastric Carcinogenesis

Recent data show that certain mutations and overexpression in *p53* may occur quite early in gastric carcinogenesis or even in normal-appearing gastric mucosa without intestinal metaplasia, dysplasia, or gastric cancer. Consequently, reported data on *p53* gene mutations in these lesions were compiled.

The samples analyzed in the articles were from Japan, Italy, and other high risk areas for gastric cancer. Among 54 mutations described, G:C → A:T transition occurred most frequently (32 mutations, 59%). The occurrence of G:C → A:T transition was compared among the geographical areas. This type of point mutation occurred most frequently in precancerous and epicancerous lesions and early gastric cancers in these three areas, although the definition of such lesions should be matched in the future international works. The second most frequent was an A:T → G:C transition (eight mutations, 15%), and the other mutation occurred less frequently (one to three alterations, 2%–6%). It should be noted that four A:T → G:C transitions were reported in two cases with multiple mutations in the same lesions. Overall, 43 (80%) of 54 mutations were consistent with the predicted types of mutation that potentially occur from deamination of DNA bases. In particular, deamination of 5-methylcytosine results in generation of thymine (T) [4]. Because T exists naturally in DNA, a miss-pair of G:T can be altered to A:T during DNA replication. Furthermore, 80% of the observed mutations in *p53* in precancerous and pericancerous gastric mucosa and in earlier stages of gastric cancers are consistent with the predicted types of mutation due to DNA deamination induced by NO and other NO-related nitroso compounds. This study therefore offers evidence that endogenous production of reactive nitrogen species stimulated by *Helicobacter* might be involved in the pathogenesis of gastric carcinogenesis.

Conclusion: NO Is an Enemy

Gastric carcinogenesis appears to be a complex, multistep, multifactorial process; and inflammatory NO production is not the only candidate for the process. As mentioned above, several gastric carcinogens, including nitroso compounds are produced during food preservation processes of specific foods, such as fish, frequently consumed in high risk areas such as Japan. Certain vegetables and preserved foods contain nitrates that can be reduced to nitrite by oral bacteria. Intraluminal nitrate and nitrite have deserved consideration for the endogenous sources of nitroso compounds in the gastric lumen [6]. However, there are significant controversies regarding the exogenous nitrate and nitrite in gastric carcinogenesis. Bioassays of these substances have not revealed a carcinogenic effect. On the other hand, *Helicobacter* stimulates inflammatory production of NO and other species including peroxynitrite. Nitrotyrosine localizes in gastric epithelium and subepithelial inflammatory cells, demonstrating that these reactive nitrogen species are generated in these areas. Reactive nitrogen species preferentially cause point mutations at hot spots of the *p53* gene. The systematic review revealed frequent G:C → A:T transitions in the *p53* gene in precancerous tissues and early phases of gastric cancer in humans.

In conclusion, the present studies demonstrate that *H. pylori* has a potent ability to stimulate NO synthesis in macrophages and neutrophils. Because reactive nitrogen species are endogenous mutagens that also nitrate proteins in the target cells, gastric inflammation induced by *H. pylori* may be an important factor in DNA damage and possibly an initiator of gastric carcinogenesis. Considering these results together, we hypothesize that inflammatory production of reactive nitrogen species stimulated by the bacteria play pivotal roles in gastric carcinogenesis.

References

1. IARC Working Group (1994) IARC monograph, vol 61. IARC, Lyon, pp 1–241
2. Tsuji S, Kawano S, Tsujii M, et al (1996) *Helicobacter pylori* extract stimulates inflammatory nitric oxide production. Cancer Lett 108:195–200
3. Dixon MF, Genta RM, Yardley JH, Correal P (1996) Classification and grading of gastritis. Am J Surg Pathol 20:1161–1181
4. Wink DA, Kazimierz S, Maragos CM, et al (1991) DNA deaminating ability and genotoxicity of nitric oxide and its progenitors. Science 254:1001–1003
5. Halliwell B (1999) Oxygen and nitrogen are pro-carcinogens: damage to DNA by reactive oxygen, chlorine and nitrogen species: measurement, mechanism and the effects of nutrition. Mutat Res 443:37–52
6. Correa P (1988) A human model of gastric carcinogenesis. Cancer Res 48:3554–3560

Interaction Between *Helicobacter pylori* Infection and NSAID Use

Akiko Shiotani[1,*] and David Y. Graham[2]

Summary. Although nonsteroidal antiinflammatory drug (NSAID) use and *Helicobacter pylori* are the most common causes of peptic ulcers, it remains unclear whether there is an interaction between them. It has been suggested that *H. pylori* infection may not influence the incidence of gastroduodenal ulcers in NSAID users and may even provide some protection against the ulceration caused by NSAIDs, possibly due to stimulation of mucosal synthesis of prostaglandins by the *H. pylori* infection. Overall, the studies are consistent with the notion that, in most instances, *H. pylori* and NSAID use are separate causes of ulcers and that they respond according to the etiology. We recently showed that only intraluminal pH and not the density of *H. pylori*, polymorphonuclear leukocytes, or mucosal levels of nitric oxide or interleukin-8 was related to protection against acute NSAID damage in humans. The data are most consistent with *H. pylori* and NSAIDs being independent causes of ulcer, although there are some interactions that lead to a twofold increase in the risk of ulcer complications among NSAID users infected with *H. pylori*. The protection afforded by *H. pylori* infection against acute NSAID damage appears limited to those who have a markedly reduced ability to produce acid consistent with the effects of administration of antisecretory therapy.

Key words. NSAIDs, *Helicobacter pylori*, Gastric ulcer, Inflammation, Interleukin-8

Introduction

Nonsteroidal antiinflammatory drug (NSAID) use and *Helicobacter pylori* (*H. pylori*) are the most common causes of peptic ulcer. The risk of developing a serious, life-threatening ulcer complication has been estimated to range from 1% to 4% of chronic NSAID users per year [1]. Although previous studies reported that approximately 50%

[1] Second Department of Internal Medicine, Wakayama Medical University, 811-1 Kimiidera, Wakayama 641-0012, Japan
[2] Department of Medicine, Veterans Affairs Medical Center and Baylor College of Medicine, Houston, TX 77031, USA
* e-mail: akikoshi@wakayama-med.ac.jp

of patients with NSAID-induced ulcers were also *H. pylori*-infected [2], it remains unclear whether *H. pylori* infection and NSAID use are synergistic, additive, or independent factors for ulcer pathogenesis. It has even been suggested that *H. pylori* infection may provide some protection against the ulceration caused by NSAIDs.

H. pylori and NSAID Ulcer Healing

H. pylori eradication accelerates the rate of healing of true *H. pylori* ulcers and virtually eliminates ulcer recurrence. In contrast, eradication of *H. pylori* in chronic NSAID users with ulcers was associated with slight impairment of the rate of proton pump inhibitor-induced ulcer healing [3–5]. Importantly, these finding come from the artificial situation in which NSAIDs are continued in those with known ulcers associated with chronic NSAID use. *H. pylori* reduces the effectiveness of proton pump inhibitor therapy through loss of ammonia from the hydrolysis of urea by *H. pylori* urease and by an increase in the ability of the corpus to produce acid following healing of the gastritis, which acts to inhibit acid secretion. Thus, outside of such an artificial and somewhat contrived condition, there is no evidence for a clinically important adverse effect of *H. pylori* on ulcer healing among chronic NSAID users.

H. pylori and NSAID Ulcer Relapse

H. pylori infection is associated with a marked increase in duodenal ulcer and a marked reduction in the effectiveness of proton pump inhibitor therapy to prevent gastric ulcers in chronic NSAID users [6]. Eradication of *H. pylori* also had a minimal effect on the rate of recurrent ulcers in those with continued or recurrent NSAID use [7]. This is consistent with the original studies of the effect of *H. pylori* eradication on ulcer recurrence showing that NSAID use was the primary variable associated with ulcer recurrence following cure of the infection [8]. Overall, these observations are consistent with the notion that in most instances *H. pylori* and NSAID use are separate causes of ulcer and that they respond according to the etiology. Importantly, eradication of *H. pylori* before NSAID therapy has been shown to reduce the occurrence of NSAID-induced peptic ulcers, which is consistent with the reported twofold increase in ulcer complications among *H. pylori*-infected chronic NSAID users [9].

H. pylori and NSAID Ulcer Bleeding

Because new *H. pylori* ulcers are rare (approximately 1% per year) and ulcer bleeding occurs in only approximately 25% of those with known *H. pylori* ulcers, most studies are expected to be consistent with the results of a case-control study by Wu et al., who concluded that *H. pylori* and NSAIDs were largely independent risk factors of gastric or duodenal ulcer bleeding [10]. Nevertheless, it is likely that NSAIDs exacerbate *H. pylori* ulcers and increase the rate of bleeding; but unless the risk was huge it would be overlooked in all but the largest studies. If such a risk occurs it is likely to be in the range reported from prospective case-control studies showing that NSAID users infected with *H. pylori* have an almost twofold increased risk of a bleeding peptic ulcer compared with NSAID users without *H. pylori* [11].

Protective Role of *H. pylori* Infection Against NSAID Gastric Mucosal Damage

There is substantial evidence that suppression of gastric prostaglandins (PGs) is the fundamental mechanism responsible for the gastrointestinal toxicity of NSAIDs [12]. PG inhibition leads to decreases in epithelial mucus, secretion of bicarbonate, mucosal blood flow, epithelial proliferation, and mucosal resistance to injury [13,14]. It has been suggested that neutrophils and the vascular endothelium are important targets for both the ulcerogenic effects of NSAIDs and the cytoprotective effects of PGs [15]. The hypothesis that *H. pylori* infection might provide some protection against the ulceration caused by NSAIDs is related to the stimulation of mucosal PG synthesis by *H. pylori* infection [16–18]. This seems intuitively incorrect, as it requires an inflamed tissue to have increased resistance to acid or to the damaging effects of NSAIDs.

Role of Inflammation. Reduction of neutrophils, such as by administration of specific antineutrophil agents, reduced NSAID-induced gastric damage in laboratory animals. Taha et al. suggested that NSAID ulcers were more likely to occur in those with neutrophilic infiltration in the gastric mucosa [19]. Hamlet et al. studied *H. pylori*-negative volunteers and showed that there was an increased production of interleukin-1β (IL-1β), IL-6, and IL-8 locally in the antral mucosa in relation to aspirin-induced gastric injury [20]. The data are difficult to interpret clinically, as the authors did not provide data regarding the relation between the biopsy sites and the presence or absence of erosions, which would be expected to show infiltration with polymorphonuclear neutrophils and an increase in IL-8.

Nitric Oxide. Nitric oxide (NO)-releasing NSAIDs are associated with markedly less gastrointestinal toxicity while retaining the antiinflammatory and antipyretic activity of the parent NSAID. There has been accumulating evidence that NO plays an important role in the *H. pylori*-related gastric mucosal lesions and in gastrointestinal mucosal protection. It has been previously shown that *H. pylori*-positive patients had a significantly lower NO concentration in the gastric lumen and more nitrite/nitrate levels in the gastric juice [21].

We performed a prospective study in *H. pylori*-positive volunteers receiving naproxen to evaluate whether mucosal damage (or protection) correlated with the levels of mucosal NO or IL-8, histologic parameters including the density of *H. pylori*, polymorphonuclear cells, mononuclear cells, or luminal pH. Short-term NSAID use had no effect on mucosal IL-8 levels or nitrite levels. We did not find a relation between *H. pylori*, neutrophil density, or histological gastritis before or after NSAID administration or placebo. Only high intraluminal pH associated with severe corpus gastritis was associated with protection against severe NSAID damage.

Conclusions

Overall, the data are most consistent with *H. pylori* and NSAIDs being independent causes of ulcers with but with some interactions that lead to a twofold increased risk of ulcer complications in NSAID users infected with *H. pylori*. The protection afforded by *H. pylori* infection against acute NSAID damage appears limited to those who have a markedly reduced ability to produce acid, consistent with the effects of administration of antisecretory therapy.

References

1. Graham DY (1996) Nonsteroidal anti-inflammatory drugs, *Helicobacter pylori*, and ulcers: where we stand. Am J Gastroenterol 91:2080–2086
2. Cullen DJE, Hawkey GM, Greenwood DC, et al (1997) Peptic ulcer bleeding in the elderly: relative roles of *Helicobacter pylori* and non-steroidal anti-inflammatory drugs. Gut 41:459–462
3. Hawkey CJ, Tulassay Z, Szczepanski L, et al (1998) Randomized controlled trial of *Helicobacter pylori* eradication in patients on non-steroidal anti-inflammatory drugs: HELP NSAIDs study: Helicobacter Eradication for Lesion Prevention. Lancet 352:1016–1021
4. Chan FK, Sung JJ, Suen R, et al (1998) Does eradication of *Helicobacter pylori* impair healing of nonsteroidal anti-inflammatory drug associated bleeding peptic ulcers? A prospective randomized study. Aliment Pharmacol Ther 12:1201–1205
5. Bianchi Porro G, Parente F, Imbesi V, et al (1996) Role of *Helicobacter pylori* in ulcer healing and recurrence of gastric and duodenal ulcers in long term NSAID users: response to omeprazole dual therapy. Gut 39:22–26
6. Graham DY (2000) NSAID ulcers: prevalence and prevention. Mod Rheumatol 10:2–7
7. Hawkey CJ, Karrasch JA, Szczepanski L, et al (1998) Omeprazole compared with misoprostol for ulcers associated with nonsteroidal anti-inflammatory drugs: omeprazole versus misoprostol foe NSAID-induced ulcer management (OMNIUM) study group. N Engl J Med 338:727–734
8. Graham DY, Lew GM, Klein PD, et al (1992) Effect of treatment of *Helicobacter pylori* infection on the long-term recurrence of gastric or duodenal ulcer: a randomized, controlled study. Ann Intern Med 116:705–708
9. Chan FKL, Sung JJY, Chung SCS, et al (1997) Randomized trial of eradication of *Helicobacter pylori* before nonsteroidal anti-inflammatory drug therapy to prevent peptic ulcers. Lancet 350:975–979
10. Wu CY, Poon SK, Chen GH, et al (1999) Interaction between *Helicobacter pylori* and non-steroidal anti-inflammatory drugs in peptic ulcer bleeding. Scand J Gastroenterol 33:234–237
11. Graham DY (1989) Prevention of gastroduodenal injury induced by chronic nonsteroidal antiinflammatory drug therapy. Gastroenterology 96:675–681
12. Laine L, Sloane R, Ferretti M, et al (1995) A randomized double-blind comparison of placebo, etodolac, and naproxen on gastrointestinal injury and prostaglandin production. Gastrointest Endosc 42:428–433
13. Whittle BJR (1977) Mechanisms underlying gastric mucosal damage induced by indomethacin and bile salts, and the actions of prostaglandins. Br J Pharmacol 60: 455–460

14. Wolfe MM, Soll AH (1988) The physiology of gastric acid secretion. N Engl J Med 319:1707–1715
15. Wallace JL (1992) Non-steroidal anti-inflammatory gastropathy and cytoprotection: pathogenesis and mechanisms re-examined. Scand J Gastroenterol 27(suppl):192:3–8
16. Avunduk C, Suliman M, Gang D, et al (1991) Gastroduodenal mucosal prostaglandid generation in patients with *Helicobacter pylori* before and after treatment with bismuth subsalicylate. Dig Dis Sci 36:431–434
17. Hudson N, Balsitis M, Filipowicz F, et al (1993) Effect of *Helicobacter pylori* colonization on gastric mucosal eicosanoid synthesis in patients taking nonsteroidal anti-inflammatory drugs. Gut 34:748–751
18. Fu S, Ramanujam KS, Wong A, et al (1999) Increased expression and cellular localization of inducible nitric oxide synthase and cyclooxygenase 2 in *Helicobacter pylori* gastritis. Gastroenterology 116:1319–1329
19. Taha AS, Dahill S, Morran C, et al (1999) Neutrophils, *Helicobacter pylori*, and non-steroidal anti-inflammatory drug ulcers. Gastoenterology 116:254–258
20. Hamlet A, Lindholm C, Nillson O, et al (1998) Aspirin-induced gastritis, like *Helicobacter pylori*-induced gastritis, disinhibits acid secretion in human: relation to cytokine expression. Scand J Gastroenterol 33:346–356
21. Shiotani A, Yanaoka K, Iguchi M, et al (1999) *Helicobacter pylori* infection reduces intraluminal nitric oxide in humans. J Gastroenterol 34:668–674

Interrelations of Nonsteroidal Antiinflammatory Drugs, *H. pylori* Infection, and Gastric Damage

Seiji Futagami[1], Tetsuro Hiratsuka[1], Ken Wada[1], Atsushi Tatsuguchi[1], Taku Tsukui[1], Kazumasa Miyake[1], Yoko Shinji[1], Tadasu Iizumi[1], Kei Shinoki[1], Tomonori Akamatsu[1], Masaru Hosone[2], Choitsu Sakamoto[1], and Masafumi Kobayashi[1]

Summary. Because 50% of elderly patients in Japan have *Helicobacter pylori* infection, many NSAID-induced peptic ulcers, by chance, occur in patients who happen to be *H. pylori*-positive. Many previous studies have reported the relation between *H. pylori* and NSAIDs. Chan et al. and Bianchi et al. described increased risk for ulcers in *H. pylori*-positive NSAID users. In contrast, recent prospective studies show that the presence of *H. pylori* does not increase the risk of gastric or duodenal ulcers in arthritis patients or healthy subjects taking NSAIDs. Because many *H. pylori*-positive patients are administered NSAIDs in Japan, it is important to determine whether these offensive factors affected the gastric mucosa additively or independently. Regarding cyclooxygenase-2 (COX-2) protein, which is the target enzyme against NSAIDs, COX-2 expressed at inflammatory sites in the gastrointestinal tract presumably plays a role in the repair process of gastric damage. *H. pylori* infection elevated COX-2 protein in gastric epithelium and decreased the levels of COX mRNA in the stomachs of mice with experimentally induced gastric erosions or ulcers, although COX-2 mRNA levels were undetectable in controls. Therefore, it seems to be important to determine the role of COX-2 protein in the gastric tissues to clarify the relation between *H. pylori* infection and NSAIDs.

Key words. *Helicobacter pylori*, NSAIDs, Cyclooxygenase (COX), COX activity, COX-2 inhibitor, Mucosal injury

Helicobacter pylori is the most common cause of chronic active gastritis and peptic ulcer disease in humans and has been implicated in the development of gastric malignancy [1]. Eradication of this bacterium has been recommended for *H. pylori*-positive incurable gastric and duodenal ulcers. The most effective treatment

[1]Third Department of Internal Medicine, [2]Department of Pathology, Nippon Medical School, 1-1-5 Sendagi, Bunkyo-ku, Tokyo 113-8603, Japan

regimens currently used for eradicating *H. pylori* are combined therapies that include nitroimidazoles and macrolides. Because current treatment regimens for *H. pylori* infection do not achieve an eradication rate of 100%, theoretically the prevalence of drug-resistant *H. pylori* will increase in the population. We need to determine how to select the cases in which we should eradicate *H. pylori*-positive gastroduodenal diseases.

More than 1% of the population of the United States uses nonsteroidal antiinflammatory drugs (NSAIDs) daily, and 60 million NSAID prescriptions are written annually every year in the United States alone. The widespread usage of these drugs is anticipated to increase even further in the future because of their efficacy in the treatment of osteoarthritic and generalized aches as an ever-increasing percentage of our population becomes elderly. For example, it has been estimated that in the United States there are more than 75,000 hospitalizations and more than 7500 deaths annually among the elderly that are directly related to NSAID use. The prevalence of gastric ulcers among chronic NSAID users has been estimated at 13% and that of duodenal ulcers approximately 11% [2]. However, many patients with NSAID-realized side effects, such as epigastralgia, heartburn, and dyspepsia, could not stop taking these drugs because of the joint pain, fever, and therapy of the original diseases.

NSAIDs work by inhibiting cyclooxygenase, with a secondary reduction in the synthesis of proinflammatory prostaglandins. Evidence suggests that NSAIDs may differentially inhibit subforms of cyclooxygenase and thereby vary in their antiinflammatory and toxicity profiles [3]. The isoenzymes are known as COX-1 and COX-2. Kargman et al. showed, using Western blotting and biochemical assays, that COX-1 was identified in all gastrointestinal tissues [4]. They further found that no COX-2 immunoreactivity is seen in the dog, monkey, or human gastrointestinal tissues, in contrast to findings for COX-1, but its expression may be enhanced at sites of inflammation. COX-2 may produce prostaglandins involved in inflammation and mitogenesis. An ideal NSAID therefore would preferentially inhibit COX-2 and exert no effect on COX-1.

Celecoxib, NS-398, and rofecoxib seem to be the first cyclooxygenase inhibitors convincingly to break the prostaglandin-dependent link between efficacy and gastrotoxicity in humans. However, there are questions to be addressed before COX-2 inhibitors can be accorded the status of a major therapeutic revolution. Whether COX-2 inhibitors become harmful in the presence of gastrointestinal inflammation depends on whether COX-2 is induced to the extent that it becomes the predominant source of prostaglandins. It is important for COX-2 inhibitors to be shown directly to be safe in these conditions. Second, will COX-2 inhibitors retard ulcer healing in humans as they have in animal studies [3]?

Because 50% of elderly patients in Japan have *H. pylori* infection, many NSAID-induced peptic ulcers, by chance, occur in patients who happen to be *H. pylori*-positive. Therefore, it is important to determine whether these offensive factors affect the gastric mucosa additively or independently. Such information would be important for understanding the pathogenesis and identifying patients at particularly high risk of ulcer complications.

There have been many previous reports on the relation between *H. pylori* and NSAIDs. Chan et al. [5] and Bianchi et al. [6] described increased risk for ulcers in *H. pylori*-positive NSAID users. In contrast, several other studies have found no difference in the incidence of NSAID-induced peptic ulcers in patients who are *H. pylori*-positive compared with those who are *H. pylori*-negative. Kim et al. [7] and Loeb et al. [8] reported that they did not find an increased risk of ulcers in *H. pylori*-positive patients. The NSAID users also had less histologic evidence of gastritis, inflammation, and epithelial abnormalities typically present with *H. pylori* infection. The findings suggest that these patients' ulcers were uniquely related to NSAID use and did not require *H. pylori* for development. Prospective studies show that the presence of *H. pylori* dose not increase the risk of gastric or duodenal ulcers in arthritis patients or healthy subjects taking NSAIDs. Graham et al. [9] reported that *H. pylori* infection leads to elevation of the prostaglandin concentration, which increases cytoprotection. More recent studies have determined that higher prostaglandin production occurs in *H. pylori*-positive patients. Furthermore, the decrease in mucosal prostaglandin production associated with some NSAIDs, such as naproxen, is ameliorated by the presence of *H. pylori*; that is, the level of prostaglandin synthesis in NSAID users who are histologically positive for *H. pylori* is approximately equivalent to that of control subjects.

Helicobacter pylori and NSAIDs respectively affect the gastric mucosa via different mechanisms. For example, *H. pylori*-induced gastroduodenal diseases depend on the inflammatory responses of the host and the release of a number of virulence factors, such as urease (responsible for ammonia generation), a vacuolating cytotoxin, and *Cag A* protein. In contrast, NSAID-induced gastritis is caused by reduction of COX activity, secretion of hydromucus, and the microvasular circulation.

To determine the relation between *H. pylori* infection and NSAIDs it is important to investigate how these factors affect each other.

Regarding COX-2 protein, which is the target enzyme against NSAIDs, COX-2 expressed at inflammatory sites in the gastrointestinal tract presumably plays a role in the repair process to reverse gastric damage. *H. pylori* infection elevated the COX-2 protein in gastric epithelium [10,11]. Recently, a decrease in the levels of COX mRNA and COX protein in the stomachs of mice with experimentally induced erosions or ulcers [11]. COX-2 mRNA levels were undetectable in controls but were high during the acute stages of gastric erosions and ulcers [11]. It is important to clarify how COX-2 protein induced by *H. pylori* infection affects NSAID-related gastric damage. Further investigations to determine the roles of COX-2 proteins in the gastric mucosa are needed to clarify the relation between *H. pylori* and NSAIDs.

References

1. Dunn BE, Cohen H, Blaser MJ (1997) *Helicobacter pylori.* Clin Microbiol Rev 10: 720–741
2. Mitchell JA, Akarasereenont P, Thiemermann C, et al (1994) Selectivity of nonsteroidal antiinflammatory drugs as inhibitors of constitutive and inducible cyclooxygenase. Proc Natl Acad Sci USA 90:11693–11697
3. Mizuno H, Sakamoto C, Matsuda K, et al (1997) Induction of cyclooxygenase 2 in gastric mucosal lesions and its inhibition by the specific antagonist delays healing in mice. Gastroenterology 112:387–397
4. Kargman S, Charleson S, Cartwright M, et al (1996) Characterization of prostaglandin G/H synthase 1 and 2 in rat, dog, monkey, and human gastrointestinal tracts. Gastroenterology 111:445–454

5. Chan FK, Sung JJ, Chung SC, et al (1997) Randomised trial of eradication of *Helicobacter pylori* before non-steroidal anti-inflammatory drug therapy to prevent peptic ulcers. Lancet 350:975–979
6. Bianchi PG, Parente F, Imbesi V, et al (1996) Role of *Helicobacter pylori* in ulcer healing and recurrence of gastric and duodenal ulcers in longterm NSAID users. Reponse to omeprazole dual therapy. Gut 39:22–26
7. Kim JG, Graham DY, the Misoprostol Study Group (1994) *Helicobacter pylori* infection and development of gastric or duodenal ulcer in arthritic patients receiving chronic NSAID therapy. Am J Gastroenterol 89:203–207
8. Loeb DS, Talley NJ, Ahlquist DA, et al (1992) Long-term nonsteroidal anti-inflammatory drug use and gastroduodenal injuries: the role of *Helicobacter pylori*. Gastroenterology 102:1899–1905
9. Graham DY (1991) Nonsteroidal anti-inflammatory drugs, *Helicobacter pylori*, and ulcers: where we stand. Am J Gastroenterol 91:2080–2086
10. Romano M, Ricci V, Memoli A, et al (1998) *Helicobacter pylori* up-regulates cyclooxygenase-2 mRNA expression and prostaglandin E_2 synthesis in MKN-28 gastric mucosal cells in vitro. J Biol Chem 273:28560–28563
11. Sakamoto C (1998) Roles of COX-1 and COX-2 in gastrointestinal pathophysiology. J Gastroenterol 33:618–624

Part 10
Prevention of Disease by Modulation of Microcirculation

Microvascular Leukocyte Activation and Apoptosis in *Helicobacter pylori*-Colonized Gastric Mucosa

Hidekazu Suzuki[1,*], Kentaro Yamabe[1], Masaharu Miyazawa[1], Soichiro Miura[2], Masayuki Suzuki[3], and Hiromasa Ishii[1]

Summary. *Helicobacter pylori* (Hp) colonization evoked gastric mucosal inflammation in Mongolian gerbils. This review summarizes the time course of *H. pylori*-associated gastric oxidative injury including leukocyte activation and apoptosis. After Hp inoculation the bacteria colonized to the surface epithelium, and in the venules of the gastric mucosa large numbers of leukocytes rolling on or adhering to the vascular wall were observed by intravital microscopy. Adherent leukocytes migrated into the parenchyma, and the levels of tissue myeloperoxidase activity increased. Among the several toxic factors, monochloramine (NH_2Cl), which derived from both activated leukocyte and Hp urease, is important for genesis of gastric cellular injury, such as apoptosis. The sequential in vitro study of NH_2Cl-induced apoptosis is summarized. Futhermore, the balance in the levels of gastric mucosal apoptosis and gastric cell proliferation and the possible relevance to gastric carcinogenesis are described.

Key words. Microcirculation, Leukocyte infiltration, Free radicals, Apoptosis, Proliferation

Discovery of *Helicobacter pylori*

In 1982 Marshall and Warren were the first to culture *Helicobacter pylori* (Hp) isolated from the gastric mucosa of patients with gastritis [1]. Until that point, it had been thought almost impossible for any microorganism to survive in the acidic environment in the stomach. Although the clinical importance of Hp was recognized only 18 years ago, it is a century since spiral microorganisms were first discovered [2] and were shown to colonize the stomach. A series of experiments with *Helicobacter felis* were undertaken and reported in 1919 by Kasai and Kobayashi [3] in Kitasato Insti-

[1] Department of Internal Medicine, School of Medicine, Keio University, 35 Shinanomachi, Shinjuku-ku, Tokyo 160-8582, Japan
[2] Second Department of Internal Medicine, National Defense Medical College, Saitama, Japan
[3] National Tokyo Medical Center, Tokyo, Japan
* e-mail: hsuzuki@med.keio.ac.jp

tute, Tokyo. They demonstrated that the *Helicobacter* found in the stomach of cats and dogs could be transmitted to mice or rabbits, and that the infections were successfully eradicated by salvarsan. It was to be another 70 years before scientists again attempted to treat gastritis associated with *Helicobacter*. At the present time, the important role played by Hp infections of the gastric mucosa in the onset of gastritis and peptic ulcer disease is becoming clearer [4].

Hp Infection in the Mongolian Gerbil

An animal model was recently established for Hp-associated gastric disease by inoculating this bacterium into Mongolian gerbils [5]. It is useful for in vivo examination of Hp-associated gastric mucosa. The Mongolian gerbil was first established as an experimental animal by Tatsuji Nomura and his mother Masuko Nomura in the Central Labolatory of Experimental Animals in Japan about 30 years ago. Recently, Japanese investigators revealed the formation of gastric cancer by inoculating only Hp to this animal [6,7]. We also used this animal and reported a significant level of gastric mucosal neutrophil accumulation and an increase in lipid peroxides and total glutathione contents after Hp infection [8,9]. The exact mechanism by which Hp infection results in gastric mucosal injury is unclear, although it has been demonstrated that extracts of the bacterium can induce a number of microvascular alterations in rat gastric mucosa, including platelet aggregation and macromolecular leakage of labeled albumin [10].

The gastric microcirculation of Mongolian gerbils (MGS/Sea) inoculated with Hp [5] was visualized by intravital microscopy [11]. The leukocyte rolling velocity on the venular endothelium and the number of adherent leukocytes were calculated by the playback image analysis of a recorded VCR. In the normal, uninfected gastric mucosa of Mongolian gerbils, the mesh of a capillary network was seen between the collecting venules (Fig. 1). The epithelial cell layer that covers the surface of the gastric mucosa was observed to have a paving stone-like pattern. During the initial phase of Hp inoculation, the bacterial body moved in the mucus by flagella and adhered to the surface cells. A month after the bacterial inoculation, no conspicuous change in the gastric mucosa was seen macroscopically. However, when the gastric mucosal microcirculation was examined, a disturbance was seen to have started in the collecting venules: Neutrophils were rolling along the luminal surface of the venular endothelium or were adhering to it. Two months later, macroscopic gastric mucosal damage had appeared in the antral mucosa near its border with the gastric body. Three months after the inoculation the mucosal lesion in the antrum was covered with necrotic tissue, creating the so-called white-coated lesion (Fig. 2). There were a large number of neutrophils adherent to the venular walls, and many neutrophils had infiltrated the minute passage in the venular walls. The leukocyte rolling velocity in the mucosal and submucosal venules decreased time-dependently in the Hp group. Leukocyte adhesion along the venules increased in the Hp group and then gradually decreased 3 months later. Tissue myeloperoxidase (MPO) activity, an index of tissue-associated neutrophil accumulation, increased significantly in the gastric mucosa of Hp-inoculated gerbils [8]. In the Hp-colonized animals fed a polaprezinc-containing diet, the increase in the level of microvascular leukocyte activation and in MPO activity

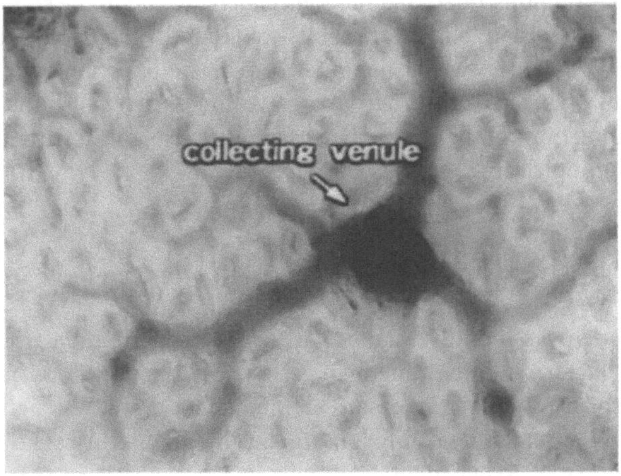

FIG. 1. Mesh of the gastric mucosal capillary network with collecting venules

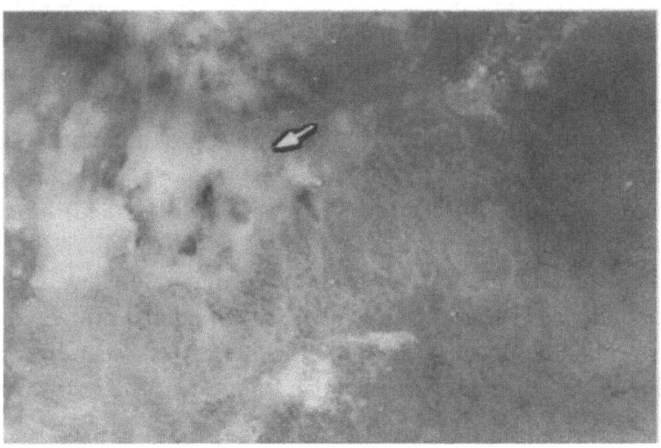

FIG. 2. Low-power view of the gastric mucosa of a Mongolian gerbil 3 months after Hp inoculation. *Arrow* indicates the necrotic, white-coated lesion

was attenuated significantly compared with that in Hp-colonized gerbils fed a chow diet [12].

Monochloramine-Induced Gastric Mucosal Apoptosis

Monochloramine (NH_2Cl) is one of the toxic oxidants generated specifically in Hp-colonized gastric mucosa. During the course of NH_2Cl generation, the enzyme in neutrophils, MPO, catalyzes oxidation of chloride by H_2O_2 to yield HOCl. Then there is an interaction between Hp-derived NH_3 and HOCl, producing NH_2Cl. We previously noted that Hp directly elicited human neutrophils and then led to the gastric mucosal injury mediated by NH_2Cl [13]. The value of luminol-dependent chemiluminescence, which depicts the contents of HOCl, a NH_2Cl precursor, is increased in Hp-colonized gastric mucosa [14]. The levels of chromatin condensation and DNA fragmentation were significantly higher in NH_2Cl-treated cells than those in NH_3- or HOCl-treated cells [15–17]. In our previous study, treatment with taurine (an NH_2Cl scavenger) significantly attenuated the NH_2Cl-evoked DNA fragmentation. The DNA fragmentation was also demonstrated in a mixture of isolated human neutrophils and NH_3 and was suppressed by neutrophil inactivation or taurine treatment [17]. Polaprezinc, a gastroprotective agent, had an inhibitory effect on NH_2Cl-induced DNA injury [18]. We recently observed the incidence of mitochondrial permeability transition (MPT) and caspase-3 activation in NH_2Cl-exposed gastric cells before the manifestation of DNA fragmentation [19], suggesting that one of the upstream pathways in Hp-associated apoptosis might be through MPT.

Gastric Epithelial Apoptosis and Proliferation

Evidence for induction of apoptosis by Hp has been obtained recently from two studies. One involved induction of apoptosis in cultured gastric epithelial cells in vitro [20,21]. The other is identification of apoptotic cells in tissue sections from Hp-infected patients [22–24]. The increased number of apoptotic cells decreases to normal following eradication of Hp, suggesting that Hp is responsible for the increased apoptosis [22].

In the healthy stomach there is a balance between proliferation of new epithelial cells and apoptosis of senescent cells. Hall et al. [25] showed that apoptosis may account for the bulk of gastric mucosal cell loss, and that it is a central feature in the regulation of cell number. Cell loss by shedding seems to play only a minor role. In the normal stomach, apoptosis is located at the most superficial aspects of the gastric mucosa and toward the base of the gastric gland. In Hp-colonized stomach, an enhanced level of apoptosis occurs primarily in the superficial compartment of gastric mucosa. Apoptosis is induced directly by Hp and is further up-regulated by the associated inflammatory response such as leukocyte-derived oxygen radicals [13,14,26–29]. According to the hypothetical model of Wagner et al. [20], the enhanced apoptosis causes compensatory hyperproliferation and enlargement of the proliferating zone, resulting in epithelial homeostasis—but at a higher rate of cell turnover. During a hyperproliferative state by persistent Hp colonization, cells that are more resistant to apoptosis are eventually produced, which may lead to gastric carcinogenesis [22]. This hypothesis was supported by Lauwers et al. [30], who reported aberrant expression of antiapoptotic protein Bcl-2 in precancerous gastric lesions. Normally in the gastrointestinal tract, the topographic distribution of Bcl-2 protein is restricted to the stem cells and the proliferative zone, that is, in the lower crypt of the gastro-intestinal tract but not along the upper crypt. However, in chronic atrophic gastritis with intestinal metaplasia, Bcl-2 protein was found in the expanded proliferative zone and along the upper crypt [30].

Because *cagA*-positive strains induce extensive gastric inflammation [29] and might cause oxidant- or cytokine-induced apoptosis in an inflamed mucosa, most of the subjects reported as having an increase in apoptosis might be infected with *cagA*-positive strains. Peek et al. [31] suggested that such an apototic effect could be due to *cagA*-negative strains because their data showed increased apoptosis in biopsy specimens from patients infected with *cagA*-negative strains. In contrast, gastric mucosal proliferation was significantly correlated with the severity of acute gastritis in persons infected with *cagA*-positive vacA s1a strains of Hp. This increased proliferation was not accompanied by a parallel increase in apoptosis, suggesting that increased cell proliferation in the absence of a corresponding increase in apoptosis may explain the heightened risk for gastric carcinoma that is associated with infection by *cagA*-positive vacA s1a strains. We investigated apoptosis and cell turnover in Mongolian gerbils in which Hp infection alone caused gastric carcinoma and in mice in which the infection did not cause cancer. It was exciting to find that in Mongolian gerbils, despite increased cell turnover during the latter phase of infection, inhibition of apoptosis was prevalent [32], and that it seemed to be associated with a high incidence of gastric cancer in this animal.

To understand the pathophysiological mechanism of apoptosis caused by Hp, the direct bacterial effect and the effect of inflammatory infiltration accompanying infection must be distinguished. Experiments by Moss et al. [22] supported the former, and they reported that there was no correlation between the apoptotic index and the degree of inflammation. Moreover, Moss et al. [33] examined tissue samples of patients with chronic atrophic gastritis who had been under observation for 31 years. The tissue samples were obtained before atrophic changes occurred; and as a result of immunohistochemical assay of apoptosis and cell proliferation of the samples, Moss et al. showed that the ratio between cell proliferation and apoptosis was not related to the forthcoming atrophic changes.

Chronic inflammation in the gastric mucosa progresses to atrophy of gastric glands and then to intestinal metaplasia. Many issues remain unclear as to the development of intestinal metaplasia. Correa et al. [34] performed thorough histological examinations of a group of patients at high risk for gastric cancer and reported that most gastric carcinomas follow a regular pathway: normal gastric mucosa, chronic gastritis, chronic atrophic gastritis, intestinal metaplasia, and dysplasia.

Hp Infection and Telomerase

At the end of eukaryotic chromosomes there is a telomere DNA, a six-basepair repeat sequence (5′-TTAGGG-3′), that perform roles similar to that of the plastic cylinder at the end of shoe laces; that is, it prevents fusion with other chromosomes and protects against degradation by exonuclease. Telomere length reduction is seen in intestinal metaplasia and gastric carcinoma; and telomerase is the only enzyme capable of synthesizing the telomere DNA. The enzyme consists of human telomerase RNA (hTR), a template RNA that is complementary in sequence with the telomere DNA, and protein subunits. Most gastric carcinoma is positive for telomerase activity regardless of tissue type and grading, and telomerase activities were found in intestinal metaplasia and adenoma as well. Hp infection seems to be associated with telomerase reactivation.

The Hp density increases in parallel with the grade of intestinal metaplasia, hTR expression, and telomerase positivity. It is possible that chronic inflammation induces chronic regenerative activity, thereby causing mutation in gastric mucosa. Reactive oxygen species and reactive nitrogen species produced in Hp-infected gastric mucosa causes active tissue regeneration and genetic toxicity by inducing infiltraion of neutrophils. Moreover, because telomere reduction was seen in intestinal metaplasia, it is possible to say that stem cell hyperplasia or already immortalized cells in intestinal metaplasia exist [35]. hTR expression was detected in all grades of intestinal metaplasia. Factors that induce the expression remain unclear; but during chronic inflammation and tissue regeneration stem cells are affected, the expression was induced, and telomerase activity might be increased in precancerous gastric mucosa. Telomerase positivity was found in incomplete-type intestinal metaplasia, and the activity increased in parallel with the grading [36]. Also, there was a difference in timing between telomerase reactivation and hTR expression during carcinogenesis of differentiated type gastric carcinoma [36].

Epilogue

As Hp has learned how to survive in the gastric lumen over millions of years, we should not be surprised if the effects of this unique bacterium on gastric cell apoptosis prove to be subtle and complex. Further investigations are needed to detect the apoptosis inducers in Hp-colonized mucosa and to determine the beneficial aspects of gastric epithelial apoptosis in the Hp-colonized gastric mucosa for regulating gastric mucosal cell turnover and preventing gastric carcinogenesis.

Acknowledgments. This study is supported by a Grant-in-Aid for Scientific Research C (11670531) from the Ministry of Education, Science, and Culture of Japan by Keio University Medical School Faculty and Alumni Grants and by a grant from Uehara Memorial Foundation.

References

1. Marshall BJ, Warren JR (1984) Unidentified curved bacilli in the stomach of patients with gastritis and peptic ulceration. Lancet 1:1311–1315
2. Bizzozero G (1893) Ueber die schlauchformigen dursen des magendarmkanals und die beziehungen ihres epithels zu dem obertflachenepithel der schleimhaut. Arch Mikr Anat 42:82–152
3. Kasai K, Kobayashi R (1919) The stomach spirochete occurring in mammals. J Parasitol 6:1–10
4. NIH Consensus Conference (1994) *Helicobacter pylori* in peptic ulcer disease: NIH consensus development panel. JAMA 272:65–69
5. Hirayama F, Takagi S, Kusuhara H, et al (1996) Induction of gastric ulcer and intestinal metaplasia in Mongolian gerbils infected with *Helicobacter pylori.* J Gastroenterol 31:755–757
6. Watanabe T, Tada M, Nagai H, et al (1998) *Helicobacter pylori* infection induces gastric cancer in Mongolian gerbils. Gastroenterology 115:642–648
7. Honda S, Fujioka T, Tokieda M, et al (1998) Development of *Helicobacter pylori*-induced gastric carcinoma in Mongolian gerbils. Cancer Res 58:4255–4259
8. Suzuki H, Mori M, Seto K, et al (1999) *H. pylori*-associated gastric pro- and anti-oxidant formation in Mongolian gerbils. Free Radic Biol Med 26:679–684
9. Suzuki H, Mori M, Seto K, et al (1999) Ethanol intake preceding *Helicobacter pylori* inoculation promotes gastric mucosal inflammation in Mongolian gerbils. J Gastroenterol Hepatol 14:1062–1069

10. Kalia N, Bardhan KD, Reed MW, et al (2000) Mechanisms of *Helicobacter pylori*-induced rat gastric mucosal microcirculatory disturbances in vivo. Dig Dis Sci 45: 763–772
11. Suzuki H, Schmid-Schönbein GW, Suematsu M, et al (1994) Impaired leukocyte-endothelial cell interaction in spontaneously hypertensive rats. Hypertension 24: 719–727
12. Suzuki H, Mori M, Seto K, et al (2001) Polaprezinc attenuates the *H. pylori*-induced gastric mucosal leukocyte activation in Mongolian gerbils: A study using intravital microscopy. Aliment Pharmacol Ther 15 (in press)
13. Suzuki M, Miura S, Suematsu M, et al (1992) *Helicobacter pylori*-associated ammonia production enhances neutrophil-dependent gastric mucosal cell injury. Am J Physiol 263:G719–G725
14. Suzuki H, Miura S, Imaeda H, et al (1996) Enhanced levels of chemiluminescence and platelet activating factor in urease positive gastric ulcers. Free Radic Biol Med 20:449–454
15. Suzuki H, Mori M, Suzuki M, et al (1997) Extensive DNA damage induced by monochloramine in gastric cells. Cancer Lett 115:243–248
16. Naito Y, Yoshikawa T, Fujii T, et al (1997) Monochloramine-induced cell growth inhibition and apoptosis in a rat gastric mucosal cell line. J Clin Gastroenterol 25: S179–S185
17. Suzuki H, Seto K, Mori M, et al (1998) Monochloramine (NH_2Cl) induced DNA fragmentation in gastric cell line, MKN 45. Am J Physiol 275:G712–G716
18. Suzuki H, Mori M, Seto K, et al (1999) Polaprezinc, a gastroprotective agent: attenuation of monochloramine-evoked gastric DNA fragmentation. J Gastroenterol 34(suppl 11):43–46
19. Suzuki H, Nagahashi S, Seto K, et al (1999) Mitochondrial permeability transition and caspase-3 activation in monochloramine (NH_2Cl) induced gastric epithelial apoptosis. Gastroenterology 116:A512
20. Wagner S, Beil W, Westermann J (1997) Regulation of gastric epithelial cell growth by *Helicobacter pylori*: evidence for a major role of apoptosis. Gastroenterology 113: 1836–1847
21. Chen G, Sordillo EM, Ramey WG, et al (1997) Apoptosis in gastric epithelial cells is induced by *Helicobacter pylori* and accompanied by increased expression of BAK. Biochem Biophys Res Commun 20:626–632
22. Moss SF, Calam J, Agarwal B (1996) Induction of gastric epithelial apoptosis by *Helicobacter pylori*. Gut 38:498–501
23. Mannick EE, Bravo LE, Zarama G (1996) Inducible nitric oxide synthase, nitrotyrosine, and apoptosis in *Helicobacter pylori*: effect of antibiotics and antioxidants. Cancer Res 56:3238–3243
24. Jones NL, Shannon PT, Cutz E (1997) Increase in proliferation and apoptosis of gastric epithelial cells early in the natural history of *Helicobacter pylori* infection. Am J Pathol 151:1695–1703
25. Hall PA, Coates PJ, Ansari A, et al (1994) Regulation of cell number in the mammalian gastrointestinal tract: the importance of apoptosis. J Cell Sci 107: 3569–3577
26. Suzuki M, Miura S, Suematsu M, et al (1993) *Helicobacter pylori* elicits gastric mucosal cell damage associated with neutrophil-derived toxic oxidants. Eur J Gastroenterol Hepatol 5:S35–S39
27. Davies GR, Simmonds NJ, Stevens TRJ, et al (1994) *Helicobacter pylori* stimulates antral mucosal reactive oxygen metabolite production in vivo. Gut 35:179–185
28. Davies GR, Rampyon DS (1994) *Helicobacter pylori*, free radicals and gastroduodenal disease. Eur J Gastroenterol Hepatol 6:1–10

29. Suzuki H, Suzuki M, Mori M, et al (1998) Augmented levels of gastric mucosal leukocyte activation by infection with *cagA* gene-positive *Helicobacter pylori*. J Gastroenterol Hepatol 13:294–300
30. Lauwers GY, Scott GV, Hendricks J (1994) Immunohistochemical evidence of aberrant bcl-2 protein expression in gastric epithelial dysplasia. Cancer 73:2900–2904
31. Peek RMJ, Moss SF, Tham KT, et al (1997) *Helicobacter pylori* $CagA^+$ strains and dissociation of gastric epithelial cell proliferation from apoptosis. J Natl Cancer Inst 89:863–868
32. Suzuki H, Nagahashi S, Seto K, et al (2000) Attenuated apoptosis in *H. pylori*-colonized gastric mucosa of Mongolian gerbils. Gastroenterology 118(suppl 2):A746
33. Moss SF, Valle J, Abdalla AM (1999) Gastric cellular turnover and the development of atrophy after 31 years of follow-up: a case-control study. Am J Gastroenterol 94:2109–2114
34. Correa P, Cuello C, Duque E (1976) Gastric cancer in Colombia. III. Natural history of precursor lesions. J Natl Cancer Inst 57:1027–1035
35. Tahara E (1998) Molecular mechanism of human stomach carcinogenesis implicated in *Helicobacter pylori* infection. Exp Toxic Pathol 50:375–378
36. Kuniyasu H, Domen T, Hamamoto T (1997) Expression of human telomerase RNA is an early event of stomach carcinogenesis. Jpn J Cancer Res 88:103–107

Alteration of Gastric Microcirculatory Architecture During Healing of Acetic Acid-Induced Ulcer and *Helicobacter pylori* Infection

MASAHIKO NAKAMURA[1,*], HIDENORI MATSUI[1], KANJI TSUCHIMOTO[2], and HIROMASA ISHII[3]

Summary. Inflammatory stimulation has been shown to bring about various microcirculatory alterations. To clarify the microcirculatory changes, a fundamental understanding of the microcirculatory architecture is important. Our histochemical studies using intraaortic injection of agar containing FITC-dextran clearly showed the existence of a functional precapillary sphincter and revealed the structure of the collecting venules. In addition, the formation of an arteriovenous anastomosis (AVA) in the regenerated gastric mucosa and its inhibition by basic fibroblast growth factor (bFGF) were demonstrated during acetic acid-induced gastric ulcer healing. *Helicobacter pylori*-induced microcirculatory changes, such as angiogenesis and myofibroblast proliferation, were also shown to have a close relation with inflammatory processes.

Key words. Gastric microcirculation, Acetic acid-induced ulcer, *Helicobacter pylori*, Arteriovenous anastomosis, Myofibroblast

Introduction

The gastric mucosa microcirculatory system has been shown to be reactive to various stimuli via alteration of the vascular permeability from the collecting venules, angiogenesis, and so on. The microcirculatory architecture and its regulation have been investigated by various methods, including dye injection methods and cast studies [1], but the precise structure and interaction of the microvascular structure with the gastric gland and surrounding mesenchymal cells of the connective tissues remain to be clarified. We have devised a method to reconstruct the microvascular network by utilizing the injection of agar mixed with fluorescein isothiocyanate (FITC)-dextran of various molecular sizes, immunohistochemistry, and confocal laser microscopic

[1] Center for Basic Research, Kitasato Institute, 5-9-1 Shirokane, Minato-ku, Tokyo 108-8642, Japan
[2] Kitasato Institute Hospital, Minato-ku, Tokyo, Japan
[3] Department of Internal Medicine, School of Medicine, Keio University, Shinjuku-ku, Tokyo, Japan
* e-mail: nakamura-m@kitasato.or.jp

observations [2]. In the present study, microcirculatory alteration has been demonstrated during inflammatory processes induced by acetic acid in rats and *Helicobacter pylori* (Hp)-induced gastric damage in Mongolian gerbils.

Gastric Microcirculatory Architecture and Relation to Intramucosal Smooth Muscle Cells

The gastric microcirculatory system is composed of arterioles, metarterioles, true capillaries, collecting venules, venules, and lymphatics (Fig. 1). The existence of a precapillary sphincter and arteriovenous anastomosis remains to be clarified.

Based on physiological studies, a so-called precapillary sphincter was proposed to regulate the mucosal microcirculation, but few anatomical observations have substantiated its existence. In our observations, the arterioles have been found to be divided into several capillaries after penetrating the muscularis mucosae. Just before the transition to capillaries, swelling of vascular smooth muscle cells into the arteriolar lumen was observed, and this structure coincides with the possible functional precapillary sphincter, which would be one of the regulators of the gastric mucosal microcirculation.

The collecting vessels are long postcapillary venules consisting of a single endothelial layer with no covering by vascular smooth muscle cells. By histochemical observations using rhodamine-phalloidin, the nonvascular smooth muscle cells were found to surround the collecting venules from just above the muscularis mucosae to the neck portion of the gastric glands, corresponded to the generative zone of the fundic gland [3].

Existence of the Arteriovenous Anastomosis

In the control gastric mucosa, few arteriovenous anastomoses (AVAs) have been found to exist in the stomach [4], although AVAs were reported to open during burn injury [5], with hypertensive gastropathy induced by chronic liver dysfunction [6], and with various agents including L-dopa [7], and calcium antagonists [8].

By infusing agar containing FITC-dextran, shunting from the arterioles to the venules was clearly shown in the basal portion of the gastric mucosa 1 week after acetic acid-induced gastric mucosal injury, suggesting that opening of the AVAs might be related to the formation of ischemia in the upper part of the gastric mucosa and exacerbation of the ulcerative lesion (Fig. 2). On the other hand, bFGF administration after acetic acid-induced ulcer provocation prevented the formation of AVAs in the gastric mucosa.

Significance of Myofibroblasts in Hp-Induced Gastric Mucosal Damage

In Hp-treated Mongolian gerbil fundic mucosa there was an increase of endothelial cells and myofibroblasts, shown by the PR 2D3 antibody [9], 3 months after induction of the Hp infection (Fig. 3), suggesting their interaction with the inflammatory process.

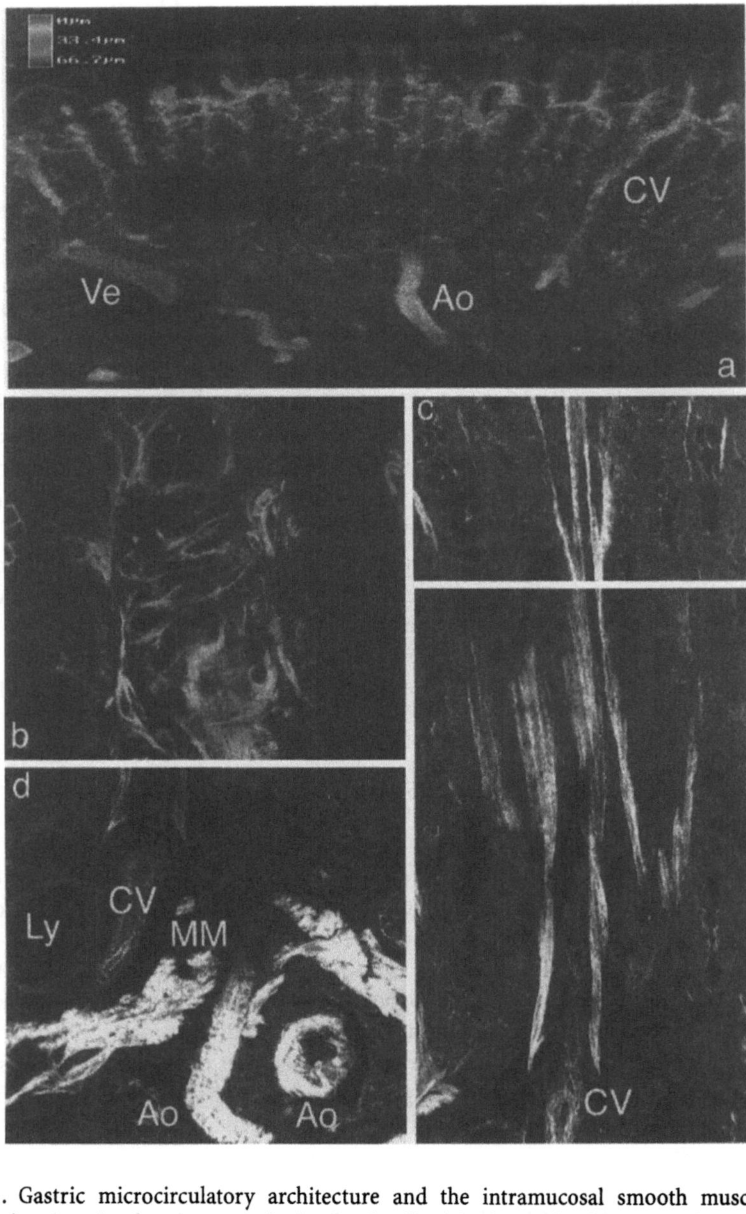

FIG. 1. Gastric microcirculatory architecture and the intramucosal smooth muscle cells. **a** Gastric microcirculatory system is clearly visualized in the rat fundic mucosa by intraaortic injection of agar containing fluorescein isothiocyanate (FITC)-dextran. *Ao*, arteriole; *Ve*, venule; *CV*, collecting venule. **b** In the tip portion of the gastric mucosa, the collecting venules are found to run tortuously. **c** Collecting venules (*CV*) are shown to be surrounded by the nonvascular smooth muscle cells. **d** In the basal portion of the gastric mucosa, arterioles (*Ao*), collecting venules (*CV*) and lymphatics (*Ly*) are clearly visualized near the muscularis mucosae (*MM*)

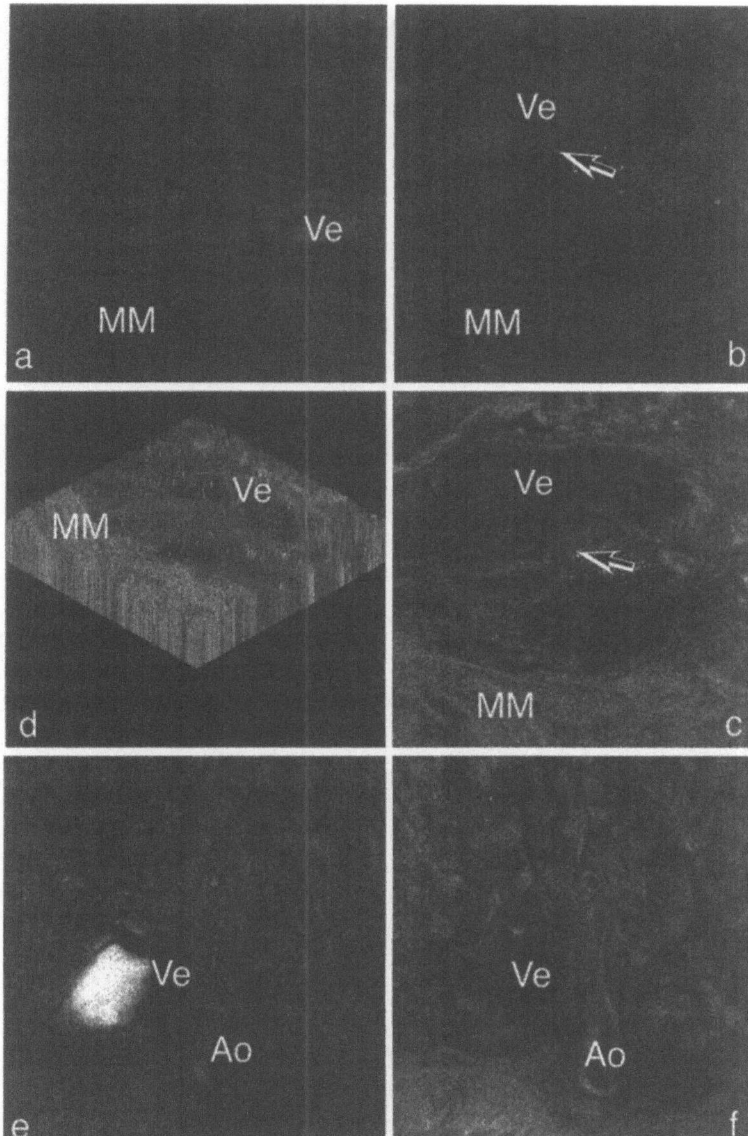

FIG. 2. Microvascular network of the regenerated gastric mucosal layer after acetic acid treatment. **a–d** Arteriovenuous anastomosis (*arrows*) is clearly seen just above the muscularis mucosae (*MM*) between the metarteriole and venules (*Ve*). **e,f** Formation of an arteriovenous anastamosis is not recognized after addition of basic fibroblast growth factor. (**a,b** FITC-dextran fluorescence. **c** Stained with rhodamine-phalloidin. **d** Three-dimensional reconstruction. **e** FITC-dextran fluorescence. **f** Stained with rhodamine-phalloidin)

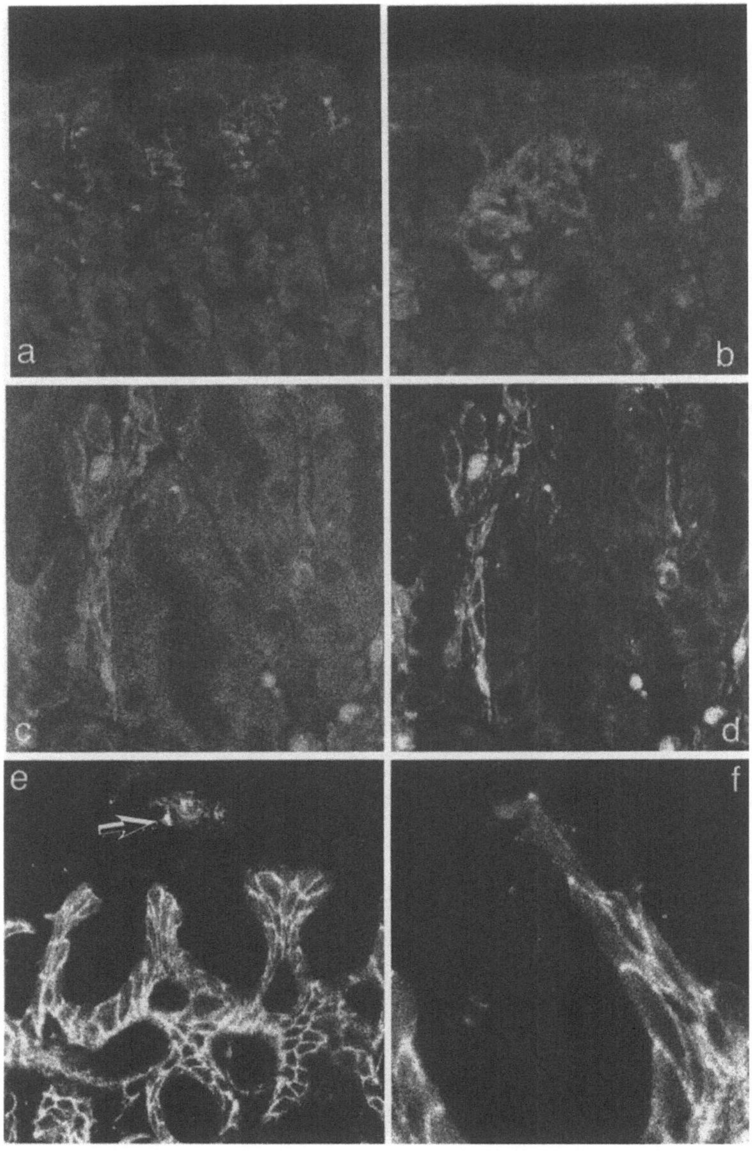

FIG. 3. Immunoreactivities of factor VIII, myofibroblast (shown by the PR 2D3 antibody), and *Helicobacter pylori* (Hp). **a,b** Endothelial cells are markedly increased in the tip of the gastric mucosa. **c,d** Myofibroblasts are also increased in the lamina propria mucosae from the tip to the base of the gastric mucosa. **e,f** In the tip, Hp immunoreactivity (*arrow*) is clearly observed

Conclusions

The existence of a functional precapillary sphincter and the structure of the collecting venules was shown by intraaortic injection of agar containing FITC-dextran. In addition, the formation of AVAs in the regenerated gastric mucosa and their inhibition by bFGF were clearly shown during acetic acid-induced gastric ulcer healing. Hp-induced microcirculatory changes, such as angiogenesis and myofibroblast proliferation, were clearly shown to have a close relation with the inflammatory processes.

References

1. Reeves JB (1919) A study of the arteries supplying the stomach and duodenum and their relation to ulcer. Coll Papers Mayo Clin 11:3
2. Nakamura M, Kitajima M, Tsuchiya M (1993) Alteration of gastric microcirculation in ulcer healing and recurrence: significance of autonomic nervous regeneration and mesenchymal cell. Gastroenterol Jpn 28:139–144
3. Nakamura M, Kishikawa H, Oda M (1999) Localization of non-vascular smooth muscle cell and myofibroblast in rat fundic mucosa: their relation to microcirculatory system. Microcirc Annu 15:125–126
4. Gorczyca J, Litwin JA, Nowogrodzka-Zagorska M, et al (1999) Architecture of blood vessels in human fetal gastric corpus: a corrosion casting study. Anat Anz 181:353–358
5. Kitajima M, Shimizu A, Sakai N, et al (1991) Gastric microcirculation and its regulating factors in stress. J Clin Gastroenterol 13:S9–S17
6. Saxena PR, Verdouw PD (1985) Tissue blood flow and localization of arteriovenous anastomoses in pigs with microspheres of four different sizes. Pflügers Arch 403:128–135
7. Nakamura M, Oda M, Yonei Y, et al (1985) Role of Arteriolovenular Anastomosis in the Pathogenesis of Gastric Ulcer. In: New trends in peptic ulcer and chronic hepatitis. Excerpta Medica, Amsterdam, pp 89–97
8. Hof RP (1989) Effects of isradipine and other calcium antagonists on arteriovenous-shunt flow in anesthetized rabbits and cats. Am J Med 86:40–49
9. Brewster CE, Howarth PH, Djukanovic R, et al (1990) Myofibroblasts and subepithelial fibrosis in bronchial asthma. Am J Respir Cell Mol Biol 3:507–511

Cyclooxygenase and Colon Cancer

Masahiko Tsujii[1,*], Shingo Tsuji[1], and Sunao Kawano[2]

Summary. Epidemiological studies suggest that nonsteroidal antiinflammatory drugs (NSAIDs) might have antineoplastic properties in colon cancer. A major target of NSAIDs is cyclooxygenase (COX). An inducible isoform, COX-2, is overexpressed in tumor tissues in colon. With colon cancer, expression of COX-2 is up-regulated in tumor epithelial cells, whose K-*ras* is frequently mutated. To investigate the role of COX-2 expression in intestinal epithelial cells, we prepared COX-2 overexpressing cells by stable transfection. COX-2 expression enhanced resistance to apoptosis and production of angiogenic factors. In colon polyps, overexpression of COX-2 is located not in tumor epithelial cells but in stromal cells. To elucidate the role of COX-2 activity in stromal cells on tumor growth, growth of xenografts in COX-2 knockout mice (COX-$2^{-/-}$) was investigated. We found that tumor growth was markedly attenuated in COX-$2^{-/-}$ but not in COX-$1^{-/-}$ or wild-type mice. A decrease in vascular density was observed in tumors grown in COX-$2^{-/-}$ mice when compared with those in wild-type mice. Because COX-2 is expressed in stromal fibroblasts, we evaluated COX-$2^{-/-}$ fibroblasts and found a reduction in their ability to produce VEGF. Expression of COX-2 in both tumor epithelial cells and stromal cells plays a pivotal role in cancer development.

Key words. Cyclooxygenase-2, Colon cancer, Apoptosis, Angiogenesis, VEGF

Introduction

There are three independent lines of research indicating that nonsteroidal antiinflammatory drugs (NSAIDs) alter the biology of colorectal carcinogenesis. First, epidemiological studies indicate a 50% reduction in mortality from colorectal cancer in individuals taking NSAIDs compared with those not taking these agents [1]. Second, familial adenomatous patients who take sulindac have a significant reduction in adenoma size and number [2]. Third, these drugs inhibit tumor formation in rodent

[1] Department of Internal Medicine and Therapeutics, Osaka University Graduate School of Medicine, [2] Department of Clinical Laboratory Sciences, School of Allied Health Sciences, Osaka University Medical School, 2-2 Yamadaoka, Suita, Osaka 565-0871, Japan
* e-mail: tsujii@medone.med.osaka-u.ac.jp

models of chemical-induced colon carcinogenesis. The cellular basis for the antitumor activity of these drugs, however, is still unkown.

One possibility involves altered metabolism of arachidonic acid, as NSAIDs are widely believed to have antiinflammatory activity by inhibiting the cyclooxygenase (COX) enzyme. Many studies have noted elevated levels of prostaglandins in colorectal carcinoma tissue when compared with normal colonic mucosa.

There are at least two isoforms: COX-1 and COX-2. COX-1 is constitutively expressed in most cases. The expression of COX-2 is regulated by a variety of mitogens and cytokines. According to the results from the Northern blotting analysis, there was no significant difference in COX-1 expression between colon cancer tissue and normal adjacent colon mucosa. COX-2 expression, however, was up-regulated in 86% of colorectal adenocarcinomas compared with adjacent normal colon mucosa. It was also reported that COX-2 mRNA and protein levels are elevated in colonic tumors that develop in rodents following carcinogen treatment and in intestinal adenomas taken from Min mice.

The data regarding the sublocalization of COX-2 in colon tumors are controversial. Some of them may be due to nonspecific binding of the polyclonal antibodies that were used for COX-2 immunostaining. Reports have shown that COX-2 expression is found in both the epithelial and stromal components of sporadic human colorectal cancers.

COX-2 Expression in Tumor Epithelial Cells

Elevated COX-2 expression has been reported in the epithelial component of adenomas in the multiple intestinal neoplasia (Min) mouse, azoxymethane-treated rat cancers, replication error repair—positive human carcinomas, and sporadic human colorectal cancers. COX-2 is expressed in some colon carcinoma cell lines, and its expression can be induced in cultured nontransformed intestinal epithelial cells by treatment with growth factors, which expressions are up-regulated in colon tumors. Point mutations of K-*ras* are reported in 40%–50% of colon neoplasms. COX-2 expression can be induced in cultured intestinal epithelial cells transformed by *ras* activation. There is no doubt that COX-2 expression is up-regulated in some colon cancer cells.

To clarify the mechanisms by which COX-2 is involved in tumor formation, we have investigated the phenotypic changes in intestinal epithelial cells programmed to express the COX-2 gene.

Differentiation and Apoptosis

Cellular differentiation and proliferative arrest are induced as intestinal stem cells ascend upward on the basement membrane along the crypt-villous axis toward the intestinal lumen. When the cells reach the surface of the villi, they become fully differentiated, undergo programmed cell death, and are shed into the lumen. The entire lifetime of an epithelial cell in humans is only 4–5 days. Prolonged cell survival could have significant biological consequences and affect the tumorigenic potential of epithelial cells.

Overexpression of COX-2 in cultured rat intestinal epithelial cells results in dedifferentiation and enhanced resistance to apoptosis [3]. Expression of Bcl-2 has been linked to inhibition of apoptosis in several cell types. Levels of Bcl-2 in the cultured intestinal epithelial cells were decreased before apoptosis was induced. On the other hand, in COX-2-expressing epithelial cells, Bcl-2 expression was elevated even under the conditions that could induce apoptosis in cultured intestinal epithelial cells. These results would increase the probabilty that cells expressing high COX-2 levels would have prolonged survival and be at risk for tumor progression.

Tumor Angiogenesis

The ability of a tumor to induce angiogenesis represents a fundamental element in the control of tumor growth beyond 2–3 mm in its greatest dimension. Suppression of tumor angiogenesis has become a center focus of cancer therapy. When we investigated the effects of specific and nonspecific COX-2 inhibitors on tumor angiogenesis, specific and nonspecific COX-2-specific inhibitors suppressed growth of COX-2-expressing colon cancer xenografts in athymic mice [4]. On the other hand, nonspecific COX-2 inhibitors suppressed growth of xenografts of colon cancer cells lacking COX-1 and COX-2 expression, although COX-2 specific inhibitors did not have any significant effect on it.

To explore the role of COX in angiogenesis, we have used two in vitro model systems involving co-culture of endothelial cells with colon carcinoma cells. COX-2-overexpressing cells produce prostaglandins and proangiogenic factors, and they stimulate both endothelial migration and in vitro angiogenesis. Control cells have little activity. The effect is inhibited by antibodies to combinations of angiogenic factors or by a selective COX-2 inhibitor (NS-398) and aspirin. NS-398 and aspirin inhibited production of angiogenic factors in COX-2-overexpressing cells in a dose-dependent manner. In vascular endothelial cells, expression of COX-1 and COX-2 were induced by angiogenic stimulation.

In an in vitro study using antisense oligonucleotide against COX-1 or COX-2, it was suggested that COX-1 in endothelial cells participated in angiogenesis induced by angiogenic factors from colon cancer cells. Cyclooxygenase regulates colon carcinoma-induced angiogenesis by two mechanisms: COX-2 can modulate production of angiogenic factors by colon cancer cells, and COX-1 regulates angiogenesis in endothelial cells.

COX-2 Expression in Stromal Cells

It has been found that COX-2 expression is also elevated in the subepithelial component in adenomas from the Min mouse, in carcinogen-induced colon cancers in mice, in polyps from APC716 mice, and in colorectal carcinomas from interleutin-$10^{-/-}$ (IL-$10^{-/-}$) mice. Therefore, it is possible that COX-2 in stromal fibroblasts could promote tumor growth by producing bioactive prostaglandins that have paracrine effects on nearby carcinoma cells.

We evaluated the contribution of stroma-derived COX-1 and COX-2 to tumor growth using both genetic and pharmacological approaches [5]. Lewis lung carcinoma

(LLC) cells grow rapidly as solid tumors when implanted in C57BL/6 mice. We found that tumor growth was markedly attenuated in COX-$2^{-/-}$ mice but not in COX-$1^{-/-}$ or wild-type mice. Treatment of wild-type C57BL/6 mice bearing LLC tumors with a selective COX-2 inhibitor also reduced tumor growth. A decrease in vascular density was observed in tumors grown in COX-$2^{-/-}$ mice when compared with those in wild-type mice. Because COX-2 is expressed in stromal fibroblasts of human and rodent colorectal carcinomas, we evaluated COX-$2^{-/-}$ mouse fibroblasts and found a significant reduction in their ability to produce vascular endothelial growth factor (VEGF). These data have demonstrated that efficient tumor growth requires the presence of COX-2 in the tumor stroma, and stroma-derived COX-2 may regulate intratumoral vascular density, which in turn may modulate tumor growth.

Conclusions

We showed that COX-2-expressing intestinal epithelial cells showed resistance to apoptosis and prolonged cell survival and enhancement of angiogenic factor production. It has been suggested that tumors be regarded as complex tissues. Cancer cells might make surrounding normal stromal cells serve as active collaborators, as there is cellular interaction between tumor cells and stromal cells. Our results also demonstrated that COX-1 expression in endothelial cells might be involved in tumor angiogenesis, and COX-2 expression in fibroblasts might modulate VEGF production. These results may provide some insight regarding the molecular basis for the chemopreventive effect of NSAIDs.

References

1. Giovannucci E, Egan KM, Hunter DJ, et al (1995) Aspirin and the risk of colorectal cancer in women. N Engl J Med 333:609–614
2. Giardiello FM, Hamilton SR, Krush AJ, et al (1993) Treatment of colonic and rectal adenomas with sulindac in familial adenomatous polyposis. N Engl J Med 328:1313–1316
3. Tsujii M, DuBois RN (1995) Alterations in cellular adhesion and apoptosis in epithelial cells overexpressing prostaglandin endoperoxide synthase 2. Cell 83:493–501
4. Tsujii M, Kawano S, Tsuji S, et al (1998) Cyclooxygenase regulates angiogenesis induced by colon cancer cells. Cell 93:705–716
5. Williams CS, Tsujii M, Reese J, et al (2000) Host cyclooxygenase-2 modulates carcinoma growth. J Clin Invest 105:1589–1594

Contribution of Colon Cancer Cells to Mesenchymal Cells in the Formation of Hepatic Metastasis

Nobuya Yamada[1,*], Sadatoshi Shimizu[1], Satoshi Takatsuka[1], Masakazu Yashiro[1], Tetsuji Sawada[1], Masaichi Ohira[1], Tetsuro Ishikawa[1], Hiroji Nishino[1], Kenji Kaneda[2], and Kosei Hirakawa[1]

Summary. Proliferations of cancer cells and mesenchymal cells are necessary for the formation of hepatic metastasis. Endothelial cells and hepatic stellate cells (HSCs), which exist in the extrasinusoidal space and produce extracellular matrix, are present in hepatic lobules as mesenchymal cells. In this study we investigated the contribution of colon cancer cells to endothelial cells and HSCs in the formation of hepatic metastasis. We collected serum-free conditioned medium (SFCM) of LM-H cells, which are highly liver metastatic colon cancer cells. The SFCM of LM-H cells significantly enhanced proliferation and migration of human umbilical vein endothelial cells (HUVECs) and enhanced the proliferation and migration of HSCs derived from rats. On investigating the growth factors in the SFCM of LM-H cells, we found vascular endothelial growth factor (VEGF) and platelet-derived growth factor (PDGF). The proliferation of HUVECs was inhibited by anti-VEGF antibody, and that of HSCs was inhibited by anti-PDGF antibody. The angiogenesis inhibitor TNP-470 significantly decreased the number of hepatic metastases of LM-H cells in nude mice. In conclusion, the VEGF and PDGF that colon cancer cells produce are important factors in the structural reorganization of hepatic metastasis. The angiogenesis inhibitor TNP-470 seems to be a potent agent for inhibiting hepatic metastasis of colon cancer.

Key words. Colon cancer cell, Hepatic metastasis, Mesenchymal cell, Hepatic stellate cell, Endothelial cell

Introduction

Hepatic metastasis is an important factor that regulates the prognosis of the patients with colorectal cancer. The pathogenesis of metastasis begins with the invasion of tissues and blood vessels by cells originating from a primary cancer. Following their release into the portal venous system, tumor cells are adherent to the endothelium of

[1] 1st Department of Surgery, [2] 2nd Department of Anatomy, Osaka City University Medical School, 1-4-3 Asahimachi, Abeno-ku, Osaka 545-8585, Japan
* e-mail: n-yamada@med.osaka-cu.ac.jp

the hepatic microvasculature. After their initial adhesion, cancer cells must invade the hepatic parenchyma, establish a microenvironment, escape host defense mechanisms, and finally grow into liver metastatic foci. Whether cancer cells can successfully metastasize in the liver depends not only on their cytological properties but also on the hepatic microenvironment (i.e., a supportive system of hepatic mesenchymal tissue). Neovascularization that provides the arterial blood to the metastatic foci is one of such mesenchymal reactions. Endothelial cells and hepatic stellate cells (HSCs), which exist in the extrasinusoidal space and produce extracellular matrix, are in hepatic lobules as mesenchymal cells. In this study, we investigated the contribution of colon cancer cells to the endothelial cells and HSCs to the formation of hepatic metastasis and the effect of angiogenesis inhibitor TNP-470 on hepatic metastasis in nude mice.

Contribution of Colon Cancer Cells to Endothelial Cells

We used a highly metastasizable colon carcinoma cell line LM-H [1] obtained after several in vivo passages of a human colon cancer cell line OCUC-LM1, which was previously established from a liver metastasis in our laboratory. Human umbilical vein endothelial cells (HUVECs) were purchased from Kurabou (Osaka, Japan). The proliferation of HUVECs was examined by counting cell numbers 72 h after treatment with serum-free conditioned medium (SFCM) of the LM-H cells. The proliferation of HUVECs was significantly increased by treatment with SFCM of LM-H cells compared to that without the treatment. The effect of SFCM of LM-H cells on the migration of HUVECs was determined using chemotaxis chambers with a filter membrane. The number of HUVECs that had migrated through the filter was significantly increased by treatment of LM-H with SFCM compared to those without the treatment. The numbers of migrating cells per field were as follows: control 2.7 ± 3.1 cells and SFCM/LM-H 33.0 ± 12.5 cells. Thus, SFCM of LM-H cells significantly enhanced the proliferation and migration of HUVECs [2]. The contents of growth factors and cytokines in SFCM/LM-H were measured by enzyme-linked immunosorbent assay (ELISA) analysis. The SFCM/LM-H contained a large amount of VEGF and PDGF but negligible amounts of hepatocyte growth factor (HGF), transforming growth factor (TGFα, TGFβ), epidermal growth factor (EGF), basic fibroblast growth factor (b-FGF), interleukin-1α (IL-1α), and tumor necrosis factor-α (TNFα) (Table 1). The suppressive effect of several neutralizing antibodies on the proliferation of HUVECs was investigated. The proliferation of HUVECs was significantly suppressed by pretreatment with anti-vascular endothelial growth factor (anti-VEGF) antibody in a dose-dependent manner compared with rabbit immunoglobulin (IgG). It is supposed that VEGF produced by cancer cells induced angiogenesis during the formation of hepatic metastases.

Contribution of Colon Cancer Cells to Hepatic Stellate Cells

The HSCs were isolated from the rat liver previously reported [3]. In the proliferation assay, the SFCM/LM-H preparation obtained by incubating semiconfluent LM-H cells with serum-free Dulbecco's modified Eagle medium (DMEM) for 4 days significantly

TABLE 1. Contents of growth factors and cytokines in serum-free LM-H-conditioned medium as determined by ELISA

Growth factor/cytokine	LM-H-CM content (pg/ml)
VEGF	1030
PDGF	753
HGF	0
TGFα	4.4
TGFβ	0
EGF	2.1
b-FGF	6.8
IL-1α	0
TNFα	<5.0

VEGF, vascular endothelial growth factor; PDGF, platelet-derived growth factor; HGF, hepatocyte growth factor; TGF, transforming growth factor; EGF, epidermal growth factor; b-FGF, basic fibroblast growth factor; IL, interleukin; TNF, tumor necrosis factor; ELISA, enzyme-linked immunosorbent assay

increased the number of activated HSCs at 3 days compared to serum-free DMEM. For the migration assay, the SFCM/LM-H in the lower chamber induced migration of a significantly larger number of activated HSCs to the lower surface of the filter at 6h compared to that with serum-free DMEM. The numbers of migrating cells per field were as follows: control 6.8 ± 1.3 cells and SFCM/LM-H 35.4 ± 2.5 cells. SFCM/LM-H enhanced proliferation and migration of not only HUVECs but also HSCs. Because PDGF was detected in the SFCM/LM-H among the growth factors and cytokines examined here, we investigated the suppressive effect of a neutralizing antibody against PDGF. The treatments with anti-PDGF antibody significantly inhibited the SFCM/LM-H-induced proliferation and migration of activated HSCs in vitro. It is supposed that PDGF produced by cancer cells stimulates hepatic stellate cells and assists them in producing extracellular matrix; cancer cells then form metastatic foci in cooperation with endothelial cells and hepatic stellate cells.

Effect of Angiogenesis Inhibitor TNP-470 on Hepatic Metastasis

The LM-H cells (1×10^5 cells per mouse) were injected into the spleens of nude mice on day 0. TNP-470 (30mg/kg body weight) was administered by subcutaneous injection once every third day for 4 weeks from day 0. The mice were sacrificed on day 28. The macroscopic metastatic nodules on the surfaces were counted. Treatment with TNP-470 significantly decreased the number of the hepatic nodules observed macroscopically on the surface of the liver. The average number of metastatic nodules in the liver was 78.2 ± 30.1 in the control group and 20.6 ± 16.5 in the treated group [4].

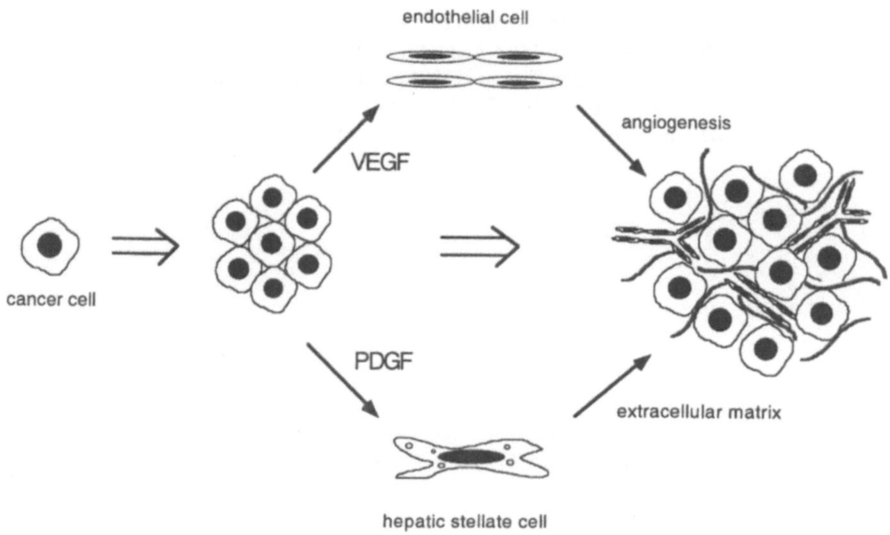

FIG. 1. Contribution of colon cancer cells to endothelial cells and hepatic stellate cells in the structural reorganization of hepatic metastasis. *VEGF*, vascular endothelial growth factor; *PDGF*, platelet-derived growth factor

Conclusions

For hepatic metastasis, colon cancer cells modify the supporting mesenchymal tissue in which they grow. We propose the mechanisms of formation of hepatic metastasis in colon cancer as summarized in Fig. 1. Colon cancer cells stimulate endothelial cells and hepatic stellate cells mediated by VEGF and PDGF, respectively. Stimulated endothelial cells and hepatic stellate cells produce various growth factors, cytokines, and matrix metalloproteinase and assist cancer cells in the structural reorganization for hepatic metastasis.

It is believed that many patients have micrometastases that cannot be detected when they are diagnosed with advanced cancer. Cancer cells can proliferate without angiogenesis to a certain extent, but they need angiogenesis to form macroscopic metastases. TNP-470 may keep cancer cells dormant and inhibit progression of micrometastases to macroscopic metastases. The angiogenesis inhibitor TNP-470 seems to be a potent agent for inhibiting hepatic metastasis of colon cancer.

References

1. Yamada N, Chung YS, Takatsuka S, et al (1997) Increased sialyl Lewis A expression and fucosyltransferase activity with acquisition of a high metastatic capacity in a colon cancer cell line. Br J Cancer 76:582–587
2. Takatsuka S, Chung YS, Yamada N, et al (1997) Characterization and purification of angiogenic factor derived from highly liver metastatic colon cancer cells. Int J Oncol 11:1035–1040

3. Kawada N, Tray-Thi TA, Klein H, et al (1993) The contraction of hepatic stellate (Ito) cells stimulated with vasoactive substances: possible involvement of endothelin-1 and nitric oxide in the regulation of the sinusoidal tonus. Eur J Biochem 213:815–823
4. Takatsuka S, Yamada N, Sawada T, et al (2000) Contribution of angiogenesis to the progression of colon cancer: possible inhibitory effect of angiogenesis inhibitor TNP-470 on tumor growth and hepatic metastasis. Int J Oncol 17:253–258

Hepatic Microcirculation in Massive Liver Necrosis and Liver Regeneration

SATOSHI MOCHIDA* and KENJI FUJIWARA

Summary. Sinusoidal endothelial cells in the liver are unique in blood coagulation regulatory function, as they express minimal anticoagulants, such as tissue factor pathway inhibitor (TFPI) and thrombomodulin. Thus, fibrin deposition can easily occur in the hepatic sinusoids when Kupffer cells or hepatic macrophages are activated to increase the activity of tissue factor, an initiator of blood coagulation cascade. Such deposition seems to be involved in the development of massive liver necrosis through microcirculatory disturbance in patients with fulminant hepatic failure and primary graft nonfunction after orthotopic liver transplantation. Anticoagulant therapies targeting the hepatic sinusoids using recombinant human TFPI and bowel decontamination with polymyxin B sulfate are promising methods to prevent these liver injuries. Endothelial cells and hepatocytes are markedly injured in massive liver necrosis with fibrin deposition in the hepatic sinusoids, suggesting that endothelial cell proliferation may be critical for sufficient liver regeneration. Vascular endothelial growth factor (VEGF) derived from activated Kupffer cells, macrophages, and stellate cells can induce capillarization of the hepatic sinusoids through vascular endothelial cell proliferation along with actions of platelet-derived growth factor and fibroblast growth factor-2. In contrast, VEGF from regenerating hepatocytes seems essential for reconstruction of the hepatic sinusoids, as sinusoidal endothelial cells can proliferate only by action of VEGF. Thus, a communication system between endothelial cells and other liver cells may play an important role in the development of and recovery from massive liver necrosis.

Key words. Massive liver necrosis, Microcirculatory disturbance, Sinusoidal endothelial cells, TFPI, VEGF

Blood Coagulation Equilibrium in the Hepatic Sinusoids

The hepatic sinusoid is a unique microcirculation system in terms of structure and function. Kupffer cells exist as resident macrophages and act as a biological filter to

---

Third Department of Internal Medicine, Saitama Medical School, 38 Morohongo, Moroyama-cho, Iruma-gun, Saitama 350-0495, Japan
* e-mail: smochida@saitama-med.ac.jp

remove gut-derived substances. Endothelial cells have a sieve-plate appearance with pores and no basement membrane in the space of Disse. Thus, circulating substances in the hepatic sinusoids can easily move to hepatocytes. Stellate cells play a role in the maintenance of such unique structures as pericytes of endothelial cells.

The regulatory mechanisms of blood coagulation equilibrium are also peculiar in the hepatic sinusoids. Kupffer cells express tissue factor, an initiator of the blood coagulation cascade, on the surface with its active domains exposed to the bloodstream [1]. In general, the cascade triggered by a tissue factor is suppressed by a tissue factor pathway inhibitor (TFPI) on endothelial cells, an anticoagulant that inhibits the catalytic activity of coagulation factor VIIa and the tissue factor on factor X. The cascade is further regulated by thrombomodulin on the cells, as thrombin is immediately inactivated by this anticoagulant even when the tissue factor produced blood coagulation. However, both TFPI and thrombomodulin expressions are minimal in endothelial cells in the hepatic sinusoids compared to that in cells in other organs [1,2]. Thus, microcirculatory disturbance due to fibrin deposition can easily develop in the hepatic sinusoids following activation of Kupffer cells, hepatic macrophages, or both [3,4]. Also, the derangement of blood coagulation equilibrium is caused by endothelial cell injury in the hepatic sinusoids [5].

Mechanisms of the Development of Massive Liver Necrosis

Massive liver necrosis develops in rats given heat-killed *Propionibacterium acnes* or that undergo 70% partial hepatectomy after intravenous administration of endotoxin [6,7]. When rats received heat-killed *P. acnes*, hepatic macrophages became activated through the cytokine network of interleukins 18 and 2 (IL-18, IL-2) and interferon-γ (IFNγ) [8]. Osteopontin, an extracellular matrix with RGD sequence, also promoted accumulation of hepatic macrophages in this model [9,10]. These macrophages are activated to produce a large amount of cytotoxic mediators such as tumor necrosis factor-α (TNFα) and superoxide anions [5,11], and they destroy endothelial cells, leading to development of fibrin deposition in the hepatic sinusoids [5,12]. In contrast, Kupffer cells became activated through bacterial translocation following 70% liver resection in rats (13). Such Kupffer cells express tissue factor after endotoxin administration in these rats and produce fibrin deposition as a result of deranged blood coagulation equilibrium in the hepatic sinusoids [3]. Hepatocyte damage occurs in both models owing to microcirculatory disturbance induced by sinusoidal fibrin deposition [3,5]. Macrophage activation and hypercoagulability are seen in patients with fulminant viral hepatitis of the acute type, suggesting that sinusoidal fibrin deposition may be responsible for massive liver necrosis in these patients.

Similar mechanisms are likely to be involved in the development of primary graft nonfunction following orthotopic liver transplantation. Sinusoidal endothelial cell injury is a major abnormal finding in rat liver after reperfusion following cold preservation in University of Wisconsin (UW) solution. Degeneration of hepatic stellate cells [14], disappearance of hepatic expression of vascular endothelial growth factor (VEGF) receptors [15], and oxygenation stress following ischemia caused such endothelial cell injury. On the other hand, tissue factor activity in Kupffer cells was markedly increased as a consequence of bacterial translocation due to portal blood congestion during the ahepatic period in rats undergoing orthotopic liver transplantation [16]. Thus, blood coagulation equilibrium was markedly deranged in the sinusoids of transplanted liver, and massive liver necrosis developed through sinusoidal fibrin deposition [4].

Therapeutic Strategies for Massive Liver Necrosis Due to Microcirculatory Disturbance

Anticoagulant therapy using antithrombin III concentrate was useful for attenuating liver injuries in rats that were fulminant hepatic failure models [6,7] and rats after orthotopic liver transplantation [4]. Similar efficacy is shown in patients with severe acute hepatitis and fulminant hepatitis of the acute type [17]. However, in patients following orthotopic liver transplantation, bleeding from the operative wound is inevitable as its adverse effect. Thus, we have developed novel anticoagulation therapies targeting the hepatic sinusoids. One is oral administration of polymyxin B sulfate to the recipients before the operation, which can attenuate tissue factor activity in Kupffer cells [16]. The other is recombinant human TFPI injected intravenously immediately after the operation, which can increase anticoagulant activity selectively in the hepatic sinusoids. This factor acted as anticoagulant by binding to heparinoids on the surface of hepatocyte microvilli in the space of Disse as well as sinusoidal endothelial cells [2,18].

Regeneration of Sinusoidal Endothelial Cells

Sinusoidal endothelial cells and hepatocytes were markedly injured during massive liver necrosis due to microcirculatory disturbance. Endothelial cell proliferation would promote liver regeneration, as the bloodstream is necessary for liver regeneration. Sinusoidal endothelial cells can proliferate in response to VEGF but not to platelet-derived growth factor (PDGF) or fibroblast growth factor-2 (FGF-2), powerful angiogenic factors.

In 70% resected rat liver, mitosis is maximal 36h after the operation in hepatocytes and at 96h in sinusoidal endothelial cells. In such liver, hepatocytes showed increased VEGF expression at the G_1 phase of the cell cycle, and the expression became more prominent after the M phase [19]. On the other hand, mRNA expression of VEGF receptors was up-regulated in the liver 72–168h after 70% resection [19]. Thus, VEGF expressed in regenerating hepatocytes may contribute to the proliferation of sinusoidal endothelial cells through VEGF receptors probably up-regulated on the cells.

When rats received carbon tetrachloride (CCl_4), liver necrosis developed 1–3 days following intoxication, and the liver became histologically normal 7 days later. In these rats VEGF was markedly expressed in activated Kupffer cells, hepatic macrophages, and stellate cells accumulating in the necrotic areas [20]. Also, regenerating hepatocytes at 7 days showed a marked increase in VEGF expression [20]. However, vascular endothelial cells proliferated in the necrotic areas, and proliferation of sinusoidal endothelial cells followed [20]. Thus, activated sinusoidal cells might induce proliferation of vascular endothelial cells leading to capillarization of the hepatic sinusoids by producing VEGF as well as PDGF and FGF-2 in these rats. It likely that VEGF derived from regenerating hepatocytes is essential for sinusoidal endothelial cell proliferation in reconstruction of the hepatic sinusoids [20].

Recently we found that the VEGF receptors flt-1 and KDR/flk-1 were expressed on hepatic stellate cells in primary culture and VEGF attenuated contraction of the cells during activation on plastic dishes [21]. Also, the porosity of sinusoidal endothelial cells in primary culture were significantly increased by addition of VEGF in a dose-related manner [22]. These data may suggest that VEGF can act as a vascular permeability factor as well as a growth factor in the liver and contribute to regulation of the hepatic microcirculation.

References

1. Arai M, Mochida S, Ohno A, et al (1995) Blood coagulation equilibrium in rat liver microcirculation as evaluated by endothelial cell thrombomodulin and macrophage tissue factor. Thromb Res 80:113–123
2. Yamanobe F, Mochida S, Ohno A, et al (1997) Recombinant human tissue factor pathway inhibitor as a possible anticoagulant targeting hepatic sinusoidal walls. Thromb Res 85:493–501
3. Mochida S, Arai M, Ohno A, et al (1999) Deranged blood coagulation equilibrium as a factor of massive liver necrosis following endotoxin administration in partially hepatectomized rats. Hepatology 29:1532–1540
4. Arai M, Mochida S, Ohno A, et al (1996) Blood coagulation in the hepatic sinusoids as a factor of liver injury following orthotopic liver transplantation in rats. Transplantation 62:1398–1401
5. Arai M, Mochida S, Ohno A, et al (1993) Sinusoidal endothelial cell damage by activated hepatic macrophages in rat liver necrosis. Gastroenterology 104:1466–1471
6. Yamada S, Ogata I, Hirata K, et al (1989) Intravascular coagulation in the development of massive hepatic necrosis induced by *Corynebacterium parvum* and endotoxin in rats. Scand J Gastroenterol 24:293–298
7. Mochida S, Ogata I, Hirata K, et al (1990) Provocation of massive hepatic necrosis by endotoxin after partial hepatectomy in rats. Gastroenterology 99:771–777
8. Toshima K, Mochida S, Ishikawa K, et al (1998) Contribution of CD14 to endotoxin-induced liver injury may depend on types of macrophage activation in rats. Biochem Biophys Res Commun 246:731–735
9. Kawashima R, Mochida S, Matsui A, et al (1999) Expression of osteopontin in Kupffer cells and hepatic macrophages and stellate cells in rat liver after carbon tetrachloride intoxication: a possible factor for macrophage migration into hepatic necrotic areas. Biochem Biophys Res Commun 256:527–531
10. Wang YH, Mochida S, Kawashima R, et al (2000) Increased expression of osteopontin in activated Kupffer cells and hepatic macrophages during macrophage migration in *Propionibacterium acnes*-treated rat liver. J Gastreoenterol 35:696–701
11. Mochida S, Ogata I, Ohta Y, et al (1989) In situ evaluation of the stimulatory state of hepatic macrophages based on their ability to produce superoxide anions in rats. J Pathol 158:67–71
12. Mochida S, Ohno A, Arai M, et al (1996) Role of adhesion molecules in the development of massive hepatic necrosis in rats. Hepatology 23:320–328
13. Mochida S, Ohta Y, Ogata I, et al (1992) Gut-derived substances in activation of hepatic macrophages after partial hepatectomy in rats. J Hepatol 16:266–272
14. Ohno A, Mochida S, Hirata K, et al (1994) Fat-storing cell abnormalities associated with endothelial cell damage after cold ischemia in UW solution. Dig Dis Sci 39: 861–865

15. Arai S, Mochida S, Ohno A, et al (1999) Decreased expressions of receptors for vascular endothelial growth factor and sinusoidal endothelial cell damage in cold preserved rat liver. Transplant Proc 31:2668–2672
16. Arai M, Mochida S, Ohno A, et al (1998) Selective bowel decontamination of recipients for prevention against liver injury following orthotopic liver transplantation: evaluation with rat models. Hepatology 27:123–127
17. Mochida S, Fujiwara K (2001) Recent advances in acute and fulminant hepatitis in Japan. Int Med (in press)
18. Mochida S, Arai S, Yamanobe F, et al (1998) Anticoagulant targeting for hepatic sinusoidal walls in prevention of hypercoagulopathy in cold preserved rat livers. Transplant Proc 30:45–48
19. Mochida S, Ishikawa K, Inao M, et al (1996) Increased expression of vascular endothelial growth factor and its receptors, *flt-1* and *KDR/flk-1*, in regenerating rat liver. Biochem Biophys Res Commun 226:176–179
20. Ishikawa K, Mochida S, Mashiba S, et al (1999) Vascular endothelial growth factor expressions in livers after partial resection and injury. Biochem Biophys Res Commun 254:587–593
21. Mashiba S, Mochida S, Ishikawa K, et al (1999) Inhibition of hepatic stellate cell contraction during activation in vitro by vascular endothelial growth factor in association with upregulation of FLT tyrosine kinase receptor family, *flt-1*. Biochem Biophys Res Commun 258:674–678
22. Funyu J, Mochida S, Inao M, et al (2001) VEGF can act as vascular permeability factor in the hepatic sinusoids, through upregulation of porosity of endothelial cells. Biochem Biophys Res Commun 280:481–485

Prevention of Hepatic Ischemia/Reperfusion Injury by Microcirculatory Regulation: Application to Liver Transplantation

Motohide Shimazu*, Go Wakabayashi, Minoru Tanabe, Shigeyuki Kawachi, Kenji Iwata, and Masaki Kitajima

Summary. We studied whether graft viability could be protected by hepatic microcirculatory regulation in rat and pig liver transplantation models. Interleukin-1 (IL-1) blockade by an IL-1 receptor antagonist rinse decreased leukocyte adhesion and increased leukocyte velocity, attenuating hepatocyte damage after liver transplantation even during prolonged cold preservation. Microcirculatory regulation by modulation of inflammatory cytokines, such as IL-1 and tumor necrosis factor, improves liver graft viability. Intraportal prostaglandin E_1 (PGE_1) perfusion alleviated microcirculatory impairment after ischemia/reperfusion by inhibiting the leukocyte-endothelium interaction. Intraportal infusion of PGE_1 also protected against hepatic ischemia/reperfusion injury and improved graft viability after liver transplantation. Intraportal PGE_1 treatment was clinically applied during living donor liver transplantation, and it appeared to be effective in maintaining graft circulation and viability.

Key words. Ischemia/reperfusion injury, Microcirculation, Cytokines, Prostaglandin E_1, Liver transplantation

Introduction

During liver transplantation the grafted liver inevitably suffers from cold and warm ischemia/reperfusion injury. We have reported that the essential mechanism of hepatic ischemia/reperfusion injury is an inflammatory response followed by microcirculatory disturbance caused by overproduction of proinflammatory cytokines [1,2]. From this point of view, we studied whether graft viability could be protected by hepatic microcirculatory regulation in rat and pig liver transplantation models.

Department of Surgery, School of Medicine, Keio University, 35 Shinanomachi, Shinjuku-ku, Tokyo 160-8582, Japan
* e-mail: shimazu@med.keio.ac.jp

Role of Proinflammatory Cytokines in Microcirculatory Disturbance After Liver Transplantation in the Rat

We studied the role of interleukin 1 (IL-1) using IL-1 receptor antagonist (IL-1ra) in microcirculatory impairment and functional disturbance of the grafted liver in rats. IL-1ra has the same affinity for the IL-1 receptor as IL-1 and evokes no signal transduction, consequently blocking IL-1. Rat liver transplantation was conducted by Kamada's cuff technique without arterial reconstruction. Inbred Lewis rats were divided into three groups based on graft preservation time and the rinse solution. Group I consisted of rats with grafts preserved for 1 h in University of Wisconsin (UW) solution and rinsed by 3 ml of lactated Ringer's solution (i.e., short preservation group). In group II the grafts were preserved for 24 h in UW solution and rinsed with 3 ml of lactated Ringer's solution (i.e., long preservation group). In group III the grafts were preserved for 24 h in UW solution and rinsed with IL-1ra (10 mg in 3 ml of lactated Ringer's solution) (i.e., long preservation with IL-1ra rinse group). At 1 and 3 h after transplantation the hepatic microcirculation was observed using intravital fluorescence microscopy following injection of two fluorescent dyes: (1) carboxyfluorescence diacetate succinimidyl ester (CFSE) to label circulating leukocytes; and (2) propidium iodide (PI) to label the nuclei of nonviable cells.

After transplantation, the number of leukocytes adhering to hepatic sinusoids or terminal venules increased in a time-dependent manner in group II compared to that in group I but did not increase in group III (Fig. 1). There were significantly more PI-positive cells at 3 h after transplantation in group II than in group I or III (Fig. 2, left). The velocity of leukocytes at 3 h after transplantation was significantly lower in group II than in group I or III (Fig. 2, right). Histological findings showed that the degeneration of hepatocytes and intravascular coagulation in group II markedly decreased in group III. Thus, IL-1 blockade by an IL-1ra rinse decreased leukocyte adhesion and increased leukocyte velocity, attenuating hepatocyte damage after liver transplantation even with prolonged cold preservation.

Efficacy of Intraportal Perfusion of PGE_1 in Hepatic Ischemia/Reperfusion

It has been reported that prostglandin E_1 (PGE_1) is an effective treatment for patients with fulminant hepatic failure [3] or primary graft nonfunction after liver transplantation [4], but the mechanism is still not clear. We studied the effects of portal perfusion with PGE_1 on microcirculatory disorders in rat ischemia/reperfusion. A rat ischemia/reperfusion model was prepared by clamping both the hepatic artery and portal vein for 60 min following portosystemic shunt by splenopexy based on the method of Meredith and Wade [5].

Animals were divided into three groups based on the type of intraportal perfusion during hepatic ischemia: group 1, untreated controls; group 2, animals perfused with lactated Ringer's solution (20 ml/kg/h); and group 3, animals perfused with PGE_1

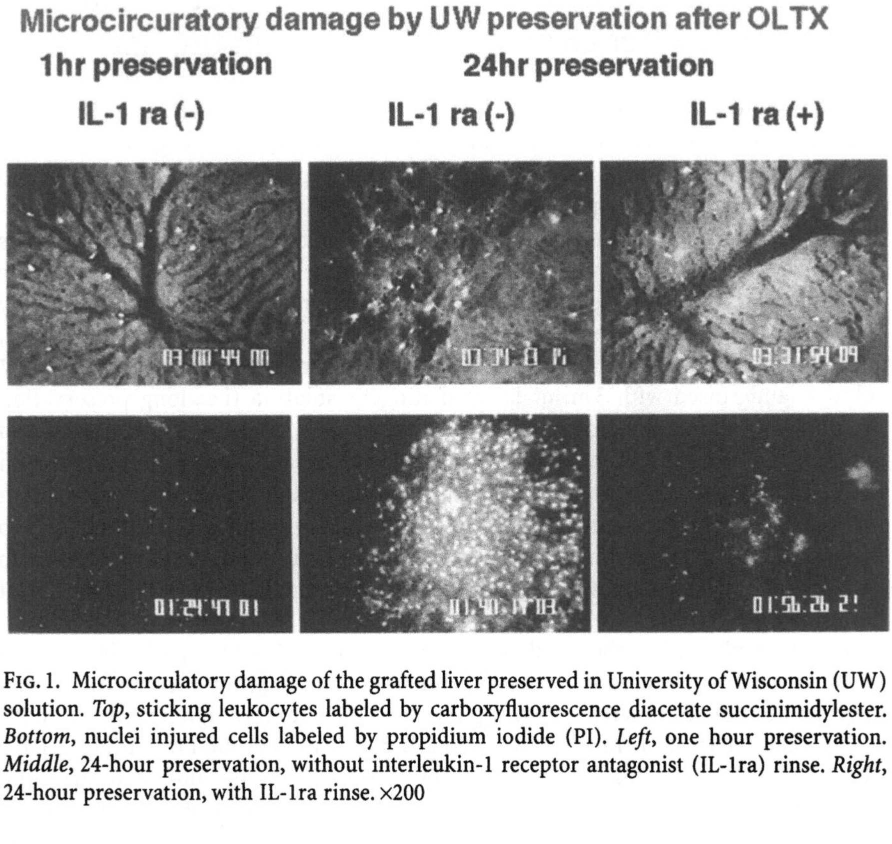

FIG. 1. Microcirculatory damage of the grafted liver preserved in University of Wisconsin (UW) solution. *Top*, sticking leukocytes labeled by carboxyfluorescence diacetate succinimidylester. *Bottom*, nuclei injured cells labeled by propidium iodide (PI). *Left*, one hour preservation. *Middle*, 24-hour preservation, without interleukin-1 receptor antagonist (IL-1ra) rinse. *Right*, 24-hour preservation, with IL-1ra rinse. ×200

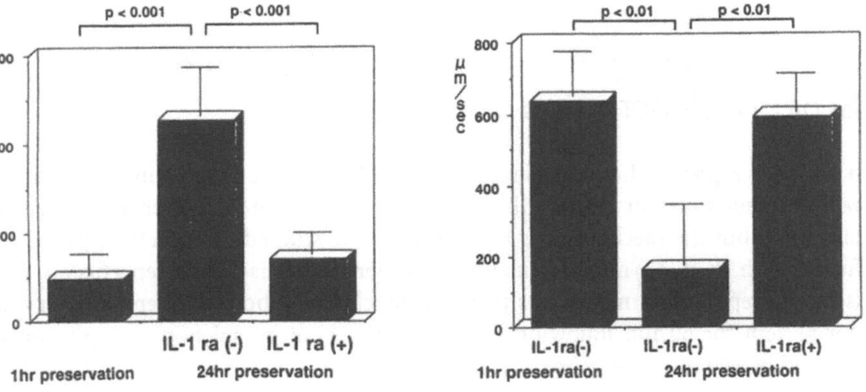

FIG. 2. *Left*, number of PI-positive cells 3h after transplantation. *Right*, velocity of leukocytes 3h after transplantation

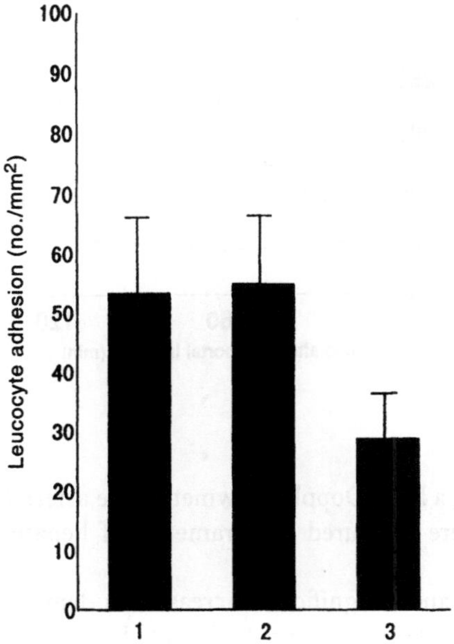

FIG. 3. Number of leukocytes adhering to hepatic sinusoidal walls and terminal venules 30 min after reperfusion. Groups 1 and 2 versus group 3; $P < 0.01$

(0.1 µg/kg/min) and lactated Ringer's solution (20 ml/kg/h). After reperfusion, the hepatic microcirculation was observed using intravital fluorescence microscopy following injection of CFSE and PI.

The number of leukocytes adhering to hepatic sinusoids and terminal venules at 30 min after reperfusion was lowest in group 3 and significantly higher in groups 1 and 2 ($P < 0.01$) (Fig. 3). Leukocyte velocity and the percentage of perfused sinusoids were significantly higher in group 3 than in the other groups. The number of PI-positive injured cells 60 min after reperfusion was significantly lower in group 3 than in the other groups ($P < 0.05$). Immunohistochemical staining of intercellular adhesion molecule-1 (ICAM-1) using anti-rat ICAM-1 monoclonal antibody (1A29) revealed that expression of ICAM-1 on hepatic sinusoidal walls was dominant in groups 2 and 3. PGE_1 treatment thus appeared to suppress sinusoidal expression of ICAM-1 during an early period of reperfusion. These findings suggest that intraportal PGE_1 perfusion alleviates microcirculatory impairment after ischemia/reperfusion by inhibiting the leukocyte–endothelium interaction.

Preclinical Study of Intraportal Infusion of PGE_1 During Porcine Liver Transplantation

In a preclinical experiment we studied the effects of intraportal infusion of PGE_1 on hepatic blood flow and graft viability after liver transplantation in pigs. Two groups of pigs underwent orthotopic liver transplantation. Group A comprised untreated controls, and group B received PGE_1 at 0.1 µg/kg/min intraportally for 2 h after vascular reconstruction of the allograft. Hepatic arterial flow (HAF) and portal venous flow (PVF) were measured by an ultrasonic transit time flowmeter; and liver

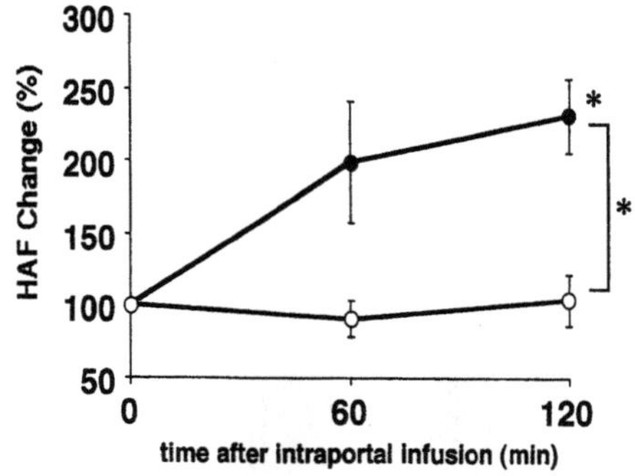

FIG. 4. Changes in hepatic arterial flow (*HAF*) in the transplanted liver after intraportal infusion of prostaglandin E_1 (PGE_1). *Open circles*, group A (untreated control group); *filled circles*, group B (intraportal PGE_1 group). *$P < 0.05$

tissue blood flow (LTBF) was measured using a laser-Doppler flowmeter. The arterial ketone body ratio (AKBR) and bile flow were measured as parameters of hepatic function.

In group B the HAF increased with time, and a significant increase was demonstrated 2h after PGE_1 infusion. In contrast, the HAF in group A did not change, and there was a significant difference in HAF between the two groups 2h after PGE_1 infusion (Fig. 4). The PVF was significantly decreased in both groups, although in group B the PVF was higher than in group A. The LTBF in group B increased with time and was significantly higher than in group A 2h after PGE_1 infusion. Group B exhibited higher AKBR and greater bile flow than group A. This study demonstrated that the intraportal infusion of PGE_1 improved hepatic allograft blood flow and appeared to improve graft viability after liver transplantation.

Clinical Application of Intraportal Infusion of PGE_1 During Living Donor Liver Transplantation

From April 1995 to November 2000 a series of 31 patients (18 children, 13 adults) underwent living donor liver transplantation at the Keio University Hospital. Indications for liver transplantation included biliary cirrhosis in 16, fulminant hepatic failure in 7, primary biliary cirrhosis in 4, and primary sclerosing cholangitis, hepatitis B cirrhosis, familial amyloid polyneuropathy, and metastatic endocrine tumor in 1 each. Of these, eight adults received intraportal infusion of PGE_1 combined with steroids to prevent microcirculatory disturbance and rejection. Of these eight, two were ABO-incompatible. After PGE_1 infusion the mean velocity of hepatic arterial flow measured by an ultrasound Doppler flowmeter increased 38% and portal venous flow 30%. Graft function was maintained, and rejection did not occurred in any of the eight, even in ABO-incompatible patients.

Conclusions

Our study suggests that microcirculatory regulation by modulating inflammatory cytokines improves liver graft viability. Intraportal infusion of PGE_1 also could protect against hepatic ischemia/reperfusion injury and improve graft viability after liver transplantation. Intraportal PGE_1 treatment was clinically applied during living donor liver transplantation, and it appeared effective for maintaining graft circulation and viability.

References

1. Shito M, Wakabayashi G, Ueda M, et al (1997) Interleukin 1 receptor blockade reduces tumor necrosis factor production, tissue injury, and mortality after hepatic ischemia-reperfusion in the rat. Transplantation 63:143–148
2. Shirasugi N, Wakabayashi G, Shimazu M, et al (1997) Up-regulation of oxygen-derived free radicals by interleukin 1 in hepatic ischemia-reperfusion injury. Transplantation 64:1398–1403
3. Abecassis M, Falk R, Blendis L (1987) Treatment of fulminant hepatic failure with a continuous infusion of ProstinVR (PGE_1). Hepatology 7:1104
4. Greig PD, Woolf GM, Sinclair SB, et al (1989) Treatment of primary liver graft nonfunction with prostaglandin E_1. Transplantation 48:447–453
5. Meredith CG, Wade DN (1981) A model of portal-systemic shunting in the rat. Clin Exp Pharmacol Physiol 8:651–652

Genetic Manipulation of Sinusoidal Endothelial Cells

Yoshiyuki Takei[1,*], Atsushi Maruyama[2], Toshihiro Akaike[2], and Nobuhiro Sato[1]

Summary. Manipulation of gene expression of sinusoidal endothelial cells (SECs) by a triplex DNA technology may lead to a new strategy to treat intractable liver diseases. The liver SEC has unique hyaluronan receptors that recognize and internalize hyaluronic acid (HA). In this study we synthesized a comb-type copolymer with HA as a side chain and evaluated its targetability to SECs through an HA receptor-mediated pathway as well as its ability to stabilize triplexes. A gene carrier system was prepared by coupling HA oligomers to poly-L-lysine (PLL) in a 1:1 weight ratio by a reductive amination reaction. The PLL-g-HA thus formed was mixed with various amounts of DNA in 154 mM NaCl at 4°C. Neither turbidity nor precipitation was observed in PLL-g-HA/DNA mixtures over the copolymer (based on PLL)/DNA charge ratio from 0 to 2, indicating that interpolyelectrolyte complex formation between PLL-g-HA and DNA exhibited minimal self-aggregation, which explains the highly soluble nature of the complex. Intravenous injection of the [^{32}P]pSV β-Gal plasmid encoding lacZ complexed to PLL-g-HA in Wistar rats demonstrated specific hepatic targeting with >90% of the injected counts taken up by the liver in 1 h. Furthermore, using an FITC-labeled DNA, it was shown that the PLL-g-HA/DNA complex was distributed exclusively in the SEC. Seventy-two hours after injection of 90 μg of pSV β-Gal in a PLL-g-HA-complexed form, a large number of SECs expressing β-galactosidase were detected. Moreover, the triplex-stabilizing efficiency of the PLL-g-HA was significantly higher than that of other oligocations such as spermine and spermidine. The PLL-g-HA/DNA carrier system permits targeted delivery of exogenous DNA selectively to the liver SECs and stabilizes triplexes.

Key words. Sinusoidal endothelial cells (SECs), Gene manipulation

[1] Department of Gastroenterology, Juntendo University School of Medicine, 2-1-1 Hongo, Bunkyo-ku, Tokyo 113-8421, Japan
[2] Department of Biomolecular Engineering, Faculty of Bioscience and Biotechnology, Tokyo Institute of Technology, 4259 Nagatsuta-cho, Midori-ku, Yokohama 226-8501, Japan
* e-mail: ytakei@med.juntendo.ac.jp

Introduction

Perturbation of gene expression of liver endothelial cells (SECs) plays an important role in liver inflammation, disturbance of the microcirculation, and tumor angiogenesis [1]. Manipulation of gene expression of the SECs may lead to a new strategy for treating intractable liver disease. To this end, we focused on triplex DNA technology employing triplex forming oligonucleotides (TFOs). TFOs can be targeted for their sequence-specific binding to the major groove of the homopurine-homopyrimidine stretch in target genes. TFOs can inhibit or enhance DNA transcription, generate site-specific mutations, cleave DNA, and induce homologous recombination [2]. However, the instability of triplex DNA under physiological conditions owing to the electrostatic repulsion between a TFO and the duplex as well as pH dependence and K^+ sensitivity, limits in vivo application of the triplex strategy. Maruyama et al. previously reported that comb-type copolymers composed of poly-L-lysine (PLL) and hydrophilic polysaccharides significantly increased the thermal stability of the triplex structure [3]. On the other hand, liver SECs have unique hyaluronan receptors that recognize and internalize hyaluronic acid (HA) [4].

In this study, we synthesized a comb-type copolymer with HA as a side chain. We then evaluated its targetability to SECs through an HA receptor-mediated pathway as well as its ability to stabilize triplexes.

Synthesis of a PLL-g-HA Comb-Type Copolymer

A gene carrier system [hyaluronate-grafted poly-(L-lysine) copolymer (PLL-g-HA)] was prepared by coupling HA to poly-L-lysine (PLL) in a 1:1 (w/w) ratio [5]. HA fragments (number-average molecular weight 1.5×10^4) were conjugated to PLL (number-average molecular weight 4.6×10^4) by reductive amination using $NaBH_3CN$ as a reductant.

The gel permeation chromatography (GPC) profile of the reaction mixture and the resulting copolymer showed that after the reaction the peak area of PLL increased whereas that of HA decreased. When HA was incubated with PLL in the presence of 10-fold molar excess of lactose or sucrose, not sucrose, the non-reducing sugar, but lactose, the reducing one, inhibited HA consumption. Therefore it can be concluded that the HA was conjugated with PLL at its reducing end through the reductive amination reaction.

PLL-g-HA/DNA Polyion Complex

DNA was mixed with the PLL-g-HA [$(\text{amino group})_{\text{copolymer}}/(\text{phosphate group})_{\text{DNA}} = 1$], and the ionic strength of the medium was gradually decreased from 1 to 0 M NaCl by step-down dialysis. The ^1H nuclear magnetic resonance (NMR) spectra of the copolymer with or without DNA were analyzed, and it was shown that the signals of ε-methylene protons of the PLL moiety in the PLL-g-HA broadened in the presence of DNA. This is likely caused by polyanion formation between the PLL moiety and DNA.

Complex formation between PLL-g-HA and DNA was further assessed with a gel retardation assay. Increasing the proportion of the PLL-g-HA copolymer in the DNA samples affected plasmid DNA migration in an agarose gel. The titration point, representing the minimum proportion of PLL-g-HA required to retard the DNA completely, occurred at around 1:1 copolymer (based on PLL)/DNA charge ratio.

Based on the results, it is postulated that the PLL-g-HA/DNA complex forms the multiphase structure in which the hydrophobic PLL-g-HA complex is surrounded by the hydrated shell of free HA. The presence of free HA chains is essential for directing the complex to the target cells.

Targetability of the PLL-g-HA/DNA Complex to SEC

To determine whether the PLL-g-HA/DNA complex was recognized by SEC HA receptors in vivo, Wistar rats were injected intravenously via the tail vein with PLL-g-HA complexed to ^{32}P-labeled pSV β-Gal (an expression plasmid encoding lacZ). One hour after-injection more than 90% of the injected radioactivity remained in the liver. Administration of the PLL-g-HA complexed to an FITC-labeled DNA revealed that the carrier–DNA complex was distributed exclusively in SECs. Polymerase chain reaction (PCR) amplification detected the presence of the transgene in the cytosolic fraction 3h after transfection only from the liver of the rats injected with PLL-g-HA/pSV β-Gal, not with pSV β-Gal alone. A large number of cells expressing β-galactosidase were detected in SECs when they were transfected with the PLL-g-HA/pSV β-Gal complex.

Evaluation of Triplex Formation

Triplex formation was analyzed by electrophoretic mobility shift assay (EMSA) using a 30-mer target duplex from rat α 1 (I) collagen gene promoter (T-1/T-2 duplex: T-1, 5′-CCTTTCCCTTCCTTTCCCTCCTCCCCCCTC-3′; T-2, 3′-GGAAAGGGAAGGAAAGGGAGGAGGGGGGAG-5′) and Pu-20 (5′-GGAAAGGGAAGGAAAGGGAGGAGGG-3′) and Py-20 (5′-CCCTTCCTTTCCCTCCTCCC-3′) as TFOs. PLL-g-HA markedly diminished K^+ inhibition of purine motif triplex formation with Pu-20 and the pH dependence of pyrimidine motif triplex formation with Py-20.

Conclusions

The PLL-g-HA/DNA carrier system permits targeted delivery of exogenous DNA selectively to liver SECs and stabilizes triplexes. The PLL-g-HA system is expected to provide a breakthrough toward the triplex-based genetic engineering of the SEC.

References

1. Gerritsen ME, Bloor CM (1993) Endothelial cell gene expression in response to injury. FASEB J 7:523–532
2. Chan PP, Glazer PM (1997) Triplex DNA: fundamentals, advantages, and potential applications for gene therapy. J Mol Med 75:267–282

3. Maruyama A, Katoh M, Ishihara T, et al (1997) Comb-type polycations effectively stabilize DNA triplex. Bioconjugate Chem 8:3–6
4. Smedsrød B, Pertoft H, Eriksson S, et al (1984) Studies in vitro on the uptake and degradation of sodium hyaluronate in rat liver endothelial cells. Biochem J 223:617–626
5. Asayama S, Nogawa M, Takei Y, et al (1998) Synthesis of novel polyampholyte comb-type copolymers consisting of a poly(L-lysine) backbone and hyaluronic acid side chains for a DNA carrier. Bioconjugate Chem 9:476–481

Controlling Tumor Microenvironment by the Antiangiogenesis Strategy

Makoto Sunamura*, Dan G. Duda, Lucian Lozonschi, Sun Libo, Kazunori Takeda, and Seiki Matsuno

Summary. Angiogenesis occurs when the balance between negative and positive regulators inclines toward the latter, allowing the tumor and metastases to develop. Studies have found that genetic alterations may correlate with the "switching" on of angiogenic phenotypes, and that numerous soluble factors, including cytokines and matrix metalloproteinases, are key regulators of angiogenesis. The insights into this complex process gained because of the rapid, comprehensive development of the study of tumor-related angiogenesis suggest that inhibition of angiogenesis may be a useful therapeutic approach. The work of our group concentrated on this strategy in a few preclinical models. A novel matrix metalloproteinase inhibitor exhibited a potent antiangiogenesis and antimetastasis effect—stronger than that found after the use of TNP-470. In another study, interleukin-12 was found to be a strong inhibitor of angiogenesis, paralleling its key role as a mediator of the immune responses. These promising results support the antiangiogenesis approach in clinical trials for gastrointestinal tract cancer and offer a broader view of the correlation between angiogenesis and carcinogenesis in the tumor microenvironment.

Key words. Tumor microenvironment, Angiogenesis, Cytokine, Interleukin-12, Matrix metalloproteinases

Introduction

Many lines of evidence have demonstrated that angiogenesis is a multistage event of paramount importance for cancer progression. Comprehensive studies have led to a thorough understanding of the dependence of tumor growth and development and metastasis on the blood supply provided by aberrant neovascularization. Interference with this process is expected to develop into a reliable strategy to control the tumor microenvironment by inducing tumor regression or dormancy using antiangiogenesis compounds. Many agents have exhibited strong effects in preclinical models, and

First Department of Surgery, Tohoku University School of Medicine, 1-1 Seiryo-machi, Aoba-ku, Sendai 980-8574, Japan
* e-mail: msun-thk@umin.ac.jp

their number increases with our understanding of the cellular events related to the "switch" to an angiogenic phenotype in tumor tissue. Several ongoing clinical trials are employing agents with different mechanisms of action that attack the formation of new vessels from the preexisting vascular network [1].

This review describes strategies focusing on control of the tumor environment using matrix metalloproteinase (MMP) inhibitors and antiangiogenic cytokines.

Matrix Metalloproteinase Inhibition

An early step in tumor angiogenesis is the breakdown of the extracellular matrix (ECM) by MMPs released mainly by stroma but also by tumor cells. Recent data have expanded the role of MMPs to the promotion and growth of tumor and metastasis [1]. A number of studies concerning the role of MMPs in tumor angiogenesis, including some studies using transgene mice [1], demonstrated the involvement of gelatinases (MMP-2, MMP-9), matrylisin (MMP-7), stromelysins (MMP-3, MMP-11), and membrane-type MMP-1. Taken together, these findings support the strategy targeting MMPs for cancer therapy.

We tested the efficiency of a new MMP inhibitor, KB-R7785, in two tumor models [2] and assessed its influence on tumor angiogenesis and metastasis. This inhibitor acts on MMP-1, MMP-3, and MMP-9; and in the model we used it proved to be a potent antiangiogenesis and antimetastasis factor.

The growth of murine C26 colon adenocarcinoma in a transparent skin chamber failed in mice administered KB-R7785 due to the limitation of expansion of tumor-related angiogenesis. In fact, the tumors appeared to be rendered dormant by the action of MMP inhibitor on angiogenesis, as shown by significantly lower functional parameters. The lung colonization model proved to be a useful model for checking this inhibitor's effects, as the administration of KB-R7785 rendered the rare metastases with less vascularity and with a high apoptotic rate. The MMP inhibitor was able to affect the functional vascular density, and it suppressed angiogenesis to a larger extent and than did a well-known antiangiogenic agent, TNP-470, tested in the same tumor model. Of course, murine models have their limitations; and such results should be evaluated cautiously in the perspective of human clinical trials. However, the clear, strong antitumor effect of this compound and the lack of side effects consistent with a number of similar results reported by many groups support the use of MMP inhibitors in clinical trials for cancer.

Controlling the Cytokine Network in the Tumor Microenvironment

Another important line of control in the treatment of tumors is the influence of the local expression of cytokines. We studied comprehensively the effect of interleukin-12 (IL-12), a key regulator of the immune system and, as we have learned from our experiments, also a potent angiogenesis inhibitor [3].

Local delivery by retrovirally transfected fibroblasts secreting stable and relatively high levels of IL-12 suppressed the tumor growth and induced immunity [4]. It also eradicated established tumors [5] and prevented the recurrence of adenocarcinoma after surgical resection [6] in mice. Interestingly, silencing of the immune response by the use of natural killer (NK) cell-depleted SCID mice revealed an additional potent effect of IL-12 on murine and human tumors: strong suppression of tumor neovascularization at an early stage and in established tumors [7]. The mechanism of this effect was interferon-γ (IFNγ)-dependent and implicated the downstream expression of IFNγ-inducible protein 10 (IP-10), both secreted by local endothelial cells. In addition, IL-12 down-regulated the expression of endothelial cell mitogens vascular endothelial growth factor (VEGF) and basic fibroblast growth factor (bFGF). Furthermore, it induced interesting histological changes, consisting of a high degree of keratinization and apoptosis and a decrease in the proliferation rate in human tumors and extensive necrosis in the murine ones.

These results confirm several lines of evidence regarding IL-12 and its potential usefulness in the treatment of cancer. Our studies also underscore the efficacy of this local delivery system to overcome the limitations incurred by the side effects of IL-12 during systemic delivery. Further studies are necessary for thoroughly understanding the tumor angiogenesis–cytokine network so we can design an appropriate treatment strategy.

Conclusions

The spectacular progress made recently in the field of tumor angiogenesis has changed our perspective of the therapeutic approach to cancer in the new millennium. Efficient strategies must take into consideration the complexity of this process and the diversity of factors implicated for each type of tumor. Nevertheless, the design of new drugs based on their antiangiogenesis effect promises to change the outcome of this disease significantly.

References

1. Nelson AR, Fingleton B, Rothenberg ML, et al (2000) Matrix metalloproteinases: biologic activity and clinical implications. J Clin Oncol 18:1135–1149
2. Lozonschi L, Sunamura M, Kobari M, et al (1999) Controlling tumor angiogenesis and metastasis of C26 murine colon adenocarcinoma by a new matrix metalloproteinase inhibitor, KB-R7785, in two tumor models. Cancer Res 59:1252–1258
3. Sunamura M, Son L, Lozonschi L, et al (2000) The anti-angiogenesis effect of IL-12 during the early growth of human pancreatic cancer in SCID mice. Pancreas 20:227–233
4. Tahara H, Zeh HJ III, Storkus WJ, et al (1994) Fibroblasts genetically engineered to secrete interleukin 12 can suppress tumor growth and induce antitumor immunity to a murine melanoma in vivo. Cancer Res 54:182–189
5. Zitvogel L, Tahara H, Robbins PD, et al (1995) Cancer immunotherapy of established tumors with IL-12. J Immunol 155:1393–1403
6. Matsumoto G, Sunamura M, Shimamura H, et al (1999) Adjuvant immunotherapy using fibroblasts genetically engineered to secrete interleukin 12 prevents recurrence after surgical resection of established tumors in a murine adenocarcinoma model. Surgery 125:257–264
7. Duda DG, Sunamura M, Lozonschi L, et al (2000) Direct in vitro evidence and in vivo analysis of the anti-angiogenesis effects of interleukin 12. Cancer Res 60:1111–1116

Pancreatic Blood Flow in Chronic Alcoholic Pancreatitis

Tsuneo Tanaka[1,*], Tatsuyoshi Fujii[2], Yasuhiro Matsugu[2], and Kiyohiko Dohi[2]

Summary. Circulatory impairment is known to be an important factor in the deterioration of acute pancreatitis. We reported a canine model of chronic ischemic pancreatitis and the first successful model resembling human chronic alcoholic pancreatitis. Using this model, we investigated the significance of pancreatic tissue blood flow. There was pancreatic tissue ischemia in a model of chronic alcoholic pancreatitis. We conclude that pancreatic tissue ischemia is an etiological factor involved in chronic pancreatitis, and that ischemia acts as an aggravating factor of chronic alcoholic pancreatitis.

Key words. Pancreatic blood flow, Chronic alcoholic pancreatitis, Ischemic pancreatitis

Introduction

Circulatory impairment is known to be an important factor in the onset and deterioration of acute pancreatitis, but there are few studies on the impairment of blood flow in chronic pancreatitis. We [1] reported an experimental model we prepared for the purpose of proving that circulatory impairment is an etiological factor of chronic pancreatitis. Although alcohol abuse is the main etiological factor of chronic pancreatitis, there has been no useful model of chronic alcoholic pancreatitis (CAP) to date. We [2] reported the first successful model resembling human CAP. Using this model, we investigated the significance of pancreatic tissue blood flow in chronic pancreatitis. Although there are various methods of measuring the amount of pancreatic tissue blood flow, we performed the measurement at various locations of the pancreas using the electrolytic blood flow meter (RBF-1) only.

[1]Department of Surgery, Hiroshima Prefectural Hospital, 1-5-54 Ujinakanda, Minami-ku, Hiroshima 734-8530, Japan
[2]Department of Surgery II, Hiroshima University School of Medicine, Hiroshima, Japan
* e-mail: juntan@ipc.hiroshima-u.ac.jp

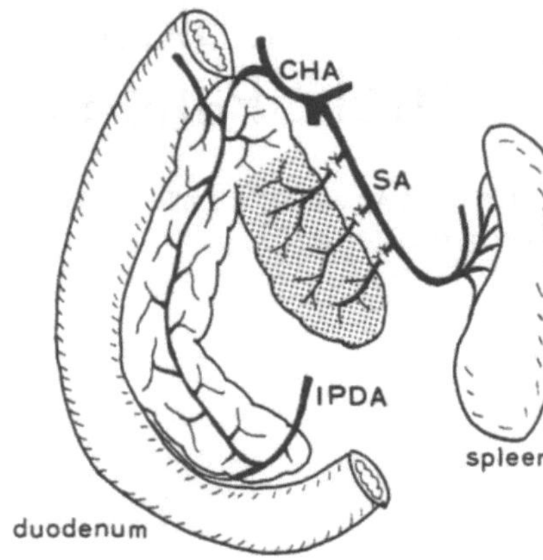

FIG. 1. Chronic ischemic pancreatitis model. *CHA*, common hepatic artery; *SA*, splenic artery; *IPDA*, inferior pancreaticoduodenal artery

Chronic Ischemic Pancreatitis

The pancreas is an organ susceptible to reduced tissue blood flow (ischemia). In fact, a sudden reduction in blood flow could result in pancreatic infarction or wide-scale pancreatic necrosis. Consequently, there has been no useful chronic pancreatitis model based on ischemia to date. We [1] reported a new experimental model we prepared based on a scheme in addition to the outline below. By ligating the branches distributed in the left pancreatic lobe from the splenic artery, the amount of tissue blood flow in the left pancreatic lobe was reduced to approximately 50% without rapid necrosis of the pancreas (Fig. 1). At 1, 2, 3, and 6 months after surgery, chronic pancreatitis could be confirmed macroscopically, histologically, and functionally. In other words, pancreatic tissue ischemia could be verified as one of the etiological factors of chronic pancreatitis. Although ischemia is a characteristic etiological factor of chronic pancreatitis, the frequency is low. Anmann and Sulser [3] called ischemia in the elderly chronic senile pancreatitis; we considered our model to correspond to this state in humans.

Chronic Alcoholic Pancreatitis

As mentioned above, alcohol is the main etiological factor of chronic pancreatitis, but, there has not been a useful experimental model of CAP to date. We [2] reported the first successful experimental model resembling human CAP, which we prepared using the method oulined below.

The pancreatic tissue blood flow in this model was measured using the electrolytic blood flowmeter (RBF-1). After 3 months laparotomy was performed again, and the investigations were carried out. The four groups were composed of mongrel dogs: The control group (group C) were dogs that underwent simple laparotomy only. In the alcohol group (group A), a gastric tube was inserted into the anterior wall of the stomach, and alcohol was administered extracorporeally; ethanol (2.0 g/kg/day) was dissolved in 100 ml of water and administered daily through the gastric tube. In the

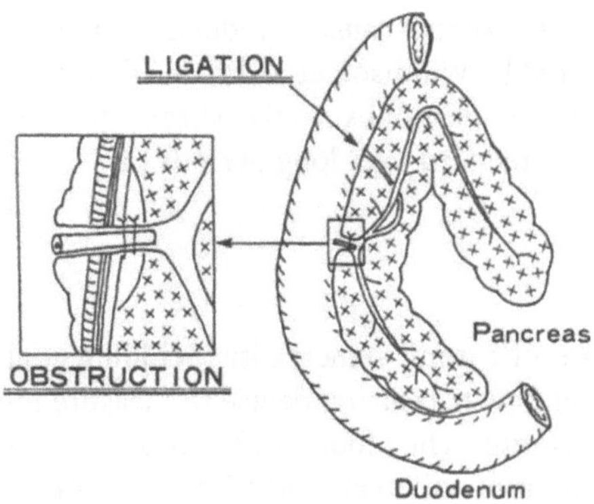

FIG. 2. Chronic alcoholic pancreatitis model

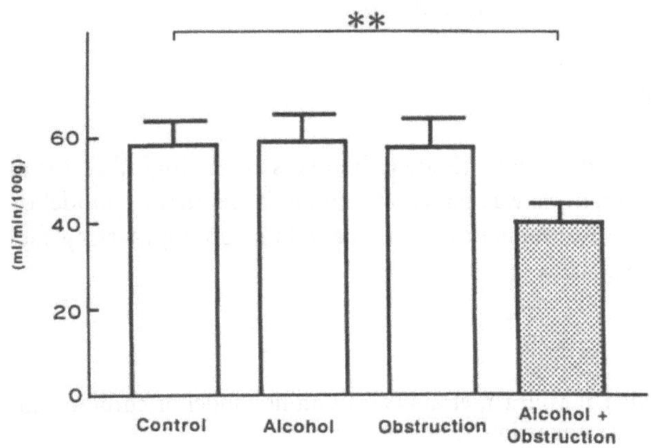

FIG. 3. Pancreatic tissue blood in each group

pancreatic duct obstruction group (group O), after ligating and isolating the minor pancreatic duct a polyethylene tube (internal diameter 0.4 mm, external diameter 1.7 mm, 10 mm long) was lodged. The alcohol administration + pancreatic duct obstruction group (group AO) consisted of groups A and O combined (Fig. 2).

The histological findings, pancreatic exocrine function tests, and analysis of the pancratic juice revealed that there was no change in groups C and A and mild obstructive pancreatitis in group O; group AO corresponded to human CAP. As shown in Fig. 3, the amount of pancreatic tissue blood flow in group C was 55.7 ± 3.4 ml/100 g/min. Compared to group C there was no difference in the amount of blood flow in groups A and O, but in group AO it was significantly low.

It is suggested that pancreatic tissue ischemia is one of the etiological factors of chronic pancreatitis; and based on the blood flow results in the CAP model (group AO), once CAP occurs it acts as a factor for aggravating pancreatic tissue ischemia. Two mechanisms are suggested for this phenomenon. One is intrapancreatic arteriolar narrowing due to pancreatic interlobular fibrosis and inflammatory cell infiltration. The other is an increase in interstitial pressure that causes a reduction in blood flow (compartment syndrome), as hypothesized by Widdison et al. [4]. Furthermore, when Widdison et al. administered alcohol to a model of obstructive chronic pancreatitis pancreatic blood flow was more potently reduced over long periods [4].

Clinical Cases

We do not measure tissue blood flow in cases of chronic pancreatitis. Schilling et al. [5] reported the use of a laser Doppler blood flow measuring device to measure the amount of pancreatic blood flow during operation. They found differences between locations in the pancreas regarding the amount of pancreatic blood flow in normal human pancreas, with the head having the highest flow followed by the body, tail, and uncus, in that order. For the CAP cases [5] there was a reduction of approximately 50% in all locations. We did not find any differences in the amount of blood flow due to the location of the pancreas in the dog.

Conclusions

We concluded that pancreatic tissue ischemia is an etiological factor of chronic pancreatitis. Moreover, there was pancreatic tissue ischemia in a model of chronic alcoholic pancreatitis. Consequently, ischemia acts as an aggravating factor of chronic alcoholic pancreatitis.

References

1. Tanaka T, Ichiba Y, Miura Y, et al (1994) Canine model of chronic pancreatitis due to chronic ischemia. Digestion 55:86–89
2. Tanaka T, Miura Y, Matsugu Y, et al (1998) Pancreatic duct obstruction is an aggravating factor in the canine model of chronic alcoholic pancreatitis. Gastroenterology 115:1248–1253
3. Ammann R, Sulser H (1976) Die senile chronische Pancreatitis: eine neue nosoligische Einheit? Schweiz Med Wochenschr 106:429–437
4. Widdison AL, Alvarez C, Schwarz M, et al (1992) The influence of ethanol on pancreatic blood flow in cats with chronic pancreatitis. Surgery 112:202–210
5. Schilling MK, Redaelli C, Reber PU, et al (1999) Microcirculation in chronic alcoholic pancreatitis: a laser Doppler flow study. Pancreas 19:21–25

Part 11
Hepatic Regeneration Update

The Role of Hepatic Oval Cells in Hepatic Regeneration: Possible Clinical Applications

SATOSHI MATSUSAKA* and AKIHIRO TOYOSAKA

Summary. Oval cells, the progeny of facultative liver stem cells, have the potential to differentiate into hepatocytes and bile epithelial cells. It has been reported that oval cells that develop in the rat 2-acetylaminofluorine/partial hepatectomy (AAF/PH) model express the c-*kit* receptor tyrosine kinase. Studies have found progenitor stem cells analogous to oval cells in diseased human liver. We investigated the role of the c-*kit* receptor tyrosine kinase in oval cell development using Ws/Ws rats, whose c-*kit* kinase activity was severely impaired owing to a small deletion in the kinase domain. The development of oval cells was remarkably suppressed in Ws/Ws rats when compared with that of +/+ rats. The present study was intended to compare the growth of hepatocytes and biliary epithelial cells in spleens given transplants of oval cell-free or oval cell-enriched isolated liver cells. The number of hepatocytes in the spleen given a transplant of oval cell-enriched liver cells was much higher than those in the spleen given a transplant of oval cell-free liver cells. Our results suggest that the c-*kit* receptor tyrosine kinase plays a crucial role in the appearance of oval cells in the rat AAF/PH model, and that intrasplenic transplantation of oval cell-enriched hepatocytes may improve survival and proliferation of hepatocytes in the spleen.

Key words. Oval cell, AAF/PH model, 2-Acetylaminofluorene/partial hepatectomy model, c-*kit* Receptor tyrosine kinase, Ws/Ws rat, Transplantation

Introduction

Mature hepatocytes proliferate after partial hepatectomy (PH), resulting in liver regeneration. When PH is performed under conditions in which the replication of mature hepatocytes is impaired, oval cells, which are thought to develop from hepatic stem cells, infiltrate into the surrounding parenchyma. Oval cells have the potential to differentiate into hepatocytes and bile epithelial cells; they have features of both fetal hepatocytes and bile epithelial cells, and express markers such as AFP and CK19.

First Department of Surgery, Hyogo College of Medicine, 1-1 Mukogawa-cho, Nishinomiya, Hyogo 663-8501, Japan
* e-mail: hcj15901@hcc1.bai.ne.jp

It has been reported that the c-*kit* receptor tyrosine kinase is expressed in oval cells [1]. Studies have found progenitor stem cells analogous to oval cells in diseased human liver [2].

We therefore studied the role of the c-*kit* receptor tyrosine kinase in oval cell development and the potential applications of oval cells in hepatocyte transplantation. Our results suggest that the c-*kit* receptor tyrosine kinase plays a crucial role in the appearance of oval cells in the rat 2-acetylaminofluorine/partial hepatectomy (AAF/PH) model, and that intrasplenic transplantation of oval cell-enriched hepatocytes may improve survival and proliferation of hepatocytes in the spleen.

Role of the *c-kit* Receptor Tyrosine Kinase in Oval Cell Development

We investigated the role of the c-*kit* receptor tyrosine kinase in oval cell development using Ws/Ws rats, which have severely impaired c-*kit* tyrosine kinase activity owing to a small deletion in the kinase domain [3]. Male Ws/Ws and +/+ rats (150–170 g) were purchased from Japan SLC (Hamamatsu, Shizuoka, Japan). For induction of oval cells, the rats were treated as described for generation of the AAF/PH model. Rats were administered AAF by gavage at a dosage of 10 mg/kg body weight daily for 4 days, and they then underwent a standard two-thirds PH on day 5. Starting from the day after PH, the rats were administered AAF at the same dosage daily for 5 days. They were killed on days 7, 9, and 13 after PH. Livers of +/+ and Ws/Ws rats were fixed in Zamboni's solution and embedded in paraffin. Serial sections (4 μm thick) were cut; one section was stained hematoxylin and eosin (Fig. 1). The number of oval cells was counted in 10 randomly selected periportal fields in each specimen stained with hematoxylin and eosin, and the result was expressed as the number of oval cells per periportal field ($0.25 \times 0.25\,mm^2$).

In the livers of +/+ rats, many oval cells were observed in the periportal areas and the surrounding parenchyma. In contrast, many fewer oval cells were observed in the livers of Ws/Ws rats. The numbers of oval cells found in Ws/Ws rats on days 7, 9, and 13 after PH were significantly reduced to 15%, 18%, and 27% of those in +/+ rats, respectively.

The proliferative activities of oval cells that developed in +/+ and Ws/Ws rats on days 7, 9, and 13 after PH were examined by [^{3}H]-thymidine incorporation and Ki-67 immunostaining. The percentage of oval cells labeled with [^{3}H]-thymidine in Ws/Ws rats was comparable with that in +/+ rats on days 7, 9, and 13 after PH. Moreover, there was no significant difference between +/+ and Ws/Ws rats in terms of the percentage of oval cells expressing Ki-67 antigen. The development of oval cells was only 15%–27% that of +/+ rats on days 7, 9, and 13 after PH. On the other hand, once oval cells appeared in Ws/Ws rats, they proliferated at a rate similar to that for +/+ rats, suggesting that the c-*kit* receptor tyrosine kinase is not essential for proliferation of oval cells.

To characterize the nature of oval cells that developed in Ws/Ws rats, liver sections of +/+ and Ws/Ws rats obtained on day 9 after PH were stained with AFP, CK19, or flt-3 RTK antibody. Oval cells of Ws/Ws rats expressed AFP, CK19, and flt-3 RTK, as was the case for +/+ rats. Thus, it is likely that the c-*kit* receptor tyrosine kinase is not

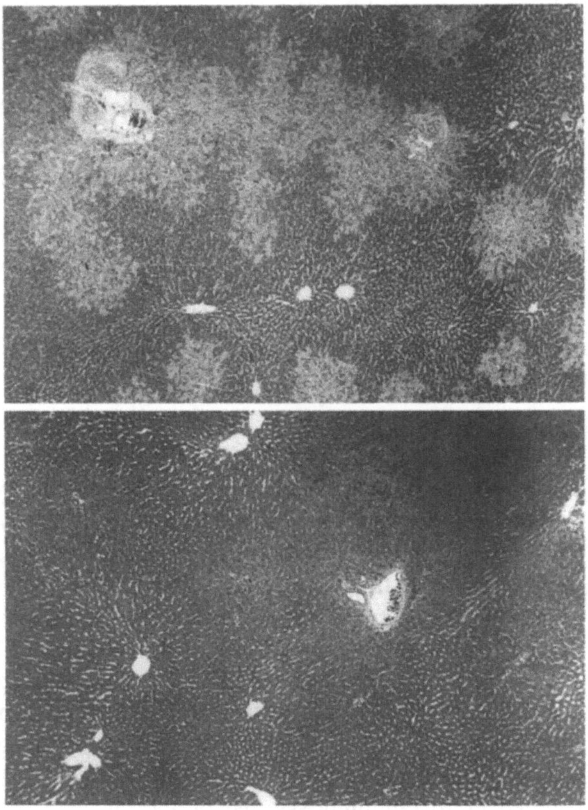

Fig. 1. Liver sections of +/+ and Ws/Ws rats on day 9 after partial hepatectomy (PH) in the 2-acetylaminofluorine (AAF)/PH model. **A** +/+ Rat. **B** Ws/Ws rat. Sections were stained with hematoxylin and eosin. Many oval cells can be seen in the section of the +/+ rat, but much fewer oval cells can be seen in the section of a Ws/Ws rat. (A, B ×30)

involved in regulating the expression of marker proteins (i.e., the phenotype of oval cells).

These results suggest that the c-*kit* receptor tyrosine kinase plays only a small role in determining the phenotype and proliferative activity of oval cells. However, the c-*kit* receptor tyrosine kinase appears to play a crucial role in the appearance of oval cells, at least in the rat AAF/PH model.

Role of Oval Cells in Rat Hepatocyte Transplantation

Orthotopic liver transplantation has become a therapeutic choice for treatment of acute or chronic liver failure and for congenital metabolic disorders, but its application is limited by organ availability. Therefore, transplantation of isolated hepatocytes could be an alternative therapy. Survival and function of isolated hepatocytes transplanted into various host organs have been examined, and the spleen and liver have been shown to be the most suitable places for transplantation. Previous studies have demonstrated that isolated adult rat hepatocytes transplanted into the spleens of syngeneic rats survive and maintain hepatocyte function for a long time. Studies have found progenitor stem cells analogous to oval cells in diseased human liver. Because liver with these cells could be the source of isolated hepatocytes for transplantation, it was of interest to examine intrasplenic transplantation of oval cell-enriched isolated liver cells [4].

Male Fisher 344 rats were purchased from Charles River Japan (Yokohama, Kanagawa, Japan) and were used for the experiments. Oval cell-free or oval cell-enriched isolated rat liver cells were transplanted into the spleens of syngeneic rats. Oval cell-free liver cells were obtained from livers of control untreated adult rats, and oval cell-enriched liver cells from livers of adult rats that had undergone AAF/PH treatment to induce oval cells. Liver cells were isolated from livers of control rats and AAF/PH-treated rats. Liver cells were isolated by collagenase digestion. Cell viability, as determined by trypan blue exclusion, was more than 85%. Isolated liver cells were stained for CK19 to estimate proportions of oval cells and biliary epithelial cells. The percentage of CK19-positive cells among liver cells isolated from AAF/PH-treated rats was 24.9% ± 1.6% (n = 5), whereas that in isolated liver cells of untreated rats was 0.12% ± 0.04% (n = 5). Isolated liver cells were suspended in Ca^{++}-free Hanks' balanced salt solution (HBSS) at 1×10^7 viable cells/0.4 ml, and 0.4 ml of the cell suspension was injected directly into the spleen of a syngeneic recipient rat. Hilar splenic vessels were clamped during intrasplenic injection, and the left branch of the portal vein was ligated after the intrasplenic injection. Recipient rats were given transplants of isolated liver cells; they were them killed at intervals of 2, 4, 8, 12, 16, 24, or 32 weeks after transplantation and their spleens removed and fixed in methacarn. To identify hepatocytes and biliary epithelial cells, the largest section of each spleen was stained with periodic acid-Schiff (PAS) (Fig. 2) and a CK19 antibody; and the numbers of PAS-positive and CK19-positive cells in these sections were counted.

The mean numbers of PAS-positive cells 2 weeks after transplantation were comparable to those in spleens given transplants of oval-cell-free liver cells. However, the numbers of PAS-positive cells in the spleens of rats transplanted with oval-cell-enriched liver cells at 4, 8, 12, 16, 24, and 32 weeks later were 2.3, 3.5, 4.5, 6.7, 6.3, and 15.1 times greater than those in spleens given transplants of oval-cell-free liver cells, respectively; these differences were statistically significant. The mean number of CK19-positive cells in spleens given transplants of oval-cell-free and oval-cell-

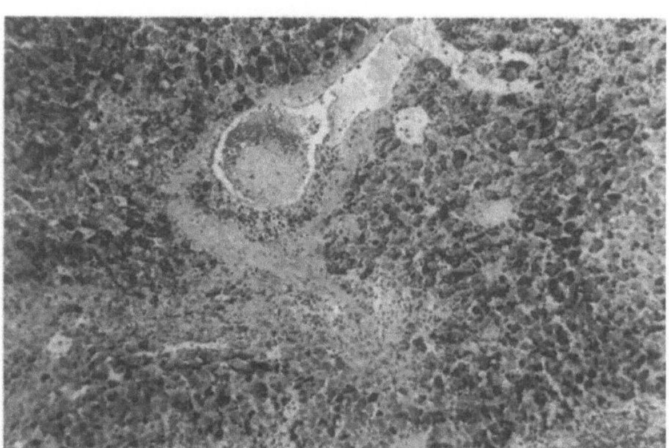

FIG. 2. Periodic acid-Schiff (PAS)-positive cells in the spleen received transplantation of isolated liver cells. A rat underwent intrasplenic transplantation of oval cell-enriched liver cells was killed 32 weeks after transplantation. (×60)

enriched liver cells increased markedly 4 weeks later and thereafter decreased rapidly with no significant differences between groups. Therefore, the initial increase in the number of biliary epithelial cells may reflect transient proliferation of contaminating bile epithelial cells or transient transformation of hepatocytes into biliary epithelial cells.

Conclusions

These results indicate an essential role of the c-*kit* receptor tyrosine kinase in the development of oval cells in the rat AAF/PH model. The c-*kit* receptor tyrosine kinase may be important in the commitment of hepatic stem cells to oval cell differentiation. Alternatively, the c-*kit* receptor tyrosine kinase may be involved in the maintenance of hepatic stem cells, and a reduction in their number may result in a decrease in the number of oval cells.

Studies have found progenitor stem cells analogous to oval cells in diseased human liver. Therefore, intrasplenic transplantation of oval cell-enriched hepatocytes obtained from these livers may improve survival and the proliferation of hepatocytes in the spleen.

References

1. Fujio K, Evarts PR, Hu Z, et al (1994) Expression of stem cell factor and its receptor, c-*kit*, during liver regeneration from putative stem cells in adult rat. Lab Invest 70:511–516
2. Roskams T, De Vos R, Eyken PV, et al (1998) Hepatic OV-6 expression in human liver disease and rat experiments: evidence for hepatic progenitor cells in man. J Hepatol 29:455–463
3. Satoshi M, Tohru T, Akihiro T, et al (1999) Role of c-kit receptor kinase in development of oval cells in the rat 2-acetylaminofluorine/partial hepatectomy model. Hepatology 29:670–676
4. Satoshi M, Akihiko T, Keiji N, et al (2000) The role of oval cells in rat hepatocyte transplantation. Transplantation 70:441–446

Hepatoma-Derived Growth Factor: Involvement in Liver Development and Regeneration

Hirayuki Enomoto*, Yoshihiko Kishima, Kenya Yoshida, and Hideji Nakamura

Summary. Hepatoma-derived growth factor (HDGF) is the first member of a new gene family that contains the HATH (homologous to the amino-terminus of HDGF) region in the N-terminal region and nuclear localization signals in the remaining parts of the sequence and traffic to the nucleus. HDGF was purified from the conditioned medium of HuH-7 hepatoma cells by DNA synthesis stimulating activity for Swiss 3T3 cells. HDGF stimulates the proliferation of endothelial cells, vascular smooth muscle cells, some hepatoma cells, and fibroblasts. HDGF is ubiquitously expressed in normal tissues, predominantly in testis, kidney, liver, heart, and brain. Recent studies have indicated that HDGF may play important roles in fetal organ development and tissue repair, such as renal glomerular formation and vascular smooth muscle cell proliferation during vascular development and neointima formation. HDGF was highly expressed in fetal liver and mainly in fetal hepatocytes with little expression in hematopoietic cells. HDGF expression in fetal hepatocytes decreased in accordance with the differentiation to mature hepatocytes. HDGF expression was significantly induced in regenerating liver after partial hepatectomy and drug-induced liver damage in adult liver. We assume that HDGF is significantly involved in liver development and regeneration.

Key words. HDGF (hepatoma-derived growth factor), HATH (homologous to the amino-terminus of HDGF) region, Fetal hepatocyte, Hepatogenesis, Liver regeneration

Introduction

To resolve clinical disorders in liver, it is important to elucidate the mechanism by which proliferation and differentiation of hepatocytes are regulated. Clarification of the molecular mechanisms of hepatogenesis and liver regeneration would give us new

Department of Molecular Medicine, Osaka University Medical School, 2-2 Yamadaoka, Suita, Osaka 565-0871, Japan
* e-mail: enomoto@imed3.med.osaka-u.ac.jp

insights into the treatment and management of acute and chronic hepatic failure, liver transplantation, the artificial liver, and so on. Furthermore, we would gain information about hepatic carcinogenesis and new tools to regulate the proliferation of hepatoma cells, as transformed cells lose the highly specific characteristics of mature hepatocytes and acquire automonous growth activity.

During liver development from the fetal stage to the newborn stage, immature hepatocytes differentiate and gain several metabolic functions specific to mature hepatocytes concomitant with a decrease in their proliferative activity. It is important to analyze this process of hepatocyte maturation during liver development so we can understand liver regeneration and malignant transformation. Indeed, recent studies have revealed that several factors, which have been supposed to be important in liver regeneration and hepatic carcinogenesis, play crucial roles in hepatogenesis.

Recently we identified a novel factor, hepatoma-derived growth factor (HDGF) from the human hepatoma-derived cell line HuH-7, which autonomously proliferates in a serum-free chemically defined medium [1]. Here we focus on this factor and its involvement in organ development and tissue repair, including the kidney, cardiovascular system, and liver.

HDGF: Novel Growth Factor in a New Gene Family

HDGF is a 26-kDa heparin-binding acidic glycoprotein consisting of 240 amino acids; it was purified from a conditioned medium of HuH-7 hepatoma cells. HDGF stimulates the proliferation of fibroblasts, endothelial cells, vascular smooth muscle cells, and some hepatoma cells, such as HuH-7, HLF, and HepG2 cells. Its primary sequence contains no signal peptide, no previously identified motif, and two putative nuclear localization signals. HDGF can traffic to the nucleus, indicating that HDGF is a unique factor belonging to the nuclear/growth factor family. HDGF was initially identified in human hepatoma-derived cells, although HDGF mRNA is ubiquitously expressed in various adult normal tissues as well as in tumor cell lines. HDGF is predominantly expressed in testis, kidney, liver, heart, brain, and skeletal muscle in adult mice and human. These findings suggest that HDGF not only significantly relates to the proliferation of cancer cells but also has some physiological functions in these normal organs.

We have found three other novel genes as well: *H*DGF- *r*elated *p*roteins (HRP). These proteins shared a highly homologous amino-terminal region consisting of about 100 amino acids, which we called HATH (homologous to the amino-terminus of HDGF) region. Lens epithelium-derived growth factor, which was reported to function as a survival factor for lens epithelium, contains a HATH region in its N-terminal region and seems to be a member of the HDGF family. We believe that HDGF and HRPs belong to a new gene family [2,3]. An HDGF family is characterized as follows: It contains a HATH region in the N-terminal region and nuclear localization signal(s) in the remaining parts of the sequence other than the HATH region, and it traffics to the nucleus.

HDGF: Involvement in Organ Development and Tissue Repair

HDGF expression is strikingly higher in fetal tissues than in adult tissues. Studies have indicated an important role of HDGF in organ development in the fetus and in tissue repair in adults. Oliver and Al-Awqati reported that an endothelial growth factor purified from the conditioned medium of a cell line of rat metanephrogenic mesenchymal cells was identical to HDGF [4]. By analyzing the expression pattern of HDGF in the developing kidney, they maintained that HDGF played an important role in glomerular capillary formation during nephron morphogenesis. Everett et al. demonstrated that HDGF was strongly expressed in proliferating vascular smooth muscle cells (SMCs) and endothelial cells in the fetus, in neointimal cells after endothelial injury, and in proliferating SMCs in human atherosclerotic lesions [5]. Exogenous HDGF and its endogenous overexpression stimulated the proliferation of vascular SMCs. These findings suggest that HDGF may regulate vascular SMC proliferation during cardiovascular development and neointimal formation.

We investigated whether HDGF was involved in liver development and regeneration. We found that HDGF was strongly expressed in immature hepatocytes of the fetal liver, and its expression was dramatically reduced near birth (Enomoto et al., in preparation) (Fig. 1). HDGF expression is reciprocal to the differentiation of hepatocytes, suggesting that HDGF is significantly related to the proliferation of hepatocytes. We also showed that HDGF was induced in two models of liver regeneration: after partial hepatectomy and with CCl_4-induced liver damage (Enomoto et al., in preparation). Endogenous overexpression of HDGF stimulates a significant increase in cell number and DNA synthesis in the hepatoblastoma-derived cell line HepG2 [Kishima Y et al., in preparation], suggesting that HDGF is involved in hepatobalst and possibly hepatocyte proliferation. We assume that HDGF plays an important role in liver development and regeneration, especially in hepatocyte proliferation.

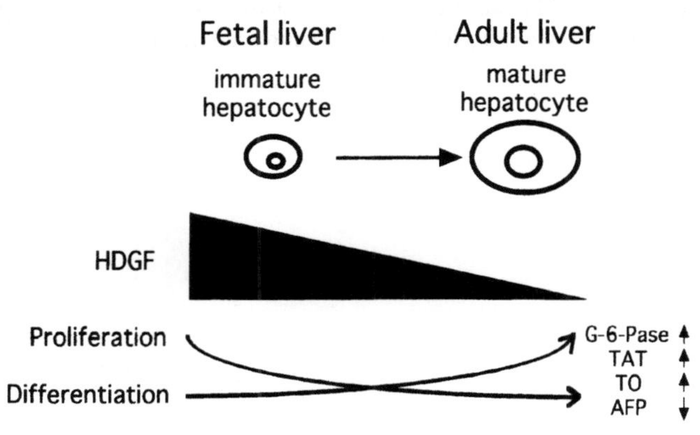

Fig. 1. Hepatoma-derived growth factor (*HDGF*) expression during hepatocyte differentiation. *G-6-Pase*, glucose-6-phosphatase; *TAT*, tyrosine aminotransferase; *TO*, tryptophan oxygenase; *AFP*, α-fetoprotein

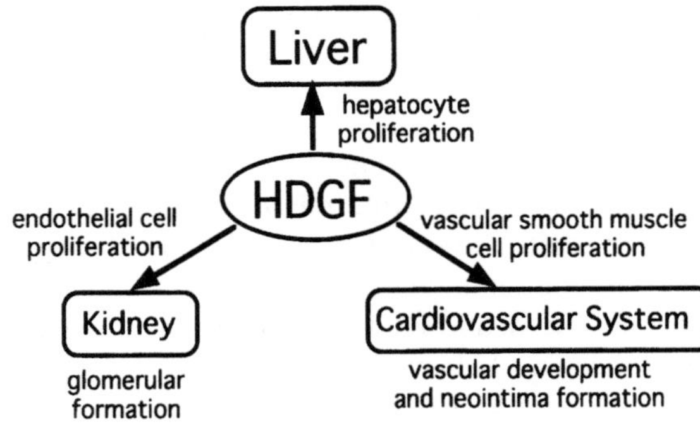

FIG. 2. Putative roles of HDGF in organ development and regeneration

Conclusions

HDGF is a novel nuclear/growth factor that belongs to a new gene family containing a HATH region in the N-terminal region and nuclear translocation signals. Studies suggest that HDGF is involved in organ development in the fetus and tissue repair in the adult, including especially the kidney, cardiovascular system, and liver (Fig. 2).

References

1. Nakamura H, Izumoto Y, Kambe H, et al (1994) Molecular cloning of complementary DNA for a novel human hepatoma-derived growth factor. J Biol Chem 269:25143–25149
2. Izumoto Y, Kuroda T, Harada H, et al (1997) Hepatoma-derived growth factor belongs to a gene family in mice showing significant homology in the amino terminus. Biochem Biophys Res Commun 238:26–32
3. Ikegame K, Yamamoto M, Kishima Y, et al (1999) A new member of a hepatoma-derived growth factor gene family can translocate to the nucleus. Biochem Biophys Res Commun 266:81–87
4. Oliver JA, Al-Awqati Q (1998) An endothelial growth factor involved in rat renal development. J Clin Invest 102:1208–1219
5. Everett AD, Lobe DR, Matsumura ME, et al (2000) Hepatoma-derived growth factor stimulates smooth muscle cell growth and is expressed in vascular development. J Clin Invest 105:567–575

Tumor Necrosis Factor and Liver Regeneration

Yasuhiro Yamada[1,2,*], Nelson Fausto[3], and Hisataka Moriwaki[1]

Summary. Liver has the remarkable ability to regenerate, but the mechanism of regeneration is still not well known. Liver resection or hepatocyte loss caused by viral or chemical injury initiates hepatocyte replication, whereas an enlarged liver mass is corrected by apoptosis. "Stem-like" cells proliferate when hepatocyte replication is blocked or delayed. Studies of the mechanisms that regulate liver growth have been done in animals subjected to partial hepatectomy (PH) or chemical injury. Liver regeneration can be divided into several phases, starting with expression of a large number of immediate early genes. Hepatocytes must be primed before they can fully respond to growth factors. Priming requires the cytokines tumor necrosis factor (TNF) and interleukin-6 (IL-6). At least four transcription factors (NF-κB, STAT3, AP-1, C/EBP) play major roles in the initiation of liver regeneration. TNF can initiate DNA replication after PH. It acts through a pathway that involves TNF receptor type 1 (TNFR-1), NF-κB, IL-6, and STAT3. We studied liver regeneration in TNFR-1, TNFR-2, and wild-type (WT) C57Bl/6 mice injected with carbon tetrachloride (CCl_4). Lack of TNFR-1 inhibited hepatocyte DNA synthesis after CCl_4 injection. TNFR-1 knockout mice had little detectable NF-κB and STAT3 binding after CCl_4 injection. In contrast, a lack of TNFR-2 did not differ significantly in WT mice regarding NF-κB and STAT3 binding, IL-6 and TNF levels, or hepatocyte replication. We conclude that a TNFR-1 signaling pathway involving NF-κB, IL-6, and STAT3 is an important component of the hepatocyte mitogenic response induced by CCl_4 injury in mouse liver.

Key words. Liver regeneration, Partial hepatectomy, Hepatic injury, Tumor necrosis factor, Transcription factors

[1] First Department of Internal Medicine, [2] Department of Laboratory Medicine, Gifu University School of Medicine, 40 Tsukasa-machi, Gifu 500-8705, Japan
[3] Department of Pathology, University of Washington School of Medicine, Box 357705, HSB-C517, Seattle, WA 98105, USA
* e-mail: yshiro@cc.gifu-u.ac.jp

Introduction

The liver has a remarkable ability to regulate its growth and mass in humans and animals. This property is particularly unique because hepatocytes, in their normal state, rarely divide; but the proliferative capacity and the ability of liver to adapt to variable metabolic demands are not lost. These properties are quickly displayed when a deficit or excess of hepatic mass occurs. Many conditions altera the liver mass, by increasing or decreasing it. Deficits are brought about by surgical removal of tissue or cell loss (functional deficit without loss of mass) caused by chemicals or viruses and, more rarely, other agents. Partial hepatectomy, resulting in removal of approximately 70% of the liver, is widely utilized for studies of liver growth in experimental animals. Segmental or lobar resections are performed in humans to remove tumors and for transplantation from living donors. For all of the conditions mentioned, quiescent hepatocytes proliferate and replicate to restore the liver functional capacity and its mass in cases of tissue resection. Functional capacity, however, is a relative rather than an absolute parameter.

The set point for growth regulation is the ratio between the liver mass and the body mass, not the liver mass alone. Liver regeneration is a multistep process with at least two critical steps: transition of the quiescent hepatocyte into the cell cycle (priming), and progression beyond the restriction point during the G_1 phase of the cycle. We propose that these steps are under separate controls: priming by tumor necrosis factor (TNF) and interleukin-6 (IL-6) family cytokines and cell cycle progression by the growth factors hepatocyte growth factor (HGF) and transforming growth factor-α (TGFα). It was thought that hepatocyte proliferative capacity during liver regeneration after hepatectomy indicated that hepatocytes divide once or twice and return to quiescence [1]. Recent experiments on the repopulation of damaged livers and serial transplantation studies have demonstrated that, on the contrary, hepatocytes have a high replication capacity, comparable to or exceeding that of precursor cells of proliferative tissues.

Molecular Mechanisms of Liver Regeneration

An understanding of the events that trigger liver regeneration has been pursued for almost a century and was given special emphasis by the description of a reproducible technique for 70% partial hepatectomy in rats by Higgins and Anderson in 1931 [2]. Study of the initiation of liver regeneration has gone through various phases, and the subject has been analyzed by physiological, biochemical, morphological, and molecular approaches. Individual gene analyses, to be meaningful, must be integrated into an understanding of the relations between liver and whole-organism functions, the interactions between parenchymal and nonparenchymal cells, and the complex network signaling that is activated during liver regeneration.

A large number of genes are either newly expressed or increase their expression after partial hepatectomy. Placing the patterns of expression of these many genes into phases facilitates our understanding the molecular events of liver regeneration. Analysis applies to liver regeneration in rats and mice and probably also to humans. However, there are interesting differences in the timing of cell cycle progression for rats and mice. Although well described, the reasons for these differences remain unclear. In rats, DNA replication after partial hepatectomy starts at approximately 14h and reaches a maximum at 24h. In mice, both the start and the peak of DNA replication are about 20h slower. The differences in the timing of DNA replication in rats and mice are a reflection of a longer G_1 phase in mice because the early events of gene activation after partial hepatectomy occur within 4h in both rodent species. There have been no reported studies of the timing of these events after partial hepatectomy in humans, but human hepatocytes in culture respond to the same growth factors as rodent cells.

Early Genes

The first phase of gene expression after partial hepatectomy, referred to as the immediate early phase, occurs rapidly after the operation and lasts approximately 4h. The proto-oncogenes *c-fos*, *c-jun*, and *c-myc* were the first genes to be identified in this group [3,4]. As many as 70 genes participate in the immediate early response to partial hepatectomy [5]. These genes do not share a common function and include, among others, transcription factors, tyrosine phosphatases, and secreted and intracellular metabolic proteins [6]. It is a difficult and important challenge to determine which among these many genes play essential roles in hepatocyte replication, but substantial progress has been made in the identification of some of these genes.

Transcription Factors Activated After Partial Hepatectomy

Transcription factors are proteins that bind specific recognition sites in genes to initiate or enhance their transactivation. Thus, transcription factors can propagate signals by activating many genes, and interactions between transcription factors provide another level of regulation for transactivating specific genes. An important advance in understanding liver regeneration was the finding that the transcription factors NF-κB, AP-1, C/EBP, and STAT3 are activated after partial hepatectomy [7–9]. Activation of these factors does not require protein synthesis, being dependent instead on posttranslation mechanisms. Several reviews have discussed these factors in detail. Here, only the role NF-κB and STAT3 may play in cytokine signaling for hepatocyte replication is highlighted.

Originally identified in B lymphocytes ("nuclear factor for the kappa chain of B cells"), NF-κB is found in almost every cell type, including hepatocytes and nonparenchymal cells. After partial hepatectomy, NF-κB is activated rapidly, within 30min. The activation is transient and is no longer present after 5h [7]. The transcription factor STAT3 is also activated after partial hepatectomy, but the activation is slower than that of NF-κB and the mechanism of activation entirely different. STAT3 is detectable in the liver 1–2h after partial hepatectomy, and the activation lasts 4–6h, as determined by gel shift assays [8]. So far, seven mammalian STAT genes have been cloned. STAT3 is activated mainly by interleukin-6 (IL-6) type cytokines. STAT3 is phosphorylated and translocated to the nucleus, where it regulates expression of a large number of genes, including those involved in inflammation, the acute-phase response, and proliferation.

Growth Factors HGF and TGFα

The expression of immediate early and delayed genes in liver regeneration does not lead to DNA replication unless the cells can progress through the cell cycle. This is accomplished by growth factors such as HGF and TGFα [10].

Liver Regeneration as a Multistep Process: Priming and Cell Cycle Progression

Given the enormous complexity of gene expression in the regenerating liver, it is essential to know how the process starts and how the transcription factor and gene activation events are regulated and coordinated. We hypothesized that gene activation (priming) is required for hepatocytes to go from quiescence to the G_1 phase of the cell cycle. During early G_1, the cells fully respond to growth factors and can then progress through the cell cycle, overcome the G_1 restriction point, and undergo DNA replication. Among the transcription factors activated after partial hepatectomy, we selected NF-κB for study. When searching for agents that could trigger NF-κB activation as an initiating event for liver regeneration, we found that TNF was a potent liver NF-κB inducer in animals [7]. TNF is a multifunctional cytokine that signals through two distinct receptors, TNFR-1 (p55) and TNFR-2 (p75). In the liver it acts as a mediator of the acute-phase response and is a cytotoxic agent in many types of hepatic injury. Akerman et al. [11] showed that administration of anti-TNF antibodies inhibited liver regeneration after partial hepatectomy in rats, suggesting that TNF may be necessary for hepatocyte proliferation.

We approached this problem by studying liver regeneration after partial hepatectomy or CCl_4 injury in knockout mice deficient in TNFR-1 or TNFR-2 [12–14]. Mice lacking functional TNFR-2 showed completely normal DNA replication and liver mass gain after partial hepatectomy, although activation of AP-1 and C/EBP was delayed. Regeneration after CCl_4 injury was also normal in these animals, indicating that TNFR-2 signaling is not essential for these growth processes. In contrast, lack of signaling through TNFR-1 greatly inhibited DNA replication after partial hepatectomy and caused significant mortality after the operation. In TNFR-1 knockouts, activation of NF-κB and STAT3 was severely inhibited, and AP-1 activation was decreased. TNF and IL-6 increase in the blood quickly after partial hepatectomy in normal animals. TNF also increases in TNFR-1 knockouts, but there is only a small change in IL-6. A single injection of IL-6 reversed the defect in liver regeneration in TNFR-1 knockouts and restored STAT3 activation. Cressman et al. [15], working with IL-6 knockout mice, showed that liver regeneration is impaired in these animals and that an IL-6 injection corrected the deficits in DNA replication and STAT3 activation after partial hepatectomy.

The work with TNFR-1 and IL-6 knockout mice and with anti-TNF antibodies demonstrates that TNF signaling through TNFR-1 is required for liver regeneration after partial hepatectomy. This signaling pathway follows the sequence TNF → TNFR-1 → NF-κB → IL-6 → STAT3. The same pathway is involved in regeneration of the liver after CCl_4 injury. The regenerative response of TNFR-1 knockout mice after CCl_4 administration was much slower than that of normal animals, but no increased mortality was apparent. The proliferative and antiapoptotic effect of these cytokines takes place only under special conditions, such as those existing after partial hepatectomy.

Future Perspectives

Knowledge about the proliferative capacity of hepatocytes and the mechanisms of liver regeneration has evolved rapidly during the last few years. In great part, but not exclusively, these advances are based on the development of genetically engineered mice in which specific genes are inserted or inactivated. We now know that mature hepatocytes have astounding proliferative capacity, and that both proliferation and apoptosis can be triggered by a single agent (TNF). The overall view of liver regeneration brought about by recent studies is that it is a multistep growth process with at least two limiting steps, regulated by different mediators.

The advances in our knowledge of hepatocyte replication described above have obvious clinical applications. Hepatocyte transplantation for treatment of liver or metabolic disease has a much brighter prospect with the knowledge that these cells may remain proliferative for a long time and that they can be stimulated to proliferate by growth factors. Infusion of growth factors preceded by administration (intrahepatic if possible) of TNF could greatly increase the effect of HGF, TGFα, or epidermal growth factor (EGF) on the growth of small transplanted livers and the repopulation of hepatocytes after massive acute injury. Finally, the hepatoprotective effects of HGF and the antiapoptotic role of IL-6 and other cytokines are topics that remain to be explored for potential clinical applications.

References

1. Fausto N (1996) Hepatic regeneration. In: Zakim D, Boyer TD (eds). Hepatology: a textbook of liver disease. Saunders, Philadelphia, pp. 32–58
2. Higgins GM, Anderson RM (1931) Experimental pathology of the liver. I. Restoration of the liver of the white rat following partial surgical removal. Arch Pathol 12:186–202
3. Thompson NL, Mead JE, Braun L, et al (1986) Sequential protooncogene expression during rat liver regeneration. Cancer Res 46:3111–3117
4. Morello D, Fitzgerald MJ, Babinet C, et al (1990) c-Myc, c-fos, and c-jun regulation in the regenerating livers of normal and H2K/c-myc transgenic mice. Mol Cell Biol 10:3185–3193
5. Haber AH, Mohn KL, Diamond RH, et al (1993) Induction patterns of 70 genes during nine days after hepatectomy define the temporal course of liver regeneration. J Clin Invest 91:1319–1326
6. Taub R (1996) Transcriptional control of liver regeneration. FASEB J 10:413–427
7. FitzGerald M, Webber E, Donovan J, et al (1995) Rapid DNA binding by nuclear factor κB in hepatocytes at the start of liver regeneration. Cell Growth Differ 6:417–427
8. Cressman DE, Diamond RH, Taub R (1995) Rapid activation of the Stat3 transcription complex in liver regeneration. Hepatology 21:1443–1449
9. Diehl AM, Yang SQ (1994) Regenerative changes in C/EBPα C/EBPβ expression modulate binding to the C/EBP site in the c-fos promoter. Hepatology 19:447–456
10. Fausto N, Laird AD, Webber EM (1995) Role of growth factors and cytokines in hepatic regeneration. FASEB J 9:1527–1536

11. Akerman P, Cote P, Yang SQ, et al (1992) Antibodies to tumor necrosis factor-α inhibit liver regeneration after partial hepatectomy. Am J Physiol 263:G579–G585
12. Yamada Y, Fausto N (1998) Deficient liver regeneration after carbon tetrachloride injury in mice lacking type 1 but not type 2 tumor necrosis factor receptor. Am J Pathol 152:1577–1589
13. Yamada Y, Kirillova I, Peschon JJ, et al (1997) Initiation of liver growth by tumor necrosis factor: Deficient liver regeneration in mice lacking type I tumor necrosis factor receptor. Proc Natl Acad Sci USA 94:1441–1446
14. Yamada Y, Webber EM, Kirillova I, et al (1998) Analysis of liver regeneration in mice lacking type 1 or type 2 tumor necrosis factor receptor: Requirement for type 1 but not type 2 receptor. Hepatology 28:959–970
15. Cressman DE, Greenbaum LE, DeAngelis RA, et al (1996) Liver failure and defective hepatocyte regeneration in interleukin-6-deficient mice. Science 274:1379–1383

Heparin-Binding EGF-Like Growth Factor: Hepatotrophic Factor in Liver Regeneration

SHINICHI KISO*, SHINJI TAMURA, and SUMIO KAWATA

Summary. The role of heparin-binding epidermal growth factor-like growth factor (HB-EGF) as a hepatotrophic factor in liver regeneration is discussed. HB-EGF is a member of the EGF family that binds to the EGF receptor (EGF-R) and is a potent mitogen for hepatocytes. Levels of HB-EGF mRNA were increased during rat liver regeneration, starting at an early phase (1.5 h) after partial hepatectomy, well before the production of hepatic hepatocyte growth factor (HGF) or transforming growth factor-α (TGFα) mRNA. The induction of HB-EGF mRNA level was detected in non-parenchymal cells, mainly Kuppfer cells and sinusoidal endothelial cells, after partial hepatectomy but was negligible in the hepatocytes. Hepatic HB-EGF may play an important role in the early stages of liver regeneration after partial hepatectomy via a paracrine mechanism. HB-EGF also increases in the regenerating rat liver after injury from hepatotoxins such as CCl_4 and D-galactosamine. In addition, when mice were injected with exogenous HB-EGF, the labeling index in the liver after hHB-EGF injection was low but significantly increased compared to control mice, indicating that exogenous hHB-EGF stimulated DNA synthesis in hepatocytes in vivo. In human subjects, plasma HB-EGF levels increased, reaching maximal levels approximately 5–7 days after gross hepatectomy (lobectomy and segmentectomy). These results indicate that HB-EGF serves as a hepatotrophic factor in vivo.

Key words. Heparin-binding epidermal growth factor-like growth factor (HB-EGF), Liver regeneration, Hepatectomy, HGF, TGFα

Introduction

A number of growth factors have been implicated in the regulation of liver growth after partial hepatectomy and toxic liver injury [1,2]. Among there are hepatocyte growth factor (HGF), transforming growth factor-α (TGFα), epidermal growth factor (EGF), acidic fibroblast growth factor (aFGF), and TGFβ [1,2].

Department of Internal Medicine and Molecular Science, Graduate School of Medicine, Osaka University (B5), 2-2 Yamadaoka, Suita, Osaka 565-0871, Japan
* e-mail: kiso@imed2.med.osaka-u.ac.jp

The purification of heparin-binding EGF-like growth factor (HB-EGF), a member of the EGF family, was initially reported from a conditioned medium of U-937 macrophage-like cells [3]. The coding sequence of human HB-EGF cDNA predicts a precursor molecule that contains 208 amino acids and is comprised of a signal peptide, a hydrophilic domain with an affinity for heparin, an EGF-like domain, and a transmembrane domain [4]. Cleavage of the precursor protein yields a mature protein containing at least 86 amino acids and comprised of an EGF-like domain and a basic region that is responsible for heparin binding. HB-EGF binds to the EGF receptor (EGF-R) and is a potent mitogen for vascular smooth muscle cells and fibroblasts [5]. In this paper, we summarize the role of HB-EGF as a hepatotrophic factor in liver regeneration.

Effects of HB-EGF on DNA Synthesis of Hepatocytes in Primary Culture

HB-EGF was found to stimulate DNA synthesis of hepatocytes in primary culture in a dose-dependent manner at least up to 30 ng/ml [6,7]. The maximal stimulation by HB-EGF accounted for more than 80% of that induced by HGF [6,7]. The in vitro interaction between HB-EGF and HGF on DNA synthesis of hepatocytes in primary culture was investigated, and the data show that HB-EGF stimulates DNA synthesis in hepatocytes additively to the hepatotrophic effect of HGF [6].

Changes in HB-EGF, HGF, and TGFα mRNA Levels in Regenerating Rat Liver After Partial Hepatectomy

To examine the role of HB-EGF as a hepatotrophic factor in liver regeneration in vivo, the regulation of HB-EGF gene expression during liver regeneration after partial hepatectomy was investigated [8]. The level of HB-EGF mRNA in regenerating liver increased 1.5 h after partial hepatectomy, reaching a maximum at 6 h (prior to the peak of DNA synthesis after partial hepatectomy) [8]. HB-EGF mRNA levels increased in nonparenchymal cells (mainly Kuppfer cells and sinusoidal endothelial cells) but not in hepatocytes 6 h after partial hepatectomy [8]. These findings suggest that HB-EGF might play an important role as a hepatotrophic factor during the early stage of regenerating liver via a paracrine mechanism.

Expression of HB-EGF in Rat Liver Injured by Treatment with Hepatotoxins

To clarify the role of HB-EGF in liver regeneration after liver injury, the expression of HB-EGF in rat liver injured by treatment with the hepatotoxins such as CCl_4 or D-galactosamine was investigated. HB-EGF mRNA levels were significantly increased in rat liver injured by hepatotoxins [9]. These increases in HB-EGF levels appeared to play a role in hepatocyte replication in the injured rat liver, as they had for rat liver regeneration after partial hepatectomy.

Effects of Exogenous Human HB-EGF on DNA Synthesis in Normal Mouse Liver Hepatocytes

The mitogenic effects and activation of transcription factors caused by exogenous human HB-EGF (hHB-EGF) were examined in mouse liver [10]. The mean labeling index for hepatocytes of hHB-EGF-injected mice was 2.6%, a significant increase over that for saline-injected controls (< 0.01%). By exogenous hHB-EGF injection, the activation of transcription factors such as nuclear factor (NF)-κB and activator factor (AP)-1 was observed in the liver as the result of injecting exogenous hHB-EGF. Intravenously injected hHB-EGF had a limited but clearly measurable effect on DNA synthesis in mouse liver hepatocytes. HB-EGF may serve as a hepatotrophic factor in vivo.

Interaction Between HB-EGF and Other Growth Factors (HGF and TGFα)

HB-EGF was added to isolated hepatocytes and nonparenchymal liver cells in primary culture to test the possibility that HB-EGF is a mediator of the production of HGF and TGFα in the regenerating liver. Expression of the HGF gene in nonparenchymal liver cells and of the TGFα gene in hepatocytes was induced to a significant extent by adding HB-EGF to the medium. These results suggest that HB-EGF may be a mediator for expression of the HGF and TGFα gene in the regenerating liver after partial hepatectomy. Indeed HGF gene expression in the liver was found to be induced in the exogenously hHB-EGF-injected mice, as evidenced by Northern blot analysis [10].

Human Plasma HB-EGF Levels in Patients After Partial Hepatectomy as Determined with an Enzyme-Linked Immunosorbent Assay

In 14 patients who underwent a partial hepatectomy, plasma HB-EGF levels were measured serially after surgery [11]. In the case of patients who had undergone gross hepatectomy (lobectomy and segmentectomy), plasma HB-EGF levels were increased, reaching maximal levels approximately 5–7 days after surgery. In the case of patients who had undergone minor hepatectomy (subsegmentectomy), plasma HB-EGF levels did not increase. The maximal plasma HB-EGF levels were significantly higher in patients whose volume of remaining liver (%ILV) increased more than 20% compared to those who had a %ILV of less than 20% (32.4 ± 19.6 vs. 7.4 ± 2.7 pg/ml; $p < 0.05$).

Expression of HB-EGF During Hepatocarcinogenesis

As mentioned above, the HB-EGF gene is mainly expressed in Kuppfer cells and sinusoidal endothelial cells, but not in hepatocytes in regenerating rat liver after partial hepatectomy. However, in the fibrotic rat liver HB-EGF was observed in some of the hepatocytes [12]. It has been reported that glutathione S-transferase P (GST-P) is expressed when hepatocytes undergo neoplastic transformation. Immunohistochemical localization of HB-EGF and GST-P protein in fibrotic liver revealed a similar pattern. Therefore, the possibility that HB-EGF is produced in transformed hepatocytes during hepatocarcinogenesis cannot be excluded [12]. We reported that the expression of HB-EGF can occur in human hepatocellular carcinoma (HCC) [13]. It has been reported that expression of HB-EGF mRNA in the liver was low during the acute and chronic hepatitis stages, and it was markedly increased at the hepatoma stage in LEC (Long-Evans with cinnamon-like coat color) rats, which spontaneously develop acute hepatitis at 12–16 weeks of age, followed by chronic hepatitis and eventually hepatoma [14]. Thus, HB-EGF may also play a role in the development or progression of HCC.

Conclusions

HB-EGF may be an important growth factor, produced during an early phase rather than HGF, in the regenerating rat liver after partial hepatectomy via a paracrine mechanism. Plasma HB-EGF levels were increased in patients who had undergone gross hepatectomy. Plasma HB-EGF may be a marker for liver regeneration after partial hepatectomy in humans. Furthermore, during hepatocarcinogenesis the expression of HB-EGF may occur as hepatocytes are transformed to a neoplastic phenotype. HB-EGF may also play a role in the development or progression of HCC.

References

1. Michalopoulos GK, DeFrances MC (1997) Liver regeneration. Science 276:60–66
2. Fausto N, Laird AD, Webber EM (1995) Liver regeneration. 2. Role of growth factors and cytokines in hepatic regeneration. FASEB J 9:1527–1536
3. Higashiyama S, Abraham JA, Miller J, et al (1991) A heparin-binding growth factor secreted by macrophage-like cells that is related to EGF. Science 251:936–939
4. Thompson SA, Higashiyama S, Wood K, et al (1994) Characterization of sequences within heparin-binding EGF-like growth factor that mediate interaction with heparin. J Biol Chem 269:2541–2549
5. Higashiyama S, Lau K, Besner GE, et al (1992) Structure of heparin-binding EGF-like growth factor: multiple forms, primary structure, and glycosylation of the mature protein. J Biol Chem 267:6205–6212
6. Ito N, Kawata S, Tamura S, et al (1994) Heparin-binding EGF-like growth factor is a potent mitogen for rat hepatocytes. Biochem Biophys Res Commun 198:25–31
7. Kiso S, Kawata S, Tamura S, et al (1994) Alteration in growth regulation of hepatocytes in primary culture obtained from cirrhotic rats: poor response to transforming growth factor-β1 and interferons. Hepatology 20:1303–1308
8. Kiso S, Kawata S, Tamura S, et al (1995) Role of heparin-binding epidermal growth factor-like growth factor as a hepatotrophic factor in rat liver regeneration after partial hepatectomy. Hepatology 22:1584–1590
9. Kiso S, Kawata S, Tamura S, et al (1996) Expression of heparin-binding EGF-like growth factor in rat liver injured by carbon tetrachloride or D-galactosamine. Biochem Biophys Res Commun 220:285–288
10. Kiso S, Kawata S, Tamura S, et al (1999) Effects of exogenous human heparin-binding epidermal growth factor-like growth factor on DNA synthesis of hepatocytes in normal mouse liver. Biochem Biophys Res Commun 259:683–687

11. Yamada A, Kawata S, Tamura S, et al (1998) Plasma heparin-binding EGF-like growth factor levels in patients after partial hepatectomy as determined with an enzyme-linked immunosorbent assay. Biochem Biophys Res Commun 246:783–787
12. Kiso S, Kawata S, Tamura S, et al (1999) Expression of heparin-binding epidermal growth factor-like growth factor in the hepatocytes of fibrotic rat liver during hepatocarcinogenesis. J Gastroenterol Hepatol 14:1203–1209
13. Inui Y, Higashiyama S, Kawata S, et al (1994) Expression of heparin-binding epidermal growth factor in human hepatocellular carcinoma. Gastroenterology 107:1799–1804
14. Miyoshi E, Higashiyama S, Nakagawa T, et al (1996) High expression of heparin-binding EGF-like growth factor in rat hepatocarcinogenesis. Int J Cancer 68:215–218

Effects of Growth Stimulatory and Inhibitory Factors on Signal Transduction of Cultured Rat Hepatocyte and the Regulation of Cyclin D1 Transcription

A. Moriuchi*, A. Ido, S. Hirono, T. Nakama, M. Ochiai, T. Hori, K. Hayashi, and H. Tsubouchi

Summary. Signal transductions induced by growth factors, such as hepatocyte growth factor (HGF) and epidermal growth factor (EGF), and the growth inhibitory factor such as transforming growth factor-β (TGFβ), have been successfully identified as being transduced to cell cycle molecules such as cyclin and cyclin-dependent kinase. Signal transduction in hepatocytes cultured with several growth-stimulatory and growth-inhibitory factors remains unclear. In addition, transcriptional factors regulating cyclin D1 gene expression, which are induced by growth factors, were not identified. In this study, we found that both HGF and EGF additively enhanced mitogen-activated protein kinase (MAPK) activity, and cyclin D1 and cyclin E gene expression resulted in increases in DNA synthesis in primary cultured rat hepatocytes with an additive manner. We also found that TGFβ1 inhibited cyclin E gene expression with no effect on HGF- and/or EGF-induced MAPK activity and cyclin D1 gene expression, resulting in complete inhibition of HGF- and/or EGF-induced DNA synthesis. We isolated the rat cyclin D1 genome containing –5 kb 5′-flanking region and found two possible regions responsible for transcriptional factors in the cyclin D1 promoter.

Key words. HGF, EGF, TGFβ, Signal transduction, Cyclin D1

Introduction

Hepatocyte growth factor (HGF), transforming growth factor (TGF)-α and heparin-binding epidermal growth factor-like growth factor (HB-EGF) are likely to play an important role in liver regeneration as hepatotrophic factors. The specific receptor for HGF is c-Met, and TGFα and HB-EGF share the epidermal growth factor receptor

Department of Internal Medicine II, Miyazaki Medical College, Kiyotake, Miyazaki 889-1692, Japan

* e-mail: kaito@post.miyazaki-med.ac.jp

(EGFR). The proliferative signal in both receptors is mediated by the Ras/MAPK system or phosphatidyl inositol 3-kinase. On the other hand, both TGFβ and activin terminate liver cell growth. Although the effects of each growth factor and each growth inhibitory factor have been reported, the details of their interactions in signal transduction are still unknown. In addition, growth factor-induced transcriptional factor for the cyclin D1 gene remains unclear. In the present study, we examined the signal transduction of rat hepatocytes cultured with HGF, EGF, or both and the effects of TGFβ on HGF- and/or EGF-stimulated signal transduction. We also isolated rat cyclin D1 gene and analyzed transcriptional activity using the 5′-flanking region of the gene.

Tyrosine Phosphorylation of c-Met and EGFR in Rat Hepatocytes Cultured with HGF, EGF, or Both in the Presence and Absence of TGFβ1

Rat hepatocytes in primary culture were incubated with HGF, EGF, or both in the presence and absence of TGFβ1. DNA synthesis was enhanced markedly in the primary cultured rat hepatocytes that were treated simultaneously with HGF and EGF. TGFβ1 completely suppressed HGF- or EGF-induced DNA synthesis (or both). The tyrosine phosphorylation of c-Met and EGFR was measured by Western blot analysis. The tyrosine phosphorylation of c-Met and EGFR was induced in primary cultured rat hepatocytes treatment with HGF and EGF, respectively. Addition of TGFβ1 did not affect HGF- and/or EGF-induced tyrosine phosphorylation of c-Met and EGFR.

MAPK Activity in Rat Hepatocytes Cultured with HGF or EGF in the Presence and Absence of TGFβ1

The Ras/MAPK system is thought to be a main pathway of HGF- and EGF-induced signal transduction for cell proliferation, and two mammalian MAPKs (ERK1 and ERK2) are ubiquitously expressed in vertebrates. We measured MAPKs (ERK1 plus ERK2) activity in rat hepatocytes cultured with HGF, EGF, or both in the presence and absence of TGFβ1, using the MAPK assay kit. MAPK activity in rat hepatocytes cultured with HGF and EGF was increased, and MAPK in rat hepatocytes cultured with a combination of HGF and EGF was higher than that with HGF or EGF alone. MAPK activity induced by HGF, EGF, or both in primary cultured rat hepatocyte was not influenced by the presence of TGFβ1.

Expression of Cyclin D1 and Cyclin E mRNAs in Rat Hepatocytes Cultured with HGF or EGF in the Presence and Absence of TGFβ1

The cell cycle is regulated by cyclins, cyclin-dependent kinase (Cdk), and Cdk inhibitors. The progression of cell cycles requires Cdk activation. Cyclin D1, the most important G1 cyclin, is associated with Cdk4 and Cdk6 and is related to progress at

TABLE 1. Effects of growth factors on signal transduction and expression of G1 cyclin in cultured rat hepatocytes

Parameter	Growth factors			
	HGF	EGF	HGF EGF	HGF EGF TGFβ1
Phosphorylation of c-Met/EGFR	+/−	−/+	+/+	+/+
MAPK activity	+	+	++	+/+
Cyclin D1 mRNA expression	+	+	++	++
Cyclin E mRNA expression	+	+	+	−

HGF, human growth factor; EGF, epidermal growth factor; TGFβ1, transforming growth factor β1

the G_1/S checkpoint. Association of cyclin E with Cdk2 is required for G_1/S transition. Thus, we examined the expression of cyclin D1 and cyclin E mRNAs in rat hepatocytes cultured with HGF, EGF, or both in the presence and absence of TGFβ1. The levels of cyclin D1 and cyclin E mRNAs in primary cultured rat hepatocytes were increased by HGF and EGF treatment. The cyclin D1 mRNA levels in rat hepatocytes cultured with a combination of HGF and EGF was greater than those in rat hepatocytes cultured with HGF or EGF alone. Addition of TGFβ1 did not affect the cyclin D1 mRNA level in rat hepatocytes cultured with HGF, EGF, or both. However, the addition of TGFβ1 significantly suppressed the cyclin E mRNA level in rat hepatocytes that had been previously increased by HGF and EGF treatment. These findings indicate that TGFβ1 inhibits cell growth between cyclin D1 and cyclin E in the HGF- and EGF-induced proliferative signal transduction. TGFβ1 induces Cdk inhibitors, such as p21, p15, and p16, which are potentially involved in the inhibitory effect on cell growth. We summarize these results in Table 1.

Isolation and Transcriptional Regulation of Rat Cyclin D1 Gene

The mechanism of growth factor-induced transcriptional regulation of cyclin D1 remains unclear. To analyze transcriptional factors of cyclin D1, which is induced by growth factors such as HGF, we isolated the rat cyclin D1 gene containing a −5 kb 5′-flanking region relative to the cap site and exons 1, 2, and 3. Transcriptional activity was found in two regions (−0.8 kb and −60 bp) upstream of the rat cyclin D1 gene in dRLh84 rat hepatoma cells by a transient transfection assay.

Conclusions

Simultaneous treatment with HGF and EGF synergistically enhanced MAPK activity, cyclin D1 mRNA, and cyclin E mRNA in rat hepatocytes in primary culture, resulting in additive enhancement of DNA synthesis. However, TGFβ1 suppressed HGF- and

EGF-induced cyclin E mRNA expression in cultured rat hepatocytes, with no effects on MAPK activity or cyclin D1 mRNA expression; and it completely inhibited HGF- and EGF-induced DNA synthesis. We isolated the rat cyclin D1 genome containing a −5 kb 5′-flanking region and found two possible regions responsible for the transcriptional factor in the cyclin D1 promoter.

References

1. Jo M, Stolz DB, Esplen JE, et al (2000) Cross-talk between epidermal growth factor receptor and c-Met signal pathways in transformed cells. J Biol Chem 275:8806–8811
2. Fausto N (2000) Liver regeneration. J Hepatol 32(Suppl 1):19–31
3. Talarmin H, Rescan C, Cariou S, et al (1999) The mitogen-activated protein kinase kinase/extracellular signal-regulated kinase cascade activation is a key signaling pathway involved in the regulation of G(1) phase progression in proliferating hepatocytes. Mol Cell Biol 19:6003–6011
4. Geng Y, Whoriskey W, Park MY, et al (1999) Rescue of cyclin D1 deficiency by knockin cyclin E. Cell 97:767–777

Significance of the Relation Between Hepatocyte Growth Factor and Transforming Growth Factor-α in Hepatocyte Proliferation

TOMOAKI TOMIYA[1,*] and KENJI FUJIWARA[2]

Summary. Transforming growth factor-α (TGFα) and hepatocyte growth factor (HGF) can stimulate DNA synthesis in hepatocytes in vitro and in vivo. These factors are thought to play significant roles in liver regeneration. The expression of HGF and TGFα mRNA has been reported to increase sequentially in regenerating rat liver. We studied the significance of the relation between these factors in liver regeneration. Serum levels of HGF increased before a detectable increase of serum TGFα when measured in patients who had undergone partial hepatectomy and those suffering from acute hepatitis. Similarly, hepatic and circulating levels of HGF increased prior to an increase in TGFα levels in rats after partial hepatectomy and in rats with acute liver injury induced by CCl_4 treatment. In cultured rat hepatocytes, TGFα levels and DNA synthesis increased in response to HGF addition to the medium. However, DNA synthesis by hepatocytes was suppressed when TGFα activity was reduced by the addition of either antisense TGFα mRNA oligonucleotide or anti-TGFα rabbit immunoglobulin G to the medium. Furthermore, the number of mitotic hepatocytes was decreased by the administration of anti-TGFα antibody to rats after partial hepatectomy even though these rats showed increased hepatic HGF levels. Together, these finding suggest that the interaction between the activities of HGF and TGFα may play a role in the regulation of hepatocyte proliferation.

Key words. TGFα, HGF, Hepatocyte proliferation, Anti-TGFα antibody, Antisense TGFα mRNA oligonucleotide

Introduction

Many agents act as mitogens for hepatocytes in vitro. The expression of several of these mitogens is reported to increase in the regenerating rat liver. The increases in

[1] Department of Gastroenterology, Faculty of Medicine, The University of Tokyo, 7-3-1 Hongo, Bunkyo-ku, Tokyo 113-8655, Japan
[2] Third Department of Internal Medicine, Saitama Medical School, 38 Morohongo, Moroyama-cho, Iruma-gun, Saitama 350-0495, Japan
* e-mail: tomiya-lim@h.u-tokyo.ac.jp

their expression are generally uniform regardless of the models of liver regeneration examined, suggesting a significant relation between these factors. Furthermore, previous in vitro experiments showed a possible communication between growth factors in regulating cell proliferation. The secretion of transforming growth factor-α (TGFα) by cultured rat hepatocytes has been reported to be enhanced by the addition of epidermal growth factor (EGF), TGFα, or hepatocyte growth factor (HGF) to the medium. In addition, TGFα mRNA expression is stimulated by TGFα in human colon carcinoma cells and by HGF in human pancreatic cancer cells. The mitogenic effects of HGF and TGFα have been shown to be additive in cultured fetal and adult hepatocytes.

A communication between HGF and the TGFα/EGF receptor systems has now been reported in rat liver epithelial cells. The TGFα/EGF receptor and c-*met*, the HGF receptor, are tyrosine kinases that autophosphorylate, as well as phosphorylate, to activate other enzymes. The src-homology regions of activated c-*met* and the TGFα/EGF receptor are reported to bind to different downstream signal transduction elements, suggesting that HGF and TGFα, via their receptors, stimulate unique targets. These observations highlight the significance of overlapping growth factor activities and the communication between growth factors in cell growth, suggesting the importance of further research. HGF and TGFα can stimulate hepatocyte proliferation in vivo and in vitro, and they are thought to play critical roles in liver regeneration. Here, we report the significance of the relation between HGF and TGFα in hepatocyte proliferation.

Serum HGF and TGFα Levels in Patients After Partial Hepatectomy and in Patients with Acute Hepatitis

We examined serum HGF and TGFα levels in patients who demonstrated liver regeneration under different clinical conditions [1–4]. In patients that had undergone partial hepatectomy the serum HGF levels increased, reaching maximum levels within 7 days after surgery. The serum HGF levels in these patients returned to preoperative levels 28 days after surgery. Serum TGFα levels also increased within 28 days in patients after partial hepatectomy and reached maximum levels later than the serum HGF levels. The TGFα levels at 28 days remained significantly higher than those before surgery. The maximum levels achieved in each case correlated significantly with the resected volume of the liver and the increased volume of the remaining liver 28 days after surgery.

In patients suffering from acute hepatitis, serum HGF levels reached the maximum level earlier than the maximum serum TGFα levels (mean ± SD of the period between the onset of the symptoms to the day when serum levels reached the maximum: 20 ± 17 days for HGF versus 29 ± 20 days for TGFα; $P < 0.05$). In these patients the maximum serum HGF levels were positively correlated with the maximum serum TGFα levels. In addition, serum TGFα levels were correlated with maximum serum alanine aminotransferase (ALT) levels. Considering that the extent of liver regeneration is dependent on the degree of the liver damage, serum TGFα levels may correlate with the degree of liver regeneration in patients with acute hepatitis.

Together, these results suggest that serum TGFα levels were increased in relation to the extent of liver regeneration, and after the increase of serum HGF levels in the patients.

TGFα and HGF Levels After Partial Hepatectomy and After Intoxication with CCl_4 in Rats

To confirm a relation between the increase in both HGF and TGFα levels and hepatocyte proliferation during liver regeneration in humans, we examined the circulating and hepatic levels of both HGF and TGFα in two different rat models of liver regeneration [5]. Partial hepatectomy induces a compensatory hyperplasia of the remaining liver with minimal necrosis. In contrast, intoxication with CCl_4 induces a compensatory hepatic hyperplasia following liver necrosis due to direct damage to hepatocytes.

The mitotic index of hepatocytes was unchanged until 18h after partial hepatectomy, then increased to a maximum level by 24h. By approximately 120h, the mitotic index had decreased to preoperative levels, although a small increase was noted at 72h. Hepatic and plasma levels of HGF were significantly increased at 6h after the partial hepatectomy, reached the maximum levels around 18h, and returned to preoperative levels at 48h. Hepatic and serum levels of TGFα were significantly increased at 12h after the partial hepatectomy, reached the maximum at 24h. Thereafter it decreased in a manner similar to the hepatocyte mitotic index.

In rats treated with CCl_4, serum ALT levels increased to peak levels on day 1 after intoxication. Hepatic and plasma levels of HGF increased in a manner similar to the serum ALT. The hepatocyte mitotic index and the hepatic and serum levels of TGFα peaked on day 3 after CCl_4 intoxication.

Together, these findings show that the hepatic and circulating HGF levels are increased in rats during liver regeneration, followed by increased TGFα levels in the liver and blood that is closely related to hepatocyte proliferation. These observations are consistent with the results obtained in the study described above using patients who had undergone partial hepatectomy or suffered from acute hepatitis.

Effect of Inhibiting TGFα Activity on DNA Synthesis in Rat Hepatocytes Cultured in the Presence of HGF

To clarify the significance of the relation between the increases of HGF and TGFα on hepatocyte proliferation, we examined the effect of inhibiting the action of TGFα on DNA synthesis in rat hepatocytes cultured in the presence of HGF. When HGF was added to the medium at increasing concentrations, cultured rat hepatocytes increased their TGFα content in a dose-related manner. A similar dose-related response was observed in DNA synthesis by hepatocytes treated with HGF. The addition of antisense TGFα mRNA oligonucleotides to the medium reduced these increases in TGFα expression and DNA synthesis. The increase in DNA synthesis by cultured hepatocytes in the presence of HGF was also reduced by the addition of anti-TGFα rabbit immunoglobulin G (IgG), which did not recognize other ligands for the TGFα/EGF receptor, such as EGF or HB-EGF. These observations suggest that TGFα expression by cultured hepatocytes is stimulated by HGF, and that the suppression of TGFα activity reduces the increase in DNA synthesis by hepatocytes in the presence of HGF.

Effect of Anti-TGFα Rabbit IgG on Hepatocyte Proliferation After Partial Hepatectomy in Rats

To examine whether suppression of TGFα activity reduces hepatocyte proliferation in vivo, we administered the anti-TGFα antibody to rats after partial hepatectomy. The rats showed increased hepatic and circulating levels of HGF and TGFα after partial hepatectomy, as mentioned above. Partially hepatectomized rats treated with either normal rabbit IgG or anti-TGFα rabbit IgG increased hepatic HGF levels in a manner comparable to that obtained when rats were dosed with the vehicle alone. However, the increased mitotic index of hepatocytes observed 24 h after partial hepatectomy was suppressed by administration of anti-TGFα rabbit IgG compared with rats administered normal rabbit IgG. These results suggest that the specific suppression of TGFα activity in hepatocytes during liver regeneration may reduce the regenerative proliferation of hepatocytes in rats.

Conclusions

When hepatic and circulating levels of HGF were increased during liver regeneration, they were followed by increases in hepatic and serum levels of TGFα. HGF stimulated TGFα production by cultured rat hepatocytes. Furthermore, the mitogenic activity of HGF on rat hepatocytes was, at least in part, dependent on endogenous TGFα. Together, these findings suggest that the relation between HGF and TGFα activities may play a role in the regulation of hepatocyte proliferation.

References

1. Tomiya T, Nagoshi S, Fujiwara K (1992) Significance of serum human hepatocyte growth factor levels in patients with hepatic failure. Hepatology 15:1–4.
2. Tomiya T, Tani M, Yamada S, et al (1992) Serum hepatocyte growth factor levels in hepatectomized and nonhepatectomized surgical patients. Gastroenterology 103:1621–1624
3. Tomiya T, Fujiwara K (1993) Serum levels of transforming growth factor-α in patients after partial hepatectomy as determined with an enzyme-linked immunosorbent assay. Hepatology 18:304–308
4. Tomiya T, Fujiwara K (1996) Liver regeneration in fulminant hepatitis as evaluated by serum transforming growth factor α levels. Hepatology 23:253–257
5. Tomiya T, Ogata I, Fujiwara K (1998) Transforming growth factor α levels in liver and blood correlate better than hepatocyte growth factor with hepatocyte proliferation during liver regeneration. Am J Pathol 153:955–961

Part 12
Hepatic Fibrosis Research and Its Application to Therapy

Transcriptional Regulation of Type I Collagen Gene Expression by Transforming Growth Factor-β and Smad Proteins

Yutaka Inagaki[1,*], Tomoyuki Nemoto[2], and Atsuhito Nakao[3]

Summary. Increased production of type I collagen is a common hallmark of fibrotic diseases in various organs including the liver. This increase is exerted mainly at the level of transcription, and transforming growth factor-β (TGFβ) is the key factor in stimulating gene transcription. We have previously shown that the −313 to −183 upstream sequence of α2(I) collagen gene (*COL1A2*) is essential for basal and TGFβ-stimulated transcription in skin fibroblasts and hepatic stellate cells. We designated this region the TGFβ-responsive element (TbRE) and revealed that a ubiquitous *trans*-activator Sp1 and unknown nuclear factor(s) bind to this region to mediate the stimulatory effect of TGFβ. Experiments using transgenic mice harboring the −313 *COL1A2* promoter have revealed that the promoter is activated in a cell type-specific manner during hepatic fibrogenesis in vivo. Smad proteins have been recently identified as mediators of intracellular signal transduction of TGFβ superfamily members. One of them, Smad3 is shown to bind to the TbRE and is implicated in mediating TGFβ-elicited stimulation of *COL1A2* transcription.

Key words. Collagen gene, Transcriptional regulation, Hepatic fibrogenesis, TGFβ, Smad

Introduction

Collagen represents a family of proteins involved not only in the maintenance of organ architecture and tissue integrity but also in the developmental program and tissue repair process. There is a dynamic balance between production and degradation of collagen and alteration of this equilibrium results in excessive collagen deposition or

[1] Department of Internal Medicine and Clinical Research Institute, National Kanazawa Hospital, 1-1 Shimoishibiki-machi, Kanazawa 920-8650, Japan
[2] Fourth Division, Osaka Bioscience Institute, 6-2-4 Furuedai, Suita, Osaka 565-0874, Japan
[3] Allergy Research Center, Juntendo University School of Medicine, 2-1-1 Hongo, Bunkyo-ku, Tokyo 113-8421, Japan
* e-mail: inagaki@kinbyou.hosp.go.jp

inadequate tissue integrity. Irrespective of the initial stimuli, fibrosis in various organs including liver is caused by a chronic, uncontrolled inflammatory/repair process leading to excessive deposition of collagen and other components of extracellular matrix (ECM).

Type I collagen, the major ECM component in fibrotic liver is a heterotrimer composed of coordinately expressed two α1 chains and one α2 chain. They are encoded by distinct genes, *COL1A1* and *COL1A2*, respectively, and transforming growth factor-β1 (TGFβ1: henceforth referred to as TGFβ) is a key factor in stimulating gene expression mainly at the level of transcription. Recently, a family of proteins termed Smad has been identified as intracellular mediators of TGFβ signal transduction. This chapter gives a brief summary of our work, which is aimed at clarifying the molecular pathogenesis underlying hepatic fibrogenesis.

Regulation of *COL1A2* Transcription by TGFβ

Hepatic stellate cells (HSCs) are considered to be the major source of collagen in fibrotic liver. We have previously identified the *COL1A2* upstream sequence spanning from −313 to −183 that mediates the stimulatory effect of TGFβ on gene transcription in skin fibroblasts [1] and HSCs [2]. We designated this region the TGFβ-responsive element (TbRE). Within the TbRE are at least two sites of DNA–protein interaction, box 3A and box B. TGFβ modifies the interaction between a ubiquitous *trans*-activator Sp1 bound to box 3A and unknown factor(s) bound to box B, which in turn increases the binding of Sp1 to box 3A (Fig. 1) [1,4].

TGFβ treatment of primary cultures of skin fibroblasts markedly stimulated *COL1A2* transcription and increased binding of both Sp1 and box B-bound factors [1]. By contrast, *COL1A2* transcription in activated HSC clones derived from a cirrhotic liver had less response to exogenous TGFβ, and their nuclear extracts contained large amounts of Sp1 and cofactors bound to the TbRE in an untreated condition [2]. TGFβ treatment did not affect protein binding to the TbRE in the cells [2], suggesting that *COL1A2* transcription in activated HSCs is already stimulated and exhibits low responsiveness to exogenous TGFβ.

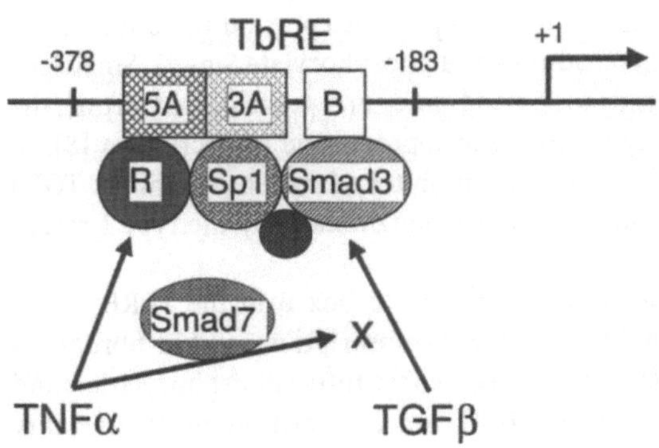

FIG. 1. *cis*-Acting DNA elements and *trans*-acting nuclear factors modulating *COL1A2* transcription and their regulation by transforming growth factor-β (*TGFβ*) and tumor necrosis factor-α (*TNFα*). A recent study [3] showed that CCAAT/enhancer binding protein β is the major component of the box *5A*-bound complex. *TbRE*, TGFβ-responsive element; *R*, repressor protein(s) bound to box *5A*

Activation of *COL1A2* Promoter During Hepatic Fibrogenesis

The results of cell transfection and DNA binding assays using cultured HSCs may not be fully applicable to hepatic fibrogenesis in vivo. We therefore sought further confirmation in transgenic mice harboring *COL1A2* upstream sequences containing the TbRE. Transgenic mouse lines were generated using the −313 to +58 *COL1A2* promoter linked to a bacterial β-galactosidase gene (*LacZ*) [5].

Following repeating carbon tetrachloride (CCl_4) injections, the *COL1A2* promoter seemed to be activated mainly in mesenchymal cells located in necrotic areas and around fibrous septa. Because *LacZ* expression driven by the −313 *COL1A2* promoter was rather weak, the identity of the *LacZ*-expressing cells was further confirmed by isolating parenchymal and nonparenchymal cell fractions and by culturing HSCs. The results indicated that the *COL1A2* promoter was utilized only in nonparenchymal cells, and that the activity was significantly higher in the cells from CCl_4-treated mice than in those from untreated animals [5]. Interestingly, TGFβ treatment increased the promoter activity and the amount of endogenous *COL1A2* mRNA in HSCs from untreated, but not CCl_4-treated, mice [5]. We concluded that the −313 *COL1A2* promoter is activated in a cell type-specific manner during hepatic fibrogenesis in vivo and confirmed that increased *COL1A2* transcription in activated HSCs does not respond to exogenous TGFβ.

Increased collagen gene expression and insensitiveness to TGFβ were mimicked during the activation process of primary culture of HSCs to myofibroblasts [6]. It has been also reported that *COL1A2* transcription level in cultured scleroderma fibroblasts is higher than in normal skin fibroblasts obtained from the same patients, and that administration of exogenous TGFβ into culture media does not increase *COL1A2* transcription in the disease cells [7]. It appears that increased collagen gene transcription, which does not respond to exogenous TGFβ, is the common feature of pathologically activated collagen-producing cells.

Role of Smad Proteins in *COL1A2* Transcription

Smad proteins play critical roles in mediating intracellular signals of TGFβ superfamily members. Following TGFβ binding to the type II receptor on the cell surface, type I and type II receptors form a heterodimer and phosphorylate Smad2, Smad3, or both. Phosphorylated Smad2/3 bind to Smad4 and are translocated from the cytoplasm to the nucleus, where they stimulate or repress gene transcription [8]. In contrast to those Smads, Smad7 is known as an inhibitory Smad, as it inhibits TGFβ signaling by interfering with phosphorylation of Smad2/Smad3 by the type I receptor kinase [9].

It has been recently reported that Smad3 can bind to box B in the TbRE and is implicated in mediating TGFβ-stimulated *COL1A2* transcription in skin fibroblasts (Fig. 1) [10,11]. Our preliminary data demonstrated constitutive phosphorylation and nuclear localization of Smad3 in an activated HSC clone, correlating the abnormality in TGFβ/Smad signaling with pathologically activated collagen gene transcription in HSCs.

We have previously shown that the counterrepression of *COL1A2* transcription by tumor necrosis factor-α (TNFα) is mediated through the TbRE, as well as by increasing the amount of repressor protein(s) bound to the immediately upstream box 5A (Fig. 1) [12]. This original observation has been supported by a recent study demonstrating induction of inhibitory Smad7 and suppression of TGFβ/Smad signaling by TNFα/NF-κB [13].

References

1. Inagaki Y, Truter S, Ramirez F (1994) Transforming growth factor-β stimulates α2(I) collagen gene expression through a *cis*-acting element that contains an Sp1 binding site. J Biol Chem 269:14828–14834
2. Inagaki Y, Truter S, Greenwel P, et al (1995) Regulation of the α2(I) collagen gene transcription in fat-storing cells derived from a cirrhotic liver. Hepatology 22:573–579
3. Greenwel P, Tanaka S, Penkov D, et al (2000) Tumor necrosis factor alpha inhibits type I collagen synthesis through repressive CCAAT/enhancer-binding proteins. Mol Cell Biol 20:912–918
4. Greenwel P, Inagaki Y, Hu W, et al (1997) Sp1 is required for the early response of α2(I) collagen to transforming factor-β1. J Biol Chem 272:19738–19745
5. Inagaki Y, Truter S, Bou-Gharios G, et al (1998) Activation of proα2(I) collagen promoter during hepatic fibrogenesis in transgenic mice. Biochem Biophys Res Commun 250:606–611
6. Dooley S, Delvoux B, Lahme B, et al (2000) Modulation of transforming growth factor β response and signaling during transdifferentiation of rat hepatic stellate cells to myofibroblasts. Hepatology 31:1094–1106
7. Kikuchi K, Hartl CW, Smith EA, et al (1992) Direct demonstration of transcriptional activation of collagen gene expression in systemic sclerosis fibroblasts: insensitivity to TGF-β1 stimulation. Biochem Biophys Res Commun 187:45–50
8. Nakao A, Imamura T, Souchenlnytskyi S, et al (1997) TGF-β receptor-mediated signalling through Smad2, Smad3 and Smad4. EMBO J 16:5353–5362
9. Nakao A, Afrakhte M, Moren A, et al (1997) Identification of Smad7, a TGFβ-inducible antagonist of TGF-β signalling. Nature 389:631–635
10. Chen S-J, Yuan W, Mori Y, et al (1999) Stimulation of type I collagen transcription in human skin fibroblasts by TGF-β: involvement of Smad 3. J Invest Dermatol 112:49–57
11. Chen S-J, Yuan W, Lo S, et al (2000) Interaction of Smad3 with a proximal Smad-binding element of the human α2(I) procollagen gene promoter required for transcriptional activation by TGF-β. J Cell Physiol 183:381–392
12. Inagaki Y, Truter S, Tanaka S, et al (1995) Overlapping pathways mediate the opposing actions of tumor necrosis factor-α and transforming growth factor-β on α2(I) collagen gene transcription. J Biol Chem 270:3353–3358
13. Bitzer M, von Gersdorff G, Liang D, et al (2000) A mechanism of suppression of TGF-β/SMAD signaling by NF-κB/RelA. Genes Dev 14:187–197

Clinical Usefulness of Plasma MMP-9 Assay Compared with the Plasma MMP-2 Assay in Patients with Chronic Liver Disease

Yoshikazu Murawaki*, Yujiro Ikuta, Kinya Okamoto, Masahiko Koda, and Hironaka Kawasaki

Summary. Gelatinases [matrix metalloproteinases (MMP-2 and MMP-9)] are involved in liver fibrosis through degradation of the basement membrane. Recently we showed that the serum MMP-2 assay was useful for diagnosing liver cirrhosis (LC). Our present aim was to examine the clinical usefulness of the plasma MMP-9 test for liver fibrosis compared to the plasma MMP-2 test. We measured the plasma MMP-9 and MMP-2 concentrations in 35 patients with chronic hepatitis (CH), 28 patients with LC, and 21 healthy controls. The plasma MMP-9 and MMP-2 levels were significantly increased in patients with LC but not in patients with CH. The liver MMP-9 and MMP-2 concentrations was significantly higher in cirrhotic livers than in noncirrhotic livers. The plasma MMP-9 and MMP-2 levels were strongly correlated with blood markers for assessing fibrosis and were closely related to the histological degree of liver fibrosis, but these relations were weaker for the plasma MMP-9 test than for the plasma MMP-2 test. Receiver operating curve analysis showed that the plasma MMP-9 test was inferior to the plasma MMP-2 test for diagnosing LC.

Key words. MMP-9, MMP-2, Gelatinase A, Gelatinase B, Liver cirrhosis

Introduction

Matrix metalloproteinase-2 (MMP-2) (gelatinase A) and MMP-9 (gelatinase B) are involved in liver fibrosis through degradation of the basement membrane [1]. Recently we reported that the serum MMP-2 level was increased in patients with liver cirrhosis (LC) owing to overproduction in the cirrhotic liver, and that the serum MMP-2 assay was a useful test for diagnosing LC [2]. Although MMP-9 has substrate profiles similar to those of MMP-2, MMP-9 has some properties different from MMP-2 in terms of the activation mechanism of proenzymes, inhibition by tissue inhibitor of metalloproteinases (TIMP), and stimulating factors [3,4]. The aim of the present study

Second Department of Internal Medicine, Tottori University School of Medicine, Yonago, Tottori 683-8504, Japan
* e-mail: murawaki@grape.med.tottori-u.ac.jp

was to examine the clinical usefulness of the plasma MMP-9 test in chronic liver disease compared with that of the plasma MMP-2 test.

Materials and Methods

Patients. The subjects of this study were 21 healthy controls, 11 patients with minimal chronic hepatitis (CH), 13 patients with mild CH, 11 patients with moderate CH, and 28 patients with LC. Informed consent was obtained from each subject before blood collection was performed.

Assays for MMP-9 and MMP-2. The MMP-9 and MMP-2 concentrations were measured with a corresponding sandwich enzyme immunoassay (Fuji Chemical Industries, Takaoka, Japan). The MMP-9 assay detects proMMP-9 and proMMP-9/TIMP-1 with the same degree of immunoreactivity but not active MMP-9 or active MMP-9/TIMPs. The MMP-2 assay detects proMMP-2 and proMMP-2/TIMP-2 with the same degree of reactivity but not active MMP-2 or active MMP-2/TIMPs.

Measurement of Liver MMP-9 and MMP-2 Content. Liver samples obtained postmortem from cirrhotic patients (n = 16) and noncirrhotic patients with malignant disease (n = 10) were rinsed with sterilized saline and frozen at –70°C until analyzed. The extraction of MMPs from the livers was carried out as described by us elsewhere [2].

Statistical Analysis. The statistical significance of differences between groups was assessed by an analysis of variance (ANOVA) and Scheffe's test. The relations were evaluated by linear regression analysis.

Results

The mean plasma MMP-9 concentration was 41% higher in the presence of minimal CH, 61% higher in mild CH, 58% higher in moderate CH, and 204% higher in LC compared with the mean of the controls. The mean plasma MMP-2 concentration was 26% higher in minimal CH, 37% higher in mild CH, 38% higher in moderate CH, and 146% higher in LC. Compared with the controls, the plasma levels of MMP-9 and MMP-2 were significantly increased in the patients with LC but not in the patients with CH (Fig. 1).

The MMP-9 and MMP-2 concentrations in the cirrhotic livers (MMP-9, 17.9 ± 13.7 ng/mg protein; MMP-2, 24.4 ± 7.4 ng/mg protein) were significantly higher than those in the noncirrhotic livers (MMP-9, 3.7 ± 1.9 ng/mg; MMP-2, 5.4 ± 1.3 ng/mg). Although these liver concentrations were positively correlated with the liver collagen content, the correlation coefficient of MMP-9 ($r = +0.379$, $P < 0.05$) was weaker than that of MMP-2 ($r = +0.705$, $P < 0.0001$).

The plasma MMP-9 and MMP-2 concentrations were significantly correlated with serum levels of 7S fragment of IV collagen (PIVNP) and hyaluronan (MMP-9: $r = 0.670$, $P < 0.0001$ for PIVNP and $r = 0.704$, $P < 0.0001$ for hyaluronan; MMP-2: $r = 0.796$, $P < 0.0001$ for PIVNP and $r = 0.827$, $P < 0.0001$ for hyaluronan). The plasma MMP-9

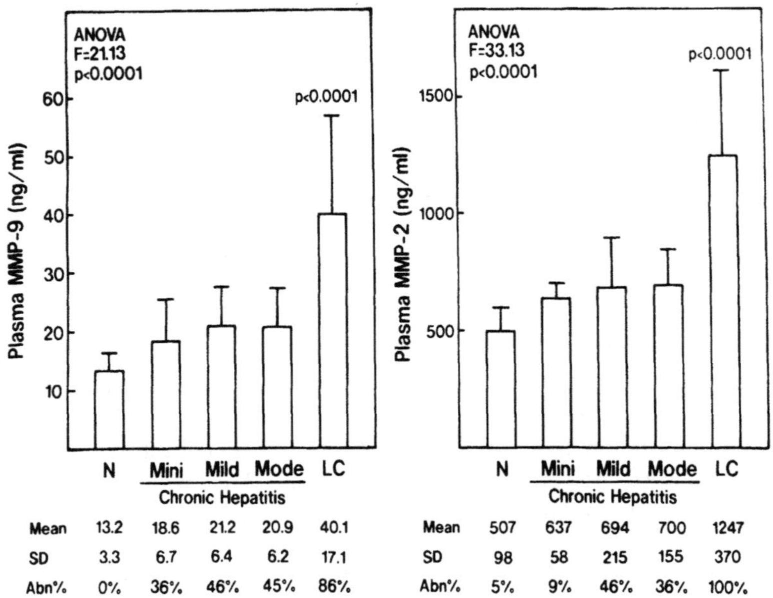

FIG. 1. Plasma levels of matrix metalloproteinases (*MMP-9, MMP-2*) in 21 controls (*N*) and 63 patients with chronic viral liver disease [11 minimal chronic hepatitis (CH) (*Mini*), 13 mild CH (*Mild*), 11 moderate CH (*Mode*), 28 liver cirrhosis (*LC*)]. *Abn%*, abnormal percentage above the normal upper limit

and MMP-2 levels were significantly related to the histological degrees of liver fibrosis (ANOVA: $F = 7.033$, $P < 0.001$ for MMP-9 and $F = 12.253$, $P < 0.0001$ for MMP-2). These relations were weaker for the plasma MMP-9 test than for the plasma MMP-2 test.

We compared the utility of the plasma MMP-9 and MMP-2 tests for diagnosing LC using receiver operating curves in CH and LC patients (Fig. 2). The best cutoff values for plasma MMP-9 and MMP-2 were 25 and 800 ng/ml, respectively. The sensitivity of the plasma MMP-9 test was 75% and the specificity 77%, whereas the sensitivity of the plasma MMP-2 test was 86% and the specificity 86%. The plasma MMP-9 test was thus less useful than the plasma MMP-2 test.

Discussion

The gelatinases MMP-2 and MMP-9 have degradative activity against native type IV collagen, so they play an important role in the remodeling and turnover of the basement membrane [1]. Although MMP-2 and MMP-9 have virtually identical substrate profiles, they also have some different properties in their activation mechanisms and in their inhibition by TIMP [3,4]. MMP-2 and MMP-9 are secreted as the corresponding proenzyme, which preferentially forms a complex with TIMP-2 or TIMP-1, respectively. ProMMP-2 is activated by the membrane type (MT) MMP family, whereas proMMP-9 is activated by serine proteinases such as plasmin or by MMP-3 and

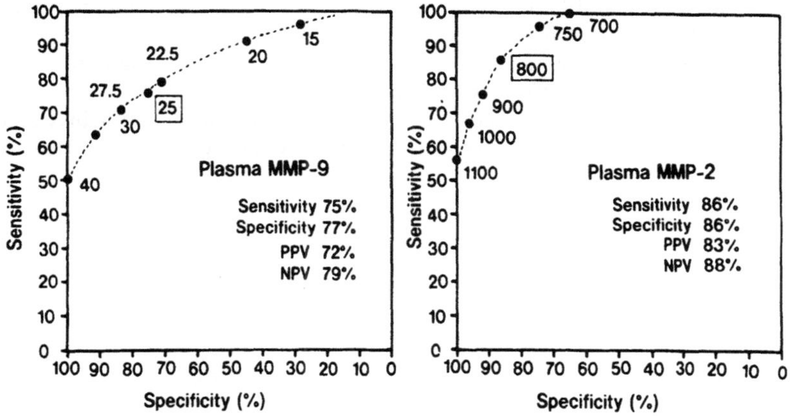

FIG. 2. Receiver operating curves of the plasma MMP-9 and MMP-2 tests for differentiating liver cirrhosis from chronic hepatitis. *PPV*, positive predictive value; *NPV*, negative predictive value

MMP-13. In this study, we found that plasma MMP-9 levels were increased in LC patients, as were plasma MMp-2 levels.

In the liver, the main cellular source of MMP-2 is hepatic stellate cells, and overexpression of MMP-2 mRNA has been demonstrated in fibrotic livers [1]. MMP-9 in the liver is produced mainly by Kupffer cells [1]. Although expression of MMP-9 mRNA is reported to be low in fibrotic livers [5], gelatin zymography analysis has shown that MMP-9 activity is increased in chronically diseased livers [1]. In the present study, similar to the MMP-2 concentration [2], the liver MMP-9 concentration was markedly increased in cirrhotic livers. Therefore, it appears that the increased plasma levels of MMP-9 and MMP-2 in cirrhotic patients can be explained by overproduction in the cirrhotic liver.

The plasma levels of MMP-9 and MMP-2 were significantly correlated with serum levels of PIVNP and hyaluronan, which are associated with the extent of liver fibrosis and might have value as a predictor of cirrhosis. In addition, these plasma levels were closely related with the histological degree of liver fibrosis. However, the relations of plasma MMP-9 were weaker than those of plasma MMP-2. These differences between the plasma MMP-9 and MMP-2 results may be due to differences of their expression in diseased livers. The gene expression pattern of MMP-9 is regulated differently from that of MMP-2; that is, expression of MMP-2 is up-regulated mainly by transforming growth factor-β1, whereas expression of MMP-2 is induced by tumor necrosis factor-α, interleukin-1, and so on [3,4]. Indeed, the plasma MMP-9 test was less accurate than the plasma MMP-2 test for diagnosing LC.

References

1. Arthur MJP (1994) Degradation of matrix proteins in liver fibrosis. Pathol Res Pract 190:825–833
2. Murawaki Y, Yamada S, Ikuta Y, et al (1999) Clinical usefulness of serum matrix metalloproteinase-2 concentration in patients with chronic viral liver disease. J Hepatol 30:1090–1098

3. Corcoran ML, Hewitt RE, Kleiner DE Jr, et al (1996) MMP-2: expression, activation and inhibition. Enzyme Protein 49:7–19
4. French DL, Ramos-DeSimone N, Rozinski K, et al (1994) Matrix metalloproteinase-9 in tumor cell invasion. Ann NY Acad Sci 732:324–334
5. Lichtinghagen R, Steinmetz C, Pehle B, et al (1999) Matrix metalloproteinases in liver and serum in chronic active hepatitis C and HCV-induced cirrhosis. Hepatol Res 14:119–134

Molecular Mechanisms of Matrix Metalloproteinase-1 Gene Expression in Hepatic Stellate Cells

Shigenari Hozawa[1,*], Haruko Suzuki[1], Sachiko Kagawa[1], Ayako Higuchi[1], Tetsu Watanabe[1], Hiromasa Ishii[2], and Isao Okazaki[1]

Summary. The molecular mechanisms of matrix metalloproteinase-1 (*MMP-1*) gene expression in hepatic stellate cells (HSCs) have not yet been clarified. Transcriptional factors that regulate *MMP-1* gene expression in other cell types are mostly associated with HSC activation. Therefore, signaling for HSC activation such as by Rho guanosine triphosphatases is thought to be closely related to *MMP-1* gene expression.

Key words. Matrix metalloproteinase-1 (*MMP-1*), Gene expression, Hepatic stellate cells, Rho family GTPases, Transcriptional factors

Introduction

Metalloproteinase-1 (MMP-1) is thought to be central to the degradation of native fibrillar collagens type I and III, which are the main extracellular matrix components of liver fibrosis. Authur et al. recently reported that collagenase activity in liver homogenate increases through the recovery phase in CCL_4 experimental hepatitis rat model [1]. Ribonuclease protection analysis demonstrated that expression of the collagenase inhibitors TIMP-1 and TIMP-2 rapidly decreased, whereas collagenase (MMP-13) mRNA expression remain at levels comparable to those at peak fibrosis. They concluded that the elevated level of collagenase activity during recovery can be explained by decreased expression of TIMPs. On the other hand, Okazaki et al. demonstrated that collagenase (MMP-13) mRNA expression was elevated during the recovery phase using both semiquantitive analysis by reverse transcriptase-polymerase chain reaction (RT-PCR), the Southern blot test, and in situ hybridization [2]. Although data from two laboratories showed a small difference in the gene expression of collagenase, both suggested that a main cellular source of collagenase (MMP-13) would be the hepatic stellate cells (HSCs).

[1] Department of Community Health, Tokai University School of Medicine, Bohseidai, Isehara, Kanagawa 259-1193, Japan
[2] Department of Internal Medicine, School of Medicine, Keio University, Shinjuku-ku, Tokyo, Japan
* e-mail: hozawas@is.icc.u-tokai.ac.jp

The molecular mechanisms of expressional regulation of MMPs in HSCs have not been reported to our knowledge. Therefore, in this review we speculate on the molecular mechanisms of MMP-1 expression in human HSCs using data from studies that used other cell lines.

Regulatory Molecular Mechanisms for Human *MMP-1* Gene Expression

Because of a low level of basal transcription and rapid turnover of MMP-1 mRNA, MMP-1 mRNA expression is often undectable even in most of the cells that express the *MMP-1* gene. Only little is known about the *cis*-acting elements that control basal transcription. The most proximal AP-1 site, located at −77 bp in the human MMP-1 promoter region, is thought to play an important role in basal transcription [3]. In addition, deletional analysis of upstream regions of the human *MMP-1* promoter has suggested that a tandem array of putative ETS family and AP-1 sites located between −2300 and −1600 bp are implicated in the basal transcription [4]. The AP-1 site located at −77 bp is also necessary for transcritional induction by various cytokines. The most proximal AP-1 site and a PEA-3 site located just upstream of the AP-1 site act in concert to regulate transcriptional induction by phorbol esters in some tumor cells and fibroblasts [5]. In addition to the proximal AP-1 site, far upstream promoter regions are suggested to be necessary for transactivation of *MMP-1* promoter activity by tumor necrosis factor-α (TNFα) and interleutin-1 (IL-1) [6]. Transcriptinal activation of the *MMP-1* gene by IL-1 in rabbit synovial fibroblasts required a dorsal-like element located at −3029 as well as an AP-1 site at −77 [7]. Our preliminary data showed that a different motif close to the dorsal-like motif is required for TNFα-induced *MMP-1* gene expression in LI90 human HSCs (unpublished data). Different mechanisms may control transcription of the *MMP-1* gene in different cells. The molecular mechanism by which transforming growth factor-β (TGFβ) suppresses *MMP-1* gene expression remains unknown, although TGFβ plays a pivotal role in hepatic fibrosis. As described for MMP-3 [8], TGFβ may act via the TGFβ inhibitory element (TIE).

Signaling Molecules Controlling HSC Activation: Association with Regulation of Human *MMP-1* Gene Expression

Activation of HSC activation is closely related to *MMP-1* gene regulation. Various extracellular stimuli, such as inflammatory cytokines, growth factors, extracellular matrix (ECM) components, oxidative stress, and mechanical stress, are reported to activate HSCs. Transcriptional factors such as c-Myb, NF-κB, Ets-1, and AP-1 have been reported to be involved in phenotypic change followed by stellate cell activation in response to various stimuli above. Among them, NF-κB, Ets-1, and AP-1 have been also reported to regulate *MMP-1* gene transcription. Other signaling molecules, which are also directly associated with HSC activation, include a small guanosine triphosphate (GTP)-binding protein of the Rho family [9] and mitogen-activated protein (MAP) kinases [10]. The Ras-related rho family GTPases have been recently reported to cause direct activation-associated changes in rat HSC morphology [9]. Rho family GTPases (Rho, Rac, Cdc42) reportedly direct the cell morphology and motility in a variety of cell types by regulating actin cytoskeleton reorganization [11,12]: Cdc42 regulates filopodia; Rac regulates membrane ruffling; and Rho is involved in cell contractility, focal adhesion, and actin stress fiber formation. In addition, Rho GTPases control other cellular events, including transcriptional regulation, membrane trafficking, cell growth, and development [13]. Rac1 was reported to be involved in *MMP-1* gene expression induced by cell shape changes in rabbit synovial fibroblasts [14]. Based on these studies, we hypothesized that Rho family GTPases may play a role in regulating cytokine-induced *MMP-1* expression in human HSCs. This hypothesis is now under investigation in our laboratory.

In rat HSCs, p38MAP kinase and JNK are activated by TNFα. Both p38MAP kinase and JNK are known to exist downstream of the Rho GTPase signaling in various cell types. However, the signaling pathways from rhoGTPases-p38MAP kinase/JNK-NFkB to *MMP-1* gene expression in HSCs are not delineated.

Singh et al. suggested that Rho family GTPases may function as molecular switches to coordinate cytoskeletal reorganization and the activation of downstream signaling cascades in HeLa cells and 293 cells [15]. If this is also true in HSCs, it is attractive for us to hypothesize that Rho GTPases may function as molecular switches to modulate signaling for HSC activation so stellate cells can adjust themselves to their microenvironment during hepatic injury.

Conclusions

It has been recently reported that even advanced fibrosis in experimental liver cirrhosis could be successfully reversed by gene therapy [16,17]. Understanding the molecular mechanisms of liver fibrolysis and *MMP-1* expressional regulation is essential to direct a therapeutic strategy for liver cirrhosis.

References

1. Iredale JP, Benyon RC, Pickering J, et al (1998) Mechanisms of spontaneous resolution of rat liver fibrosis. J Clin Invest 102:538–549
2. Watanabe T, Niioka M, Hozawa S, et al (2000) Gene expression of interstitial collagenase in both progressive and recovery phase of rat liver fibrosis induced by carbon tetrachloride. J Hepatol 33:224–235
3. James TW, Wagner R, White LA, et al (1993) Induction of collagenase and stromelysin gene expression by mechanical injury in a vascular smooth muscle-derived cell line. J Cell Physiol 157:426–437
4. Imai S, Fujino T, Nishibayashi S, et al (1994) Immortalization-susceptible elements and their binding factors mediate rejuvenation of regulation of the type I collagenase gene in similian virus 40 large T antigen-transformed immortal human fibroblasts. Mol Cell Biol 14:7182–7192
5. Gutman A, Wasylyk B (1990) The collagenase gene promoter contains a TPA and oncogene-responsive unit encompassing the PEA3 and AP-1 binding sites. EMBO J 9:2241–2246

6. Brenner DA, O'Hara M, Angel P, et al (1989) Prolonged activation of jun and collagenase genes by tumour necrosis factor-alpha. Nature 337:661–663
7. Vincenti MP, Coon CI, Brinckerhoff CE (1998) Nuclear factor κB/p50 activates an element in the distal MMP-1 promoter in IL-1b-stimulated synovial fibroblasts. Arthritis Rheum 41:1987–1994
8. Kerr LD, Miller DB, Matrisian LM (1990) TGFb1 inhibition of transin/stromelysin gene expression is mediated through a Fos binding sequence. Cell 61:267–278
9. Yee HF Jr (1998) Rho directs activation-associated changes in rat hepatic stellate cell morphology via regulation of the actin cytoskeleton. Hepatology 28:843–850
10. Reeves HL, Dack CL, Peak M, et al (2000) Stress-activated protein kinases in the activation of rat hepatic stellate cells in culture. J Hepatol 32:465–472
11. Hall A (1998) Rho GTPases and the actin cytoskeleton. Science 279:509–514
12. Tapon N, Hall A (1997) Rho, Rac and Cdc42 GTPases regulate the organization of the actin cytoskeleton. Curr Opin Cell Biol 9:86–92
13. Van Aelst L, D'Souza-Schorey C (1997) Rho GTPases and signaling networks. Genes Dev 11:2295–322
14. Kheradmand F, Werner E, Tremble P, et al (1998) Role of Rac1 and oxygen radicals in collagenase-1 expression induced by cell shape change. Science 280:898–902
15. Singh R, Wang B, Shirvaikar A, et al (1999) The IL-1 receptor and rho directly associate to drive cell activation in inflammation. J Clin Invest 103:1561–1570
16. Ueki T, Kaneda Y, Tsutsui H, et al (1999) Hepatocyte growth factor gene therapy of liver cirrhosis in rats. Nat Med 5:226–230
17. Qi Z, Atsuchi N, Ooshima A, et al (1999) Blockade of type beta transforming growth factor signaling prevents liver fibrosis and dysfunction in the rat. Proc Natl Acad Sci USA 96:2345–2349

Molecular Analysis of Stellate Cells Activation by Proteomics

NORIFUMI KAWADA*

Summary. The stellate cell is a principal producer of extracellular matrix proteins in the liver and plays a major role in the development of liver fibrosis. The molecular basis of cell activation has therefore been analyzed intensively during the past decade. To determine the total gene/protein synthesis in stellate cells, in particular the dynamic change in their expression level in response to activation, proteomics were performed. More than 150 stellate cell proteins were successfully analyzed; and in several novel findings were observed that represent activation-associated change. Thus, molecules associated with stellate cell activation, and consequently liver fibrosis, may still be undiscovered. Comprehensive understanding of the molecular basis of liver fibrosis is required.

Key words. Stellate cell, Suppression subtractive hybridization, Proteomics, Genomics

Introduction

Hepatic stellate cells, which reside in the space of Disse and are in close contact with sinusoidal endothelial cells and hepatocytes, play multiple roles in the pathophysiology of the liver [1]. Quiescent stellate cells represent a principal retinol-storing phenotype and metabolize a small amount of basement membrane-forming substratum. When liver injury occurs, they undergo transformation into myofibroblasts, eliciting active proliferation, increased extracellular matrix (ECM) production, enhanced contractility, secretion of growth factors and chemotactic proteins, and retinoid loss.

Stellate cell activation is initiated by oxidative stress induced by damaged hepatocytes; paracrine stimulation of cytokines and growth factors derived from activated Kupffer cells, endothelial cells, and infiltrating leukocytes; and early ECM changes including the production of a splice variant of cellular fibronectin (EIIIA isoform) [2,3]. Transcriptional activation by a zinc finger gene *Zf-9*, which is induced at an early stage of liver injury, enhances gene expression regulating ECM accumulation.

Third Department of Internal Medicine, Osaka City University Medical School, 1-4-3 Asahimachi, Abeno-ku, Osaka 545-8585, Japan
* e-mail: kawadanori@med.osaka-cu.ac.jp

Activated stellate cells are highly responsive to growth factors such as platelet-derived growth factor BB (PDGF/BB) and insulin-growth factor 1 (IGF-1). Expression of receptors for individual growth factors and activation of the intracellular signal cascade [e.g., tyrosine phosphorylation, mitogen-activated protein kinase (MAPK), phosphatidyl inositol 3-kinase (PI3-K)] results in DNA synthesis and proliferation [4]. Transforming growth factor-β (TGFβ), a key regulatory molecule for ECM metabolism, functions as an autocrine and a paracrine mediator. The impact of TGFβ1 in the liver fibrosis has been well documented in the TGFβ1 knockout mouse model and in the marked attenuation of the development of liver fibrosis using soluble type II TGFβ receptor [5]. Thus analysis of the molecular mechanism underlying stellate cell activation is assumed to be essential for the development of effective therapy against liver fibrosis. To obtain deeper knowledge on this subject we undertook proteomic studies.

Proteomics

The proteome (*prote*in + gen*ome*), or proteomics, refers to the total protein profile of a given cell or tissue type; proteome research basically involves the following experimental steps (Fig. 1). First, proteins are separated in two-dimensional polyacrylamide gel electrophoresis (2-D PAGE). This technique combines isoelectric focusing (IEF) in the first dimension with sodium dodecyl sulfate (SDS) PAGE in the second dimension; it is capable of separating several thousands of proteins on a single 2-D gel. Second is identification and characterization of individual proteins using mass spectrometric techniques such as matrix-assisted laser desorption ionization (MALDI) or electrospray ionization (ESI) mass spectrometry. Advances in these techniques of protein analysis using mass spectrometry has made it possible to increase the sensitivity of the analysis (less than 100 fmol of protein can be analyzed) and shorten the time for analysis (only 30 min is required for partial sequencing of one protein spot). Moreover, the tandem mass (MS/MS) method represents direct analysis of the amino acid sequence of the protein spot without any prepurification (e.g., high-performance liquid chromatography) resulting in determination of the protein by referring to a database.

In practice, samples were prepared from quiescent or activated stellate cells, intact or fibrotic liver, and conditioned medium. They were dissolved in a lysis buffer. After IEF, 2-D SDS-PAGE was performed in 9%–18% acrylamide gradient gels. Proteins were visualized by silver staining. Protein spots of interest were excised from the 2-D gels and were digested overnight at 37°C in a buffer containing trypsin. After brief purification, they were applied to a Q-TOF mass spectrometer. The MS mode was used to scan samples for detectable peptides. Subsequently, the MS/MS mode was used to fragment individual peptides; and from the resulting MS/MS spectra the amino acid sequence was determined for each peptide. Finally, the proteins were identified by the obtained amino acid sequences referring to the SwissProt and GenBank database using the GenomeNet WWW server at Kyoto University.

A total of 308 protein spots have been successfully identified, including 225 protein spots derived from stellate cell lysate and 83 spots of secreted proteins. Among the identified proteins were Cu/Zn SOD, PAI-1, ubiquitin, vimentin, and several heat shock proteins. Several proteins whose expression levels were up- or down-regulated during

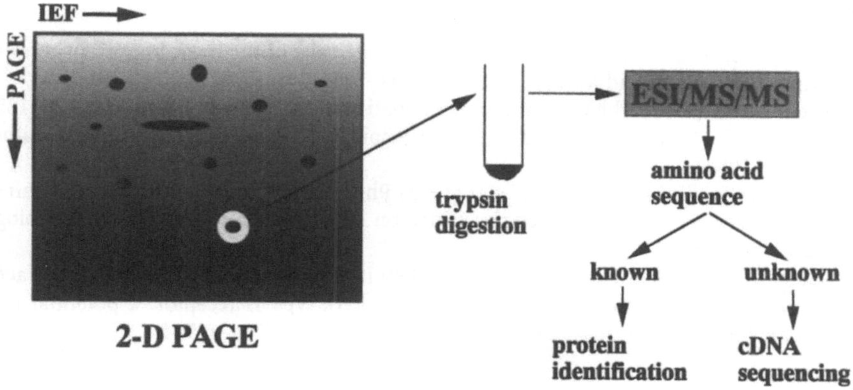

FIG. 1. **Proteome analysis.** Stellate cell proteins are lysed and separated by two-dimensional polyacrylamide gel electrophoresis PAGE, and then one protein spot is cut from the gel stained with silver staining. The protein is digested with trypsin; and after brief purification the solution is applied to electrospray ionization mass spectrometry/tandem mass method (*ESI/MS/MS*). The protein is identified by the obtained amino acid sequences against the Swiss-Prot and GenBank databases using the Genome Net WWW server. If an unknown amino acid sequence is found, cDNA is cloned using the degenerated polymerase chain reaction technique. *IEF*, isoelectric focusing

the course of stellate cell activation were identified. They included actin-binding proteins, secreted fragments of type I and III collagens, and some proteases. Surprisingly, a novel protein was successfully identified, and the cDNA has been cloned and sequenced.

Thus, the proteomics approach is highly useful for analyzing protein/gene expression of stellate cells in response to their activation in vitro and in vivo. Such a global catalogue of protein expression can offer profound understanding of stellate cell biology and the molecular mechanism of liver fibrosis.

Conclusions

We have performed three techniques—suppression subtractive hybridization, proteomics, and genomics—to profile gene expression especially in activated stellate cells and fibrotic liver tissues. Consequently, we have identified prion protein expression in activated stellate cells. Using the proteomic and genomic approaches, actin-binding proteins and nerve-associated genes have been found to be expressed in stellate cells in an up- or down-regulated manner during stellate cell activation; these represent novel findings. The results indicate that although current research and therapeutic focus are targeted to a few molecules such as TGFβ, PDGF, and HGF the cellular response to liver injury is more complicated and cannot be simplified. Hence, a global understanding of the protein and gene expression profile in stellate cells and fibrotic liver tissues is definitely required to establish a novel therapeutic strategy for liver fibrosis.

References

1. Blomhoff R, Wake K (1991) Perisinusoidal stellate cells of the liver; important roles in retinol metabolism and fibrosis. FASEB J 5:271–277
2. Friedman SL (1993) The cellular basis of hepatic fibrosis. N Engl J Med 328:1828–1835
3. Kawada N (1997) The hepatic perisiunusoidal stellate cell. Histol Histopathol 12:1069–1080
4. Marra F, Gentilini A, Pinzani M, et al (1997) Phosphatidylinositol 3-kinase is required for platelet-derived growth factor's actions on hepatic stellate cells. Gastroenterology 112:1297–1306
5. George J, Roulot D, Koteliansky VE, et al (1999) In vivo inhibition of rat stellate cell activation by soluble transforming growth factor beta type II receptor: a potential new therapy for hepatic fibrosis. Proc Natl Acad Sci USA 96:12719–12724

Tissue Inhibitor of Metalloproteinase-1: Strong Promotion of Liver Fibrosis Development in the Transgenic Mouse Model

HITOSHI YOSHIJI*, SHIGEKI KURIYAMA, and HIROSHI FUKUI

Summary. The tissue inhibitor of metalloproteinases-1 (TIMP-1) reportedly increases during liver fibrosis development, but the direct role of TIMP-1 has not been defined. To elucidate the role of TIMP-1 in liver fibrogenesis, we developed liver-targeted TIMP-1 transgenic mice under the control of albumin promoter/enhancer. A model of CCl_4-induced hepatic fibrosis was used to assess the extent of fibrosis development in TIMP-1 transgenic (TIMP-Tg) mice and control hybrid mice. With no treatment, overexpression of TIMP-1 in the liver did not induce liver fibrosis. After 4 weeks of treatment with CCl_4, however, a densitometric analysis revealed that the TIMP-Tg mice had a sevenfold increase in liver fibrosis compared to the control mice. The hepatic collagen and hydroxyproline content and serum fibrosis markers, such as 7S collagen and P-III-N-P, were also significantly increased in the TIMP-Tg mice. Furthermore, immunohistochemical analysis showed that collagen I and collagen IV accumulation was markedly increased along the sinusoidal lining in the liver of the TIMP-Tg mice with a pattern similar to that of smooth muscle α-actin (α-SMA)-positive cells. Activated hepatic stellate cells (HSCs) from TIMP-Tg mice displayed markedly increased RNA expression of procollagen I and collagen IV in response to exogenous recombinant TIMP-1. These results suggest that TIMP-1 does not by itself result in liver fibrogenesis but strongly promotes liver fibrosis development in the transgenic mice through HSC stimulation.

Key words. TIMP-1, MMP, Fibrosis, Transgenic mouse, Hepatic stellate cells

Introduction

Extensive remodeling of the extracellular matrix (ECM) has been shown during liver fibrosis development [1]. The alternation of the balance between the matrix metalloproteinases (MMP) and its inhibitor, tissue inhibitor of metalloproteinases (TIMP),

---

Third Department of Internal Medicine, Nara Medical University, Shijo-cho, Kashihara, Nara 634-8522, Japan
* e-mail: yoshijih@naramed-u.ac.jp

has been shown to play a pivotal role in liver fibrogeneis [2,3]. During liver fibrosis development TIMP-1 expression in the liver and the serum TIMP-1 level are markedly up-regulated in both humans and murine fibrosis models [4–9]. Moreover, in a rat model of reversible liver fibrosis, matrix remodeling and resolution of liver fibrosis were closely associated with a marked decrease in TIMP-1 expression [10]. Accordingly, it has been suggested that TIMP-1 plays an important role in liver fibrosis development. To date, however, the direct role of TIMP-1 in liver fibrogenesis has not been clarified. Recently, we developed liver-targeted TIMP-1 transgenic mice and examined the effect of TIMP-1 overexpression on a CCl_4-induced experimental model. In this chapter, the role of TIMP-1 in liver fibrogenesis is summarized along with the results of our studies.

Liver-Targeted TIMP-1 Transgenic Mouse

The mouse albumin enhancer/promoter was used to obtain liver-specific expression. The 3.7-kb transgene, which included TIMP-1 cDNA, β-globin chimeric intron, and SV40-late poly A region, was microinjected into the pronuclei of one-cell C57BL/6J-CBA hybrid mouse embryos; and we then we established several transgenic lines with standard transgenic technology. The human TIMP-1 (hTIMP-1) concentration in the liver measured by enzyme-linked immunosorbent assay (ELISA; Amercham Pharmacia Biotech, NJ, USA) ranged from 623.2 ± 120.4 ng/mg protein at 6 weeks to 684.6 ± 145.4 ng/mg protein at 30 weeks of age (the plasma level was 486.6 ± 134.7 ng/ml at 6 weeks and 548.8 ± 163.6 ng/ml at 30 weeks; $n = 5$).

Effect of TIMP-1 on Experimental Liver Fibrogenesis

Experimental Protocol

In the fibrosis model, 6-week-old male TIMP-Tg mice and control mice received intraperitoneal (i.p) injections of CCl_4 (1 ml/kg/body weight) twice a week. Four weeks after injection, the mice were killed and examined.

Quantitative analysis of fibrosis development was carried out with an image analyzing system. Immunohistochemical staining of collagens I and IV and smooth muscle α-actin (α-SMA) was performed. At the end of the experiment, serum samples from the TIMP-Tg mice and control mice were assessed for liver dysfunction and fibrosis markers. The hepatic hydroxyproline and collagen contents were also measured. The activated hepatic stellate cells (HSCs) were isolated from the livers of CCl_4-treated TIMP-Tg and control mice by pronase/collagenase perfusion and purified by density gradient centrifugation. The cells were treated with recombinant TIMP-1 (rTIMP-1) 500 ng/ml (Fuji Chemical, Toyama, Japan). The cells were subjected to pro (α1)-collagen-I and (α2)-collagen-IV RNA expression analysis by semiquantitative reverse transcriptase-polymerase chain reaction (RT-PCR). In each animal of the TIMP-Tg and control groups, liver samples were collected from seven mice and used for MMP-2 and TIMP-1 measurements. Total and active-form MMP-2 levels were measured by an ELISA detection kit (BIOTRAK: Amesham Pharmacia Biotech). The TIMP-1 activity was determined by reverse zymography.

TABLE 1. Effect of TIMP-1 overexpression on various fibrosis markers in animals treated with CCl_4

Mice	Fibrosis area (/mm² liver)	Hydroxyproline (μg/g wet wt)	Collagen (μg/100 g wet wt)	P-III-N-P (ng/ml)	7S Collagen (ng/ml)	Hyaluronic acid (ng/ml)
TIMP-Tg	0.21 ± 0.03*	728.4 ± 186.3*	378.6 ± 92.2**	40.4 ± 0.03*	183.9 ± 23.5*	118.9 ± 27.5*
Controls	0.03 ± 0.01	42.4 ± 14.1	299.6 ± 40.1	4.43 ± 0.65	40.6 ± 8.0	33.5 ± 6.2

Results are expressed as means ± SD ($n = 7$) from TIMP-1 transgenic mice (TIMP-Tg) and control mice
*,** Statistically significant difference as compared with the control mice (* $P < 0.001$; ** $P < 0.005$)

Enhancement on Liver Fibrosis in TIMP-Tg Mice

In CCl_4-induced liver fibrosis, Azan-Mallory staining revealed a marked increase in the extent of liver fibrosis in the TIMP-Tg mice compared to that in the control mice. Densitometric analysis showed that the fibrotic areas in the livers of the TIMP-Tg mice were sevenfold larger than those in the control Mice (Table 1) ($P < 0.001$). TIMP-Tg mice without CCl_4 treatment did not show any morphological evidence of fibrosis, suggesting that TIMP-1 overexpression itself did not have a fibrogenic effect on the liver. Once the liver fibrosis process was initiated by CCl_4, however, the fibrogenic response was much stronger in the TIMP-Tg mice than in the control mice.

Biochemical and Immunohistochemical Changes

Serum aspartate aminotransferase (AST) and alanine aminotransferase (ALT) and other parameters of liver function (albumin, total bilirubin, total bile acid) were not different between the two groups. These results suggest that the increase in fibrosis development was not a secondary response to transgenic TIMP-1-mediated liver damage. The serum concentrations of 7S collagen, P-III-N-P, and hyaluronic acid, which reflect the extent of liver fibrosis, were higher in the TIMP-Tg mice than in the control mice (Table 1). The liver hydroxyproline content in the TIMP-Tg mice was significantly higher than that in the control mice ($P < 0.001$), and there was a markedly increased accumulation of collagen in the liver of the TIMP-Tg mice ($P < 0.05$). Immunohistochemical analysis was carried out to examine the extent of collagen accumulation in the livers of the TIMP-Tg and control mice. We also assess the levels of collagen I, the main interstitial type of collagen, and collagen IV, the major structural component of the basement membrane [3]. The livers of TIMP-Tg mice showed more pronounced immunopositivity of collagens I and IV than did the control mice. Because activated HSCs express α-SMA during liver fibrosis development [11], we used serial immunostained sections to compare the localization of α-SMA with that of collagens I and IV. We found that α-SMA-immunopositive cells had a distribution pattern similar to that of collagens I and IV (i.e., along the sinusoidal lining but not in the hepatocytes).

MMP-2 Levels and TIMP-1 Bioactivity

It has been suggested that elevation of TIMP-1 expression during liver fibrosis development is closely related to MMP activities; therefore, we assayed MMP-2 protein levels in the liver lysates by ELISA. In accordance with a previous report [12], the total MMP-2 levels were increased in the CCl_4-treated fibrotic livers in both TIMP-Tg and control mice. The amount of total MMP-2 in the livers of the TIMP-Tg mice was higher than that in the control mice, regardless of CCl_4 treatment. The constitutive higher MMP-2 levels in the TIMP-Tg livers may be due to the biological feedback homeostatic mechanism in response to the transgenic TIMP-1. On the other hand, the active form of MMP-2 was decreased more significantly in the TIMP-Tg livers than in the control mice. The TIMP-1 activity, measured by reverse zymography, was 3.4-fold higher in the TIMP-Tg mice than in the control mice.

Effect of TIMP-1 on Collagen Synthesis in Activated HSCs

To further examine whether the activated HSCs were the source of collagen production in the TIMP-Tg mice, we performed in vitro experiments using activated HSCs isolated from livers of CCl_4-treated TIMP-Tg and control mice. The activated HSCs from TIMP-Tg and control mice produced comparable levels of procollagen I and collagen IV. When the activated HSCs from TIMP-Tg mice were treated with rTIMP-1 500 ng/ml, however, a significant increase in RNA expression of procollagen I (2.7-fold) and collagen IV (2.6-fold) was observed in the HSCs of the TIMP-Tg livers compared to the HSCs of the control mice, which showed no change in procollagen I or collagen IV RNA expression following treatment with rTIMP-1.

Mechanisms of TIMP-1 Promotion Activity on Liver Fibrogenesis

TIMP-1 expression has been shown to be markedly increased during liver fibrosis development in both humans and experimental animal models [4–9]. Moreover, in the rat model of reversible liver fibrosis, matrix remodeling and resolution of liver fibrosis were closely associated with a marked decrease in TIMP-1 expression [10]. Although those reports strongly suggested that TIMP-1 plays an important role in liver fibrosis, the direct role of TIMP-1 in its pathogenesis has not been elucidated.

We found that TIMP-1 significantly promoted liver fibrosis development in the transgenic mouse model. The net increase in MMP inhibitory activity by TIMP-1 overexpression is likely to lead to reduction of matrix degradation in the liver and consequently contributes to enhanced liver fibrosis development. However, this increase of MMP inhibition is not sufficient to explain the TIMP-1 direct promoting activity in liver fibrogenesis, as fibrosis was not induced only by TIMP-1 overexpression. Once the liver was initiated for liver fibrosis process by CCl_4, TIMP-1 first revealed a strong fibrogenic response. In other words, TIMP-1 seems not to be initiator but a strong promoter of liver fibrosis development. In addition, we found that the activated HSCs derived from the TIMP-Tg mice showed increased procollagen I and IV RNA expression in response to rTIMP-1. Because the activated HSCs from the control mice showed no increased response, we must assume that the HSCs from the TIMP-Tg mice had been sensitized somehow by the constitutively elevated hepatic TIMP-1 levels. We previously reported that TIMP-1 transfection of the rat mammary carcinoma cells led to an increase in collagen IV and laminin accumulation [13]. Translocation of TIMP-1 but not TIMP-2 into the nucleus further suggests that TIMP-1 can act as a transcription factor [1,14,15]. It is possible that long-term exposure of the HSCs to high levels of exogenous TIMP-1 somehow changes the phenotype.

TIMP-1 has been reported to inhibit apoptosis [1,16]. Apoptosis of HSCs and a rapid decrease in TIMP-1 expression have been suggested to contribute to resolution in the rat liver fibrosis model [12]. It is also possible that the high TIMP-1 activity in the liver microenvironment prevents apoptosis of the HSCs and thus contributes to the fibrogenic progress upon liver injury. Further studies are required to elucidate the exact mechanisms.

Conclusions

By itself, TIMP-1 expression does not result in liver fibrosis; but upon CCl_4-mediated injury it causes marked augmentation of liver fibrosis. In vitro studies of activated HSCs from TIMP-Tg mice showed a significant increase in procollagen I and collagen IV RNA expression in response to rTIMP-1. These data suggest that chronic elevation of TIMP-1 in the liver microenvironment promotes fibrogenesis through stimulation of the HSCs.

References

1. Gomez DE, Alonso DF, Yoshiji H, et al (1997) Tissue inhibitors of metalloproteinases: structure, regulation and biological functions. Eur J Cell Biol 74:111–122
2. Olaso E, Friedman SL (1998) Molecular regulation of hepatic fibrogenesis. J Hepatol 29:836–847
3. Arthur MJ (1994) Degradation of matrix proteins in liver fibrosis. Pathol Res Pract 190:825–833
4. Iredale JP (1997) Tissue inhibitors of metalloproteinases in liver fibrosis. Int J Biochem Cell Biol 29:43–54
5. Kossakowska AE, Edwards DR, Lee SS, et al (1998) Altered balance between matrix metalloproteinases and their inhibitors in experimental biliary fibrosis. Am J Pathol 153:1895–1902
6. Iredale JP, Benyon RC, Arthur MJ, et al (1996) Tissue inhibitor of metalloproteinase-1 messenger RNA expression is enhanced relative to interstitial collagenase messenger RNA in experimental liver injury and fibrosis. Hepatology 24:176–184
7. Murawaki Y, Ikuta Y, Idobe Y, et al (1997) Tissue inhibitor of metalloproteinase-1 in the liver of patients with chronic liver disease. J Hepatol 26:1213–1219
8. Benyon RC, Iredale JP, Goddard S, et al (1996) Expression of tissue inhibitor of metalloproteinases 1 and 2 is increased in fibrotic human liver. Gastroenterology 110:821–831
9. Herbst H, Wege T, Milani S, et al (1997) Tissue inhibitor of metalloproteinase-1 and -2 RNA expression in rat and human liver fibrosis. Am J Pathol 150:1647–1659
10. Iredale JP, Benyon RC, Pickering J, et al (1998) Mechanisms of spontaneous resolution of rat liver fibrosis: hepatic stellate cell apoptosis and reduced hepatic expression of metalloproteinase inhibitors. J Clin Invest 102:538–549
11. Arthur MJ, Mann DA, Iredale JP (1998) Tissue inhibitors of metalloproteinases, hepatic stellate cells and liver fibrosis. J Gastroenterol Hepatol 13(suppl):S33–S38
12. Takahara T, Furui K, Funaki J, et al (1995) Increased expression of matrix metalloproteinase-II in experimental liver fibrosis in rats. Hepatology 21:787–795

13. Yoshiji H, Buck TB, Harris SR, et al (1998) Stimulatory effect of endogenous tissue inhibitor of metalloproteinases-1 (TIMP-1) overexpression on type IV collagen and laminin gene expression in rat mammary carcinoma cells. Biochem Biophys Res Commun 247:605–609
14. Zhao WQ, Li H, Yamashita, et al (1998) Cell cycle-associated accumulation of tissue inhibitor of metalloproteinases-1 (TIMP-1) in the nuclei of human gingival fibroblasts. J Cell Sci 111:1147–1153
15. Ritter LM, Garfield SH, Thorgeirsson UP (1999) Tissue inhibitor of metalloproteinases-1 (TIMP-1) binds to the cell surface and translocates to the nucleus of human MCF-7 breast carcinoma cells. Biochem Biophys Res Commun 257:494–499
16. Guedez L, Stetler-Stevenson WG, Wolff L, et al (1998) In vitro suppression of programmed cell death of B cells by tissue inhibitor of metalloproteinases-1. J Clin Invest 102:2002–2010

Antioxidant and Antiapoptotic Activities of a Tissue-Specific Selective Estrogen Receptor Modulator, Idoxifene, in Rat Fibrotic Liver and Cultured Rat Hepatocytes

ICHIRO SHIMIZU[1,*], TOSHIHIRO OMOYA[1], YAJUN ZHOU[1], MINA ITONAGA[1], HIROSHI INOUE[1], GUANGMING LU[1], YOSHIHITO OKAMURA[2], MASAYUKI SHONO[2], HIROHITO HONDA[1], and SUSUMU ITO[1]

Summary. Idoxifene is a tissue-specific selective estrogen receptor modulator. Oxidative stress has a causative role in the development of hepatic fibrosis and apoptosis, and the Bcl-2 protein suppresses lipid peroxidation and prevents apoptosis. Although estradiol is a potent endogenous antioxidant, little information is available relative to the beneficial role of idoxifene in the liver. The antioxidant and antiapoptotic activities of idoxifene have been examined using experimental rat fibrotic livers and cultured rat hepatocytes undergoing oxidative stress. Hepatic levels of collagen and malondialdehyde were decreased and hepatic levels of superoxide dismutase and glutathione peroxidase were increased by the presence of idoxifene and estradiol in the experimental fibrosis model. The antioxidant enzyme response of cultured hepatocytes to oxidative stress was significantly improved by idoxifene in a dose-dependent manner. Idoxifene was also observed to induce Bcl-2 expression in the injured livers and hepatocytes, to have no adverse effects, and to act as an inhibitor early in the apoptotic pathway. In addition, treatment with idoxifene inhibited IκB-α degradation and NF-κB activation with attenuation of hepatocyte oxidative bursts. The hepatoprotective effect of idoxifene was somewhat greater than that observed for the same dose of estradiol. These findings suggest that idoxifene may enhance biological defense activities against oxidative stress and function as a potent antifibrosuppressant by inhibiting lipid peroxidation and preventing early apoptosis in the liver.

Key words. Hepatic fibrosis, Estradiol, Superoxide dismutase, *bcl-2*, NF-κB

---

[1]Second Department of Internal Medicine, [2]General Laboratory for Medical Research, The University of Tokushima School of Medicine, Kuramoto-cho, Tokushima 770-8503, Japan
* e-mail: shimizui@clin.med.tokushima-u.ac.jp.

Introduction

Hepatic fibrosis, or the deposition of extracellular matrix (ECM), is often associated with inflammation and cell death, which accompanies the repair processes. It is a consequence of the severe liver damage that occurs in many patients with chronic hepatitis C and B [1], progressing more rapidly in men than in women [2,3]. It is now evident that oxidative stress is a causative factor in hepatic fibrosis [1] and apoptosis [4,5]. Estradiol (E2) is a potent endogenous antioxidant that reduces lipid peroxide levels in liver and serum [6,7]. It is also well known that Bcl-2 protein suppresses apoptosis and is up-regulated by estrogen in several tissues [8–10], acting as a regulator of an antioxidant pathway, which prevents oxidative damage such as lipid peroxidation [11]. In addition, many cells have their own unique enzymatic defense systems against oxidative stress, including the production of superoxide dismutase (SOD) and glutathione peroxidase (GPx), which play a critical role in protecting the cell from oxygen-derived free radicals and other reactive oxygen species (ROS).

Our previous reports showed that the fibrotic response of livers in men was significantly stronger than that of livers in women [12], and that E2 treatment resulted in a dose-dependent suppression of hepatic fibrosis, with reduced collagen content and lower levels of procollagen type I and III mRNAs in the liver of a hepatic fibrosis model, which was induced in male rats by treatment with dimethylnitrosamine (DMN).[13] These findings may indicate the putative antifibrogenic role of E2 in the liver. However, it should be noted that the administration of estrogen per se in women poses some potential risks including breast cancer and endometrial abnormalities [14–16].

Idoxifene, or (*E*)-1-(2-{4-[1-(4-iodophenyl)-2-phenyl-1-butenyl]-phenoxy} ethyl) pyrrolidine, is one of a series of synthesized 4-substitued analogues of tamoxifen (Fig. 1) [17]. It is a tissue-specific selective estrogen receptor modulator [18] that acts in breast tissue as an estrogen antagonist through the same estrogen response element as the natural steroid hormone [19]. Idoxifene acts in bone as an estrogen agonist for osteoblasts through interaction with the osteoblast estrogen receptor [20] and shows negligible agonist activity in human endometrial cells [20]. Idoxifene was originally developed to treat advanced breast cancer [21] and to prevent postmenopausal osteoporosis. Nevertheless, little information is available relative to the beneficial role of idoxifene in the liver.

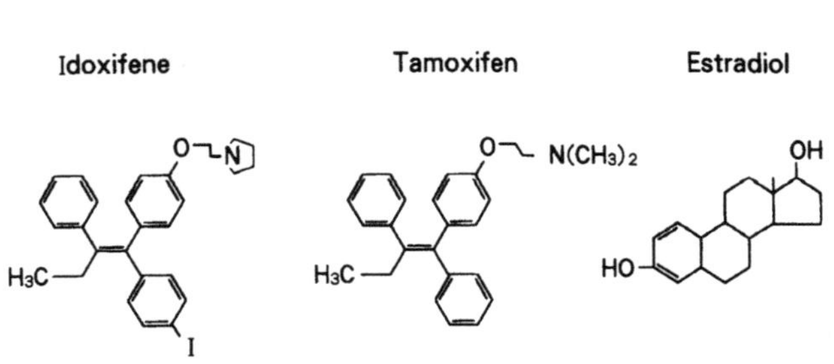

FIG. 1. Structures of idoxifene, tamoxifen, and estradiol

The present review summarizes our current knowledge of the biological functions of idoxifene as it relates to antioxidant and antiapoptotic activities in the liver in direct comparison to the natural hormone E2.

Effects of Idoxifene on Antioxidant Activities in the Liver

There is evidence that the products of lipid peroxidation modulate collagen gene expression [22,23], suggesting that lipid peroxidation is a link between liver tissue injury and fibrosis [24,25]. Although it is difficult to discriminate between the profibrogenic effect of the necrotic event and the true fibrogenic effect, which is induced by ROS, an independent stimulation of ECM deposition appears to occur at a prenecrotic stage during oxidative stress-associated liver injury [26]. It has been reported that paracrine stimuli derived from hepatocytes undergoing oxidative stress induce hepatic stellate cell proliferation and collagen synthesis [27]. Hepatic stellate cells have also been shown to be activated by the generation of ROS with Fe^{2+}/ascorbate [28] and by malondialdehyde (MDA) [29] and 4-hydroxynonenal [30], aldehydic products of lipid peroxidation. Antioxidants were observed to inhibit hepatic stellate cell activation by type I collagen [28]. We have already reported that E2 inhibited the prooxidant-enhanced lipid peroxidation in cultured rat hepatocytes, suppressed oxidative burst and type I collagen production in cultured rat hepatic stellate cells, and inhibited lipid peroxidation induced in rat liver mitochondria by Fe^{2+}/adenosine 5′-diphosphate [31]. In addition to these E2 functions, idoxifene suppressed hepatic fibrosis with reduced hepatic levels of collagen and MDA and induced hepatic levels of SOD and GPx in the DMN model of hepatic injury. Moreover, the antioxidant enzyme response of cultured hepatocytes to oxidative stress was significantly improved by idoxifene in a dose-dependent manner. Idoxifene was also observed to inhibit lipid peroxidation in rat liver mitochondrial membranes. These findings serve to clarify the fibrosuppressive and antioxidant effects of idoxifene. The antioxidant activity of idoxifene was somewhat greater than that of the same dose of E2, although the difference between the two was not statistically significant. Tamoxifen did not show such antioxidative activity in the rat hepatocytes and liver mitochondria.

Effects of Idoxifene on Antiapoptotic Activities in the Liver

A considerable body of data exists demonstrating that cellular damage, including damage to DNA, can be attributed to the presence of ROS that are by-products of the inflammatory response. In addition, nuclear factor NF-κB (NF-κB) is a key transcription factor that induces multiple genes in response to inflammation, infections, or oxidative stress [32]. Signals that induce NF-κB activity cause the dissociation and subsequent degradation of IκB-α protein [33], allowing NF-κB dimers to enter the nucleus and bind to specific sequences in the promoter regions of target genes [34].

Our resent study demonstrates that cultured rat hepatocytes respond robustly to oxidative stress with a time-dependent increase in the degradation of IκB-α and subsequent NF-κB activation and in secretion of MDA and LDH into the culture medium. Treatment with idoxifene and E2 inhibited the IκB-α degradation and NF-κB activation with attenuation of hepatocyte oxidative bursts and decreased extracellular levels of MDA and LDH in a dose-dependent manner.

Iimuro and coworkers reported that NF-κB prevents apoptosis during liver regeneration [35]. Moreover, overexpression of Bcl-2 is known to suppress lipid peroxidation and prevents apoptosis [11,36]. Therefore, Bcl-2 can protect hepatocytes from oxidative damage, leading to an increase in cellular longevity. In preliminary studies, we showed that idoxifene induces Bcl-2 expression in fibrotic livers and hepatocytes, which were in a state of oxidative stress, and acts as an inhibitor early in the apoptotic pathway. Bcl-2, which can be characterized as an anti-apoptotic, also functions as an antioxidant [11,36]. These findings suggest that idoxifene and estradiol function as apoptosis suppressants and protect hepatocytes from inflammatory cell injury (Fig. 2).

It has been reported that idoxifene differs from E2 in a tissue-specific manner. In reproductive tissues of the breast and uterus, where E2 is a potent agonist through the estrogen response element, idoxifene shows activity for estrogen antagonism, minimal agonism, or both [19,20]. In addition, idoxifene has estrogen agonism activity in the desired target tissue of bone [20]. Osborne and coworkers reported that idoxifene derivatives are much less reactive toward DNA than tamoxifen derivatives both chemically and in human and rat hepatocytes [37]. Tamoxifen is similar to idoxifene in its chemical structure (Fig. 1) and is widely used to treat estrogen receptor-positive breast cancer. However, it has been shown to form DNA adducts and to induce liver cancer in rats [38]. There is, as yet, no evidence for any such effect on human livers, and no tamoxifen adducts were detectable in human hepatocytes treated with tamoxifen [39]. These findings indicate that idoxifene should be a safer drug for hepatic protection.

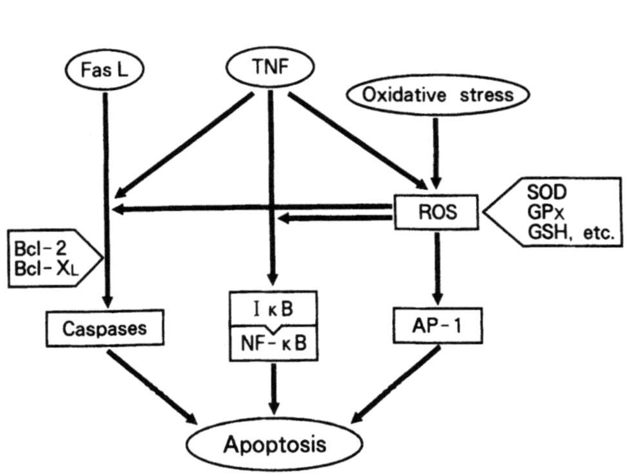

Fig. 2. Working hypothesis regarding the role of reactive oxygen species (*ROS*) in inducing apoptosis in the liver. *SOD*, superoxide dismutase; *GPx*, glutathione peroxidase; *GSH*, glutathione; *TNF*, tumor necrosis factor

Conclusions

Idoxifene has been shown to be a potent estrogen agonist in the liver; it shows no significant adverse effects and plays a protective role during hepatic oxidative damage by suppressing lipid peroxidation and apoptosis. Judging from the present data, along with earlier findings concerning its beneficial effects on breast cancer development and bone loss, this compound may be useful in developing new therapeutic strategies for the treatment of patients with hepatic fibrosis.

References

1. Shimizu I (2000) Sho-saiko-to: Japanese herbal medicine for protection against hepatic fibrosis and carcinoma. J Gastroenterol Hepatol 15(suppl):D84–D90
2. McMahon BJ, Alberts SR, Wainwright RB, et al (1990) Hepatitis B-related sequelae: prospective study in 1400 hepatitis B surface antigen-positive Alaska native carriers. Arch Intern Med 150:1051–1054
3. Poynard T, Bedossa P, Opolon P (1997) Natural history of liver fibrosis progression in patients with chronic hepatitis C. Lancet 349:825–832
4. Kurose I, Higuchi H, Miura S, et al (1997) Oxidative stress-mediated apoptosis of hepatocytes exposed to acute ethanol intoxication. Hepatology 25:368–378
5. Patel T, Gores GJ (1997) Inhibition of bile-salt-induced hepatocyte apoptosis by the antioxidant lazaroid U83836E. Toxicol Appl Pharmacol 142:116–122
6. Yoshino K, Komura S, Watanabe I, et al (1987) Effect of estrogens on serum and liver lipid peroxide levels in mice. J Clin Biochem Nutr 3:233–239
7. Lacort M, Leal AM, Liza M, et al (1995) Protective effect of estrogens and catecholestrogens against peroxidative membrane damage in vitro. Lipids 30:141–146
8. Garcia-Segura LM, Cardona GP, Naftolin F, et al (1998) Estradiol upregulates Bcl-2 expression in adult brain neurons. Neuroreport 9:593–597
9. Wang TT, Phang JM (1995) Effects of estrogen on apoptotic pathways in human breast cancer cell line MCF-7. Cancer Res 55:2487–2489
10. Gohel A, McCarthy MB, Gronowicz G (1999) Estrogen prevents glucocorticoid-induced apoptosis in osteoblasts in vivo and in vitro. Endocrinology 140:5339–5347
11. Hockenbery DM, Oltvai ZN, Yin XM, et al (1993) Bcl-2 functions in an antioxidant pathway to prevent apoptosis. Cell 75:241–251
12. Yasuda M, Shimizu I, Shiba M, et al (1999) Suppressive effects of estradiol on dimethylnitrosamine-induced fibrosis of the liver in rats. Hepatology 29:719–727
13. Shimizu I, Mizobuchi Y, Shiba M, et al (1999) Inhibitory effect of estradiol on activation of rat hepatic stellate cells in vivo and in vitro. Gut 44:127–136
14. Grady D, Rubin SM, Petitti DB, et al (1992) Hormone therapy to prevent disease and prolong life in postmenopausal women. Ann Intern Med 117:1016–1037
15. Colditz GA, Hankinson SE, Hunter DJ, et al (1995) The use of estrogens and progestins and the risk of breast cancer in postmenopausal women. N Engl J Med 332:1589–1593
16. Collaborative Group on Hormonal Factors in Breast Cancer (1997) Breast cancer and hormone replacement therapy: collaborative reanalysis of data from 51 epidemiological studies of 52705 women with breast cancer and 108411 women without breast cancer. Lancet 350:1047–1059
17. McCague R, Leclercq G, Legros N, et al (1989) Derivatives of tamoxifen: dependence of antiestrogenicity on the 4-substituent. J Med Chem 32:2527–2533
18. Treinen KA, Rehm S, Wier PJ (1998) An evaluation of the novel selective estrogen receptor modulator, idoxifene, for effects on reproduction in rats and rabbits. Toxicol Sci 41:199–207

19. Johnston SR, Boeddinghaus IM, Riddler S, et al (1999) Idoxifene antagonizes estradiol-dependent MCF-7 breast cancer xenograft growth through sustained induction of apoptosis. Cancer Res 59:3646–3651
20. Nuttall ME, Bradbeer JN, Stroup GB, et al (1998) Idoxifene: a novel selective estrogen receptor modulator prevents bone loss and lowers cholesterol levels in ovariectomized rats and decreases uterine weight in intact rats. Endocrinology 139:5224–5234
21. Quigley M, Haynes B, Dowsett M, et al (1994) Phase I clinical trial of a new antioestrogen idoxifene in advanced breast cancer. Br J Cancer 69:1187
22. Iredale JP, Murphy G, Hembry RM, et al (1992) Human hepatic lipocytes synthesize tissue inhibitor of metalloproteinases-1: implications for regulation of matrix degradation in liver. J Clin Invest 90:282–287
23. Houglum K, Brenner DA, Chojkier M (1991) d-Alpha-tocopherol inhibits collagen alpha 1(I) gene expression in cultured human fibroblasts: modulation of constitutive collagen gene expression by lipid peroxidation. J Clin Invest 87:2230–2235
24. Bedossa P, Houglum K, Trautwein C, et al (1994) Stimulation of collagen alpha 1(I) gene expression is associated with lipid peroxidation in hepatocellular injury: a link to tissue fibrosis? Hepatology 19:1262–1271
25. Houglum K, Filip M, Witztum JL, et al (1990) Malondialdehyde and 4-hydroxynonenal protein adducts in plasma and liver of rats with iron overload. J Clin Invest 86: 1991–1998
26. Pietrangelo A (1996) Metals, oxidative stress, and hepatic fibrogenesis. Semin Liver Dis 16:13–30
27. Baroni GS, D'Ambrosio L, Ferretti G, et al (1998) Fibrogenic effect of oxidative stress on rat hepatic stellate cells. Hepatology 27:720–726
28. Lee KS, Buck M, Houglum K, et al (1995) Activation of hepatic stellate cells by TGF alpha and collagen type I is mediated by oxidative stress through c-myb expression. J Clin Invest 96:2461–2468
29. Baraona E, Liu W, Ma XL, et al (1993) Acetaldehyde-collagen adducts in N-nitrosodimethylamine-induced liver cirrhosis in rats. Life Sci 52:1249–1255
30. Parola M, Pinzani M, Casini A, et al (1993) Stimulation of lipid peroxidation or 4-hydroxynonenal treatment increases procollagen (I) gene expression in human liver fat-storing cells. Biochem Biophys Res Commun 194:1044–1050
31. Omoya T, Shimizu I, Liu F, et al (1999) Estradiol enhances biological defense activities against oxidative stress and prevents hepatic fibrosis (abstract). Hepatology 30(suppl 2):490A
32. Barnes PJ, Karin M (1997) Nuclear factor-κB: a pivotal transcription factor in chronic inflammatory diseases. N Engl J Med 336:1066–1071
33. Stancovski I, Baltimore D (1997) NF-κB activation: the I κB kinase revealed? Cell 91:299–302
34. Haskill S, Beg AA, Tompkins SM, et al (1991) Characterization of an immediate-early gene induced in adherent monocytes that encodes I κB-like activity. Cell 65:1281–1289
35. Iimuro Y, Nishiura T, Hellerbrand C, et al (1998) NF-κB prevents apoptosis and liver dysfunction during liver regeneration. J Clin Invest 101:802–811
36. Kane DJ, Sarafian TA, Anton R, et al (1993) Bcl-2 inhibition of neural death: decreased generation of reactive oxygen species. Science 262:1274–1277
37. Osborne MR, Hewer A, Davis W, et al (1999) Idoxifene derivatives are less reactive to DNA than tamoxifen derivatives, both chemically and in human and rat liver cells. Carcinogenesis 20:293–297
38. Hard GC, Iatropoulos MJ, Jordan K, et al (1993) Major difference in the hepatocarcinogenicity and DNA adduct forming ability between toremifene and tamoxifen in female Crl:CD(BR) rats. Cancer Res 53:4534–4541
39. Phillips DH, Carmichael PL, Hewer A, et al (1996) Activation of tamoxifen and its metabolite alpha-hydroxytamoxifen to DNA-binding products: comparisons between human, rat and mouse hepatocytes. Carcinogenesis 17:89–94

Blockade of TGFβ Signaling: Prevention of Fibrosis/Dysfunction and Enhancement of Hepatocyte Regeneration in Injured Liver

Hikaru Ueno* and Toru Nakamura

Summary. To clarify the role of transforming growth factor-β (TGFβ) in liver fibrosis, we specifically blocked TGFβ action by adenovirus-mediated local expression of a truncated TGFβ type II receptor (AdTβ-TR), which serves as a dominant-negative receptor. Rats were intravenously injected with AdTβ-TR, AdLacZ (a control adenovirus expressing β-galactosidase), or saline and then were treated with dimethylnitrosamine (DMN) for 3 weeks. Liver fibrosis, as assessed by histology and hydroxyproline content, was markedly attenuated in AdTβ-TR-treated rats. All AdTβ-TR-treated rats remained alive, and their serum levels of hyaluronic acid and transaminases remained at low levels, whereas all the AdTβ-TR-untreated rats died of liver dysfunction. Some rats were first treated with DMN for 3 weeks; then AdTβ-TR, AdLacZ, or saline was applied followed by an additional 3-week DMN treatment. The truncated receptor was expressed mainly in the fibrotic area. Liver fibrosis progressed during the additional 3-week DMN treatment. However, in AdTβ-TR-treated rats, fibrosis remained at the level seen in rats given DMN for only 3 weeks. Electron microscopy of the AdTβ-TR-treated livers showed (1) less accumulation of extracellular matrix proteins in Disse's spaces; (2) regenerated hepatocytes; and (3) fat droplet-rich "quiescent" hepatic stellate cells. The results demonstrate for the first time that TGFβ plays a critical role in liver fibrogenesis and its progression, and that anti-TGFβ intervention could be therapeutic, not only by suppressing fibrosis but by facilitating hepatocyte regeneration.

Key words. TGFβ, Liver fibrosis, Gene transfer, Gene therapy, Adenovirus

Introduction

Many people suffer from fibrosis of their critical organs. Clarification of its pathophysiology at a molecular level and the development of effective therapy are both of clinical importance. It has been thought that transforming growth factor-β (TGFβ)

Department of Cardiology, Kyushu University School of Medicine, Fukuoka 812-8582, Japan
* Present address: Department of Biochemistry and Molecular Pathophysiology, School of Medicine, University of Occupational and Environmental Health, Kitakyushu, Fukuoka 807-8555, Japan
* e-mail: hueno@med.uoeh-u.ac.jp

Note: Most of the results have been already published in two papers [1,2]. Thus actual figures are not shown in this chapter.

may play a pivotal role in the fibroproliferative changes that follow tissue damage in many vital organs, including liver, lung, kidney, skin, heart, and the arterial wall [3–6]. However, whether TGFβ is indeed of crucial importance in fibrogenesis and in its progression, and whether inhibition of fibrosis would be therapeutic or hinder the physiological repair process after tissue injury has not yet been elucidated.

As a model of irreversible fibrosis, we focused on dimethylnitrosamine (DMN)-induced liver fibrosis [7,8], an established animal model with a pathophysiology closely resembling that of human liver cirrhosis [5,7,8]. To achieve a specific block of the action of TGFβ, we used an adenoviral vector to express a truncated type II TGFβ receptor locally that can specifically abolish all the diverse signaling by TGFβ as a dominant-negative receptor [9]. We also examined whether TGFβ is important for progression of already established fibrosis. Electron microscopic analysis gave us some important insights into the mechanisms of dysfunction in fibrotic livers.

Materials and Methods

Preparation of Adenoviruses

Replication-defective $E1^-$ and $E3^-$ adenoviral vectors expressing either a truncated human TGFβ type II receptor (AdTβ-TR) [9] or β-galactosidase (AdLacZ) [9] under a CA promoter comprising a cytomegalovirus enhancer and chicken β-actin promoter [10] were prepared as previously described [9,11].

Animal Models

Male Sprague-Dawley rats (10 weeks old) were given an intravenous infusion of AdTβ-TR (total 1.0×10^9 pfu), AdLacZ, or saline. Rats subsequently received an intraperitoneal injection of DMN [10 μg/g body weight (BW) or for the survival assay 12 μg/g BW] three times a week for 3 weeks. The liver was then either fixed with 4% buffered paraformaldehyde for histological examination or frozen immediately for extraction of hydroxyproline, the content of which was measured as previously described [12]. Biochemical parameters were measured using standard methods. Some rats were treated with DMN for 3 weeks after which either adenovirus or saline was applied followed by an additional 3-week DMN treatment.

Histological Examination

Tissue sections were either stained with Masson-trichrome or subjected to immunohistostaining using antibodies against collagen type I, fibronectin, smooth muscle α-actin, or TGF-β1. Immunoreactive materials were visualized by use of a biotinylated anti-mouse immunoglobulin G (IgG) antibody, peroxidase-labeled streptavidin, and diaminobenzidine. Some livers were fixed with 2% glutaraldehyde and then with 1% osmium tetroxide in cacodylate buffer. Ultra-thin sections were double-stained with uranium acetate and lead citrate and then examined by transmission electron microscopy.

Results and Discussion

Block of TGFβ Signaling and Prevention of Liver Fibrogenesis and Dysfunction in DMN-Treated Rats

Intraperitoneal injection of DMN for 3 weeks induced fatty degeneration of hepatocytes, activation and proliferation of hepatic stellate cells (HSCs), and matrix deposition mainly in the centrilobular area and portal tracts. The fibrotic area was intensely stained by an anti-TGF-β1 antibody. The cells in the fibrotic area were stained with an antibody against α-smooth muscle actin, indicating that they were myofibroblasts or activated HSCs. In contrast, liver fibrosis was markedly reduced in AdTβ-TR-treated rats. We measured the hydroxyproline content of the liver as a quantitative evaluation. The amount of hydroxyproline was 3.4 times higher in DMN rats infused with AdLacZ or saline than in intact rats. However, in DMN rats infused once with AdTβ-TR, the hydroxyproline content showed only a slight excess over the value seen in intact rats. Serum levels of hyaluronate, aspartate aminotransferase, and alanine aminotransferase were low in DMN rats treated with AdTβ-TR but high in DMN rats infused with saline or AdLacZ.

Fibrosis may be part of the physiological response to tissue damage. Thus, whether prevention of fibrosis is indeed beneficial is an important question. All the DMN-treated rats (for the survival studies DMN was given at 12 μg/g BW) infused with saline or AdLacZ died of liver dysfunction within 3 weeks, whereas all AdTβ-TR-treated rats remained alive throughout the study.

Our results clearly indicate that TGFβ does indeed play a central role in liver fibrogenesis and that blockade of fibrosis via anti-TGFβ intervention can be therapeutic.

Critical Role of TGFβ in the Progression of Fibrosis

After an initial 3-week DMN treatment, AdTβ-TR was infused. Immunohistostaining readily detected the truncated receptor in the fibrotic area of the livers, indicating that gene transfer was done into the activated HSCs. It is speculated that adenovirus infection may occur via the sinusoidal bloodstream, and that the septal cells and extracellular matrix (ECM) in the area are likely to serve as a barrier to the infection of hepatocytes. HSCs in the septal area are responsible for fibrosis. Taken together, adenovirus-mediated gene transfer of antifibrosis molecules such as a truncated TGFβ receptor may have a potential as antifibrosis gene therapy.

Following gene transfer an additional 3-week DMN administration was performed. DMN treatment for 6 weeks induced advanced fibrotic changes. However, in the rats that received AdTβ-TR on day 22, the degree of fibrosis remained at a level similar to that seen in the rats given DMN for only 3 weeks. These results were confirmed in a quantitative manner by measuring the hydroxyproline content of the livers. The hydroxyproline content in the AdTβ-TR-treated liver stayed at the level seen after the initial 3-week DMN treatments or even decreased slightly. The results indicate that anti-TGFβ therapy can halt the progression of fibrosis.

Blockade of TGFβ Signaling and Regeneration of Hepatocytes and HSCs with a "Quiescent" Phenotype

Electron microscopic analysis of DMN livers showed deposition of ECM proteins in Disse's spaces and degenerated hepatocytes. Only "activated" HSCs that were rich in rough endoplasmic reticulum but had lost fat droplets were seen. In striking contrast, the AdTβ-TR-treated livers showed (1) a decreased accumulation of ECM proteins in Disse's spaces; (2) regenerated hepatocytes; and (3) HSCs containing a large number of fat droplets. We found that about half of the HSCs contained such fat droplets, whereas not a single HSC of this type was found in the AdLacZ- or saline-treated livers. An association between liver diseases and the accumulation of ECM in the space of Disse has long been recognized. TGFβ is an inhibitor of the proliferation of hepatocytes in vitro [13,14], and TGFβ may induce oxidative stress leading to hepatocyte apoptosis [14]. Thus, attenuation of the action of TGFβ might well facilitate the process of hepatic regeneration and prevent hepatocyte damage from occurring. The phenotypic conversion of HSCs from "activated" to "quiescent" is important and requires further study.

It should be noted that suppression of TGFβ action for a prolonged period of time might have unfavorable consequences, such as the inflammation and tissue necrosis observed in TGFβ1 gene-disrupted mice [15]. This area also needs to be investigated carefully in future studies.

References

1. Qi Z, Atsuchi N, Ooshima A, et al (1999) Blockade of TGF-β signaling prevents liver fibrosis and dysfunction in the rats. Proc Natl Acad Sci USA 96:2345–2349
2. Nakamura T, Sakata R, Ueno T, et al (2000) Inhibition of transforming growth factor-β prevents progression of liver fibrosis and enhances hepatocyte regeneration in dimethylnitrosamine-treated rats. Hepatology 32:247–255
3. Massague J (1990) The transforming growth factor-β family. Annu Rev Cell Biol 6:597–641
4. Sporn MB, Roberts AB (1992) Transforming growth factor-β: recent progress and new challenges. J Cell Biol 119:1017–1021
5. Friedman SL (1993) The cellular basis of hepatic fibrosis. N Engl J Med 328:1828–1835
6. Border WA, Noble NA (1994) Transforming growth factor β in tissue fibrosis. N Engl J Med 331:1286–1292
7. Jenkins SA, Grandison A, Bazter JN, et al (1985) A dimethylnitrosamine-induced model of cirrhosis and portal hypertention in the rat. J Hepatol 1:489–499
8. Jezequel AM, Mancini R, Rinaldesi ML, et al (1987) A morphological study of the early stages of hepatic fibrosis induces by low doses of dimethylnitrosamine in the rat. J Hepatol 5:174–181
9. Yamamoto H, Ueno H, Ooshima A, et al (1996) Adenovirus-mediated transfer of a truncated transforming growth factor (TGF)-β type II receptor completely and specifically abolishes diverse signaling by TGF-β in vascular wall cells in primary culture. J Biol Chem 271:16253–16259
10. Niwa H, Yamamura K, Miyazaki J (1991) Efficient selection for high-expression transfectants with a novel eukaryotic vector. Gene 108:193–200
11. Miyake S, Makimura M, Kanegae Y, et al (1996) Efficient generation of recombinant adenoviruses using adenovirus DNA-terminal protein complex and a cosmid bearing the full-length virus genome. Proc Natl Acad Sci USA 93:1320–1324

12. Woessner JFJ (1961) The determination of hydroxyproline in tissue and protein samples containing small amounts of the amino acid. Arch Biochem Biophys 93:440–447
13. Carr BI, Hayashi I, Branum EL, et al (1986) Inhibition of DNA synthesis in rat hepatocytes by platelet-derived type beta transforming growth factor. Cancer Res 46:2330–2334
14. Sanchez A, Alvarez AM, Benito M, et al (1996) Apoptosis induced by transforming growth factor-β in fetal hepatocyte primary cultures. J Biol Chem 271:7416–7422
15. Shull MM, Ormsby I, Kier AB, et al (1992) Targeted disruption of the mouse transforming growth factor-β1 gene results in multifocal inflammatory disease. Nature 359:693–699

Protease Inhibitors: Suppression of Activation of Hepatic Stellate Cells by Inhibiting TGFβ Generation

Masataka Okuno[1,*], Kuniharu Akita[1], Seiji Adachi[1], Hisataka Moriwaki[1], and Soichi Kojima[2]

Summary. Transforming growth factor-β (TGFβ) plays a central role in the pathogenesis of liver fibrosis. TGFβ is secreted from hepatic stellate cells (HSCs) in a latent form and must be activated before it exerts biological functions. Several proteases, including plasmin, promote the proteolytic activation of latent TGFβ. Therefore, protease inhibitors that may inhibit TGFβ activation might be useful for therapy against liver fibrosis. We examined this idea employing rat HSC cultures. Among 20 protease inhibitors examined, we found several compounds that strongly suppressed active TGFβ generation induced by plasmin, retinoic acid, or basic fibroblast growth factor. We selected one compound (camostat mesilate) and showed its suppressing effect not only on the activation and generation TGFβ but also on transformation of HSCs. These results suggest that the compound may be useful for therapy against liver fibrosis. Experiments are now under way to examine its effect in vivo employing rat hepatic fibrosis models.

Key words. Hepatic fibrosis, Hepatic stellate cell, Plasmin, Protease inhibitor, Transforming growth factor-β

Introduction

Transforming growth factor-β (TGFβ) is the major cytokine implicated in the pathogenesis of liver fibrosis and cirrhosis [1–3]. TGFβ is produced mainly by hepatic stellate cells (HSCs) particularly in the damaged liver. Because TGFβ is secreted in a biologically latent form, it must be activated before it can bind to its cognate receptor and exert its biological function. We have demonstrated that activation of latent TGFβ is a key event in the process of liver fibrosis [4–6]. We have shown that in porcine serum-treated rats hepatic fibrosis is exacerbated following simultaneous adminis-

[1] First Department of Internal Medicine, Gifu University School of Medicine, Gifu 500-8705, Japan
[2] Laboratory of Molecular Cell Sciences, Tsukuba Research Institute, RIKEN, Tsukuba, Ibaraki 305-0074, Japan
* e-mail: mokuno@cc.gifu-u.ac.jp

tration of retinoic acid (RA) by elaborating TGFβ generation in HSCs [4]. RA upregulates expression of plasminogen activator through the nuclear RA receptor and thus increases plasmin levels on the HSC surface. This causes proteolytic release and activation of latent TGFβ constitutively produced by HSCs and stored in the adjacent extracellular matrix. The resultant active TGFβ autostimulates HSCs to produce TGFβ itself, and the resulting TGFβ exacerbates fibrosis by increasing collagen production in HSCs. Similar series of plasmin-mediated TGFβ activation were also induced by a novel isomer of RA, 9,13-di-*cis* RA generated endogenously in the fibrotic liver [5,6].

From these observations, we speculated that proteolytic release and activation of latent TGFβ is a potential target for suppression of TGFβ-mediated liver fibrosis. This idea led us to examine which protease inhibitors would effectively suppress TGFβ generation by cultured HSCs in vitro [7]. This experiment is particularly important for exploring our novel idea in vivo in the future. Rat primary HSCs, isolated and precultured for 7 days, were incubated with plasmin (Sigma, St. Louis, MO, USA) in the absence and presence of each of 20 protease inhibitors (kindly supplied by Ono Pharmaceuticals, Osaka, Japan). Thereafter, concentrations of both active and total (active plus latent) TGFβ present in the culture medium were determined by bioassays employing CCL64 mink lung epithelial cells. Unexpectedly, all protease inhibitors tested significantly suppressed activation and generation of TGFβ, suggesting that both release and activation were blocked. Similar results were obtained with HSCs stimulated by RA (Sigma) or basic fibroblast growth factor (bFGF) (Boehringer, Manheim, Germany), reagents that increase endogenous plasmin levels in the cells. Among 20 compounds examined, we selected one reagent, camostat mesilate, and examined its effect on the activation (or transformation) of HSCs. Currently, camostat mesilate is used clinically to treat pancreatitis and reflux esophagitis, and its drug safety is widely accepted from the clinical experiences. Rat primary HSCs, precultured for 1 day after isolation, were incubated with camostat mesilate and cultured for an additional 7 days in the absence or presence of the compound. Camostat mesilate suppressed morphological changes of HSCs (e.g., loss of lipid droplets from the cytoplasm) and inhibited the expression of smooth muscle α-actin, a marker of activated

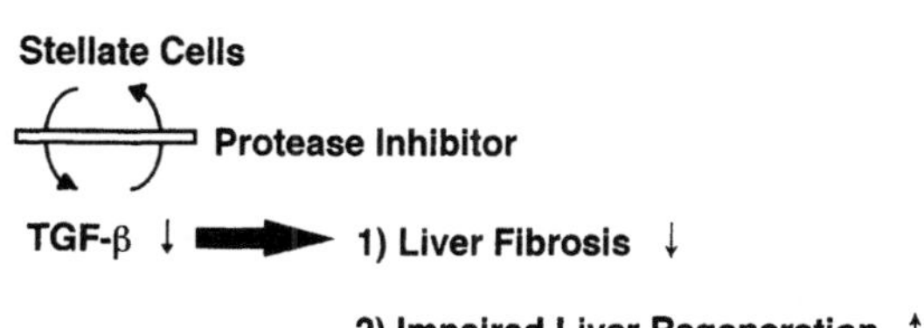

FIG. 1. Strategy for the use of protease inhibitors for the therapy against chronic liver diseases. In the damaged liver, transforming growth factor-β (*TGFβ*) is mainly secreted from hepatic stellate cells (HSCs) in a biologically latent form. Proteolytic activation of latent TGFβ is a key event in the progression of liver fibrosis. Active TGFβ stimulates HSCs to produce TGFβ itself as well as extracellular matrices. TGFβ also suppresses proliferation of hepatic parenchymal cells. Therefore, inhibition of TGFβ activation may be a target for a new therapy against liver fibrosis and impaired liver regeneration. We developed protease inhibitors for future clinical use to regulate overfunction of TGFβ in chronically damaged liver

HSCs. Thus, camostat mesilate inhibited not only the generation of active TGFβ but also transformation of HSCs.

These results suggest that a protease inhibitor or a combination of several protease inhibitors may be useful in vivo, suppressing generation of TGFβ in the liver and subsequent development of hepatic fibrosis (Fig. 1). Because several compounds including camostat mesilate are broad-spectrum inhibitors, the result suggests that these protease inhibitors blocked the activity of plasmin or plasmin-activated unknown proteases capable of generating TGFβ (or both). The present data suggest that these compounds might be beneficial for treating liver fibrosis. The idea of using protease inhibitors against hepatic fibrosis is further supported by the fact that some protease inhibitors have been used episodically as cytoprotective agents against liver damage [3]. We are now testing the idea employing rat hepatic fibrosis models [8].

References

1. Friedman SL (1993) The cellular basis of hepatic fibrosis. N Engl J Med 328:1828–1835
2. Friedman SL (2000) Molecular regulation of hepatic fibrosis, an integrated cellular response to tissue injury. J Biol Chem 275:2247–2250
3. Gressner AM (1991) Liver fibrosis: perspectives in pathobiochemical research and clinical outlook. Eur J Clin Chem Clin Biochem 29:293–311
4. Okuno M, Moriwaki H, Imai S, et al (1997) Retinoids exacerbate rat liver fibrosis by inducing the activation of latent TGFβ in liver stellate cells. Hepatology 26:913–921
5. Imai S, Okuno M, Moriwaki H, et al (1997) 9,13-di-*cis*-Retinoic acid induces the production of tPA and activation of latent TGFβ via RARα in a human liver stellate cell line, LI90. FEBS Lett 411:102–106
6. Okuno M, Sato T, Kitamoto T, et al (1999) Increased 9,13-di-*cis*-retinoic acid in rat hepatic fibrosis: implication for a potential link between retinoid loss and TGFβ mediated fibrogenesis in vivo. J Hepatol 30:1073–1080
7. Okuno M, Moriwaki H, Muto Y, et al (1998) Protease inhibitors suppress TGFβ generation by hepatic stellate cells. J Hepatol 29:1031–1032
8. Okuno M, Akita K, Moriwaki H, et al (2001) Prevention of hepatic fibrosis by the protease inhibitor, camostat mesilate, via reduced generation of active TGF-β. Gastroenterology (in press)

Plasma Transforming Growth Factor-β1: A Useful Marker for Hepatic Fibrosis in Chronic Hepatitis C

NOBUYUKI ITO* and SUMIO KAWATA

Summary. Transforming growth factor-β1 (TGFβ1) has been shown to play a pivotal role in the development of hepatic fibrosis. We have demonstrated that plasma TGFβ1 levels are elevated in patients with chronic hepatitis C and correlate with the degree of hepatic fibrosis. Interferon-α (IFNα) therapy reduced hepatic fibrosis in association with a decrease in the plasma TGFβ1 level in not only responders but also non-responders. IFNα may inhibit hepatic fibrosis independent of the results of viral clearance or suppression of necroinflammation.

Key words. IFNα, TGFβ1, Hepatic fibrosis, Chronic hepatitis C

Introduction

Evidence that transforming growth factor-β1 (TGFβ1) plays a pivotal role in hepatic fibrosis has been accumulating. TGFβ1 is produced as a latent form, which is processed to an active form that is rapidly cleared from circulation in vivo. We established an enzyme-linked immunosorbent assay (ELISA) system for measuring total (latent plus active) TGFβ1 and showed that the plasma TGFβ1 levels are elevated in patients with chronic hepatitis C [1]. We show here the usefulness of measuring plasma TGFβ1 concentrations for evaluating the degree of hepatic fibrosis in patients with chronic hepatitis C and discuss the antifibrotic effect of interferon-α (IFNα) therapy.

Plasma TGFβ1 Level: Correlation with the Degree of Hepatic Fibrosis

The factor TGFβ1 has been shown to promote fibrosis by stimulating extracellular matrix production and inhibiting matrix-degradative proteolytic enzymes in vitro. In animal models a positive correlation between TGFβ1 and procollagen I, II, and IV

Department of Internal Medicine and Molecular Science, Graduate School of Medicine, Osaka University (B-5), 2-2 Yamadaoka, Suita, Osaka 565-0871, Japan
* e-mail: nobu_ito@imed2.med.osaka-u.ac.jp

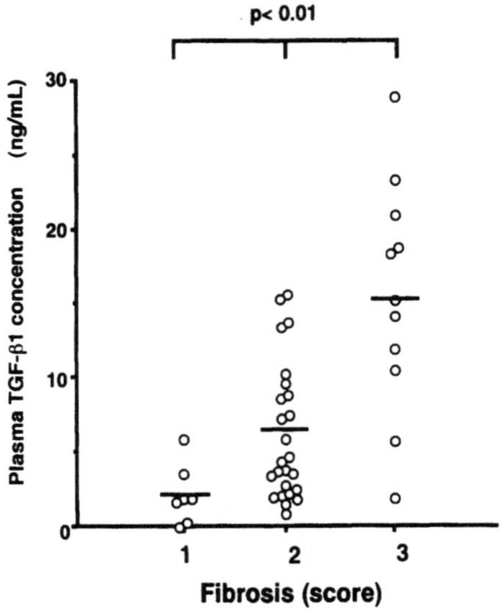

FIG. 1. Relation between plasma transforming growth factor-β1 (*TGF-β1*) levels and degree of hepatic fibrosis in patients with chronic hepatitis C before interferon-α (IFNα) therapy. Kruskal-Wallis test was used for statistical analysis. (From [5], with permission)

mRNA levels in the rat liver with carbon tetrachloride-induced hepatic fibrosis [2] and development of hepatic fibrosis in transgenic mice expressing mature TGFβ1 in the liver have been reported [3]. Although normal liver expresses a very low level of TGFβ1, TGFβ1 mRNA levels in the liver of patients with chronic hepatitis C are elevated and correlate with the fibrogenic activity [4]. In a previous study we demonstrated positive correlations of plasma TGFβ1 levels with tissue TGFβ1 content in the liver [5] and the degree of hepatic fibrosis [5] (Fig. 1). These results indicate that the plasma TGFβ1 level may be a useful marker for hepatic fibrosis.

IFNα Therapy: Inhibition of Hepatic Fibrosis

Interferon-α therapy is currently used for chronic viral hepatitis and is recognized as beneficial in sustained responders by normalizing serum aminotransferase levels, reducing hepatocellular necrosis and inflammation, and preventing hepatocarcinogenesis. Moreover, studies have demonstrated the antifibrotic effect of IFNα; significant regression of hepatic fibrosis and persistent suppression of serum markers of hepatic connective tissue turnover by IFNα therapy have been reported for chronic viral hepatitis, independent of its effects on viral replication and hepatic necroinflammation [6,7]. We have shown a reduction of hepatic fibrosis at the end of IFNα therapy in not only sustained responders (SRs) but also nonresponders (NRs) (Fig. 2a). Plasma TGFβ1 levels consistently decreased at the end of therapy both in NRs and SRs (Fig. 2b). Short-term administration of IFNα resulted in a marked reduction of the plasma TGFβ1 level (unpublished data), indicating that IFNα may inhibit hepatic fibrosis, in part, by reducing the plasma TGFβ1 level. Thus, IFNα may prevent the progression to cirrhosis by inhibiting hepatic fibrosis as well as by suppressing necroinflammation.

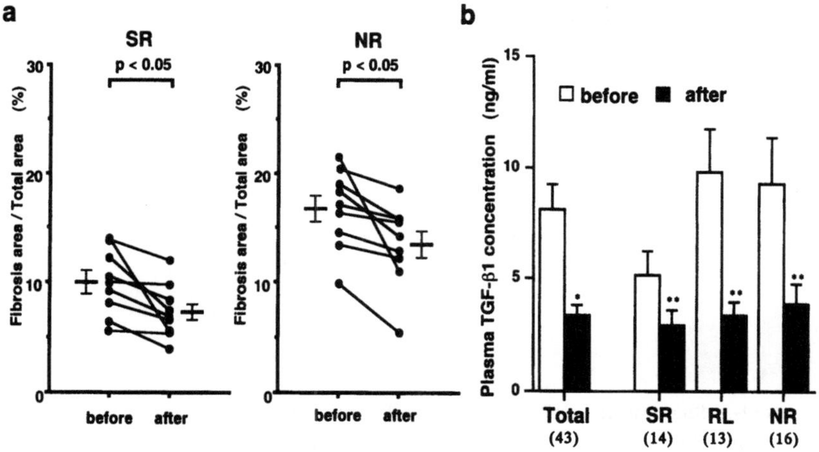

FIG. 2. **a** Changes in hepatic fibrosis estimated by morphometric analysis before and after IFNα therapy. **b** Changes in plasma TGFβ1 level before and after IFNα therapy. *SR*, sustained responder; *RL*, relapser; *NR*, nonresponder. $^{*}P < 0.01$, $^{**}P < 0.05$

Conclusions

Plasma TGFβ1 may be a useful marker for hepatic fibrosis. IFNα may prevent disease progression by inhibiting hepatic fibrosis as well as by suppressing necroinflammation.

References

1. Shirai Y, Kawata S, Tamura S, et al (1994) Plasma transforming growth factor-β1 in patients with hepatocellular carcinoma: comparison with chronic liver diseases. Cancer 73:2275–2279
2. Armendariz-Borunda J, Seyer JM, Kang AH, et al (1990) Regulation of TGFβ1 gene expression in rat liver intoxicated with carbon tetrachloride. FASEB J 4:215–221
3. Sanderson N , Factor V, Nagy P, et al (1995) Hepatic expression of mature transforming growth factor-β1 in transgenic mice results in multiple tissue lesions. Proc Natl Acad Sci USA 92:2572–2576
4. Castilla A, Prieto J, Fausto N (1991) Transforming growth factor β1 and α in chronic liver disease: effects of interferon alpha therapy. N Engl J Med 324:933–940
5. Tsushima H, Kawata S, Tamura S, et al (1999) Reduced plasma transforming growth factor-β1 levels in patients with chronic hepatitis C after interferon-α therapy: association with regression of hepatic fibrosis. J Hepatol 30:1–7
6. Manabe N, Chevallier M, Chossegros P, et al (1993) Interferon-α2b therapy reduces liver fibrosis in chronic non-A, non-B hepatitis: a quantitive histological evaluation. Hepatology 18:1344–1349
7. Teran JC, Muller KD, Hoofnagle JH, et al (1994) Decrease in serum levels of markers of hepatic connective tissue turnover during and after treatment of chronic hepatitis B with interferon-α. Hepatology 19:849–856

Key Word Index

MIX
Papier aus verantwortungsvollen Quellen
Paper from responsible sources
FSC® C105338

If you have any concerns about our products,
you can contact us on
ProductSafety@springernature.com

In case Publisher is established outside the EU,
the EU authorized representative is:
Springer Nature Customer Service Center GmbH
Europaplatz 3, 69115 Heidelberg, Germany

Printed by Libri Plureos GmbH
in Hamburg, Germany